Advances in
Oto-Rhino-Laryngology
Vol. 26

Series Editor
C. R. Pfaltz, Basel

S. Karger · Basel · München · Paris · London · New York · Sydney

Sialadenosis and Sialadenitis

Pathophysiological and Diagnostic Aspects

Volume Editors
C. R. Pfaltz, Basel
R. Chilla, Göttingen

37 figures and 30 tables, 1981

S. Karger · Basel · München · Paris · London · New York · Sydney

Advances in Oto-Rhino-Laryngology

National Library of Medicine, Cataloging in Publication

Sialadenosis and sialadenitis: pathophysiological and diagnostic aspects/volume editors, C.R. Pfaltz, R. Chilla. – Basel; New York: Karger, 1981 (Advances in oto-rhino-laryngology; v. 26)
1. Salivary Gland Diseases – diagnosis
2. Salivary Gland Diseases – physiopathology
I. Chilla, R. II. Pfaltz, C.R. (Carl Rudolf) III. Series WI 230 S562

ISBN 3–8055–1669–X

Contents

Contents

Contents

Contents

Adv. Oto-Rhino-Laryng., vol. 26, pp. 1–38 (Karger, Basel 1981)

Sialadenosis of the Salivary Glands of the Head

Studies on the Physiology and Pathophysiology of Parotid Secretion[1]

Reinhard Chilla

Department of ENT (Director: Prof. *A. Miehlke*), University of Göttingen, Göttingen, FRG

Sialadenosis and Parotid Secretion

Sialadenosis of the Salivary Glands of the Head

Besides inflammatory diseases of the salivary glands of the head (sialadenitis), salivary gland tumors and sialolithiasis, the sialadenoses form another group of salivary gland diseases. In contrast to most forms of sialadenitis, their pathogenesis has not yet been completely elucidated. *Rauch* [159] coined the terms 'sialadenosis' and 'sialosis', the first term indicating that, besides secretory disorders [dyschylia: 186], parenchymatous changes of the major salivary glands of the head are predominantly involved in the clinical picture. One of the most precise definitions was given by *Seifert* [186]. According to this author, sialadenosis is 'a non-inflammatory, parenchymatous salivary gland disease rooted in metabolic and secretory disorders of the glandular parenchyma, and, in most cases, accompanied by a recurrent, painless bilateral swelling of the salivary glands, especially of the parotid gland'. According to this definition, the Sjögren and Heerfordt syndromes are not to be counted among the sialadenoses but belong into the group of chronic inflammations of the salivary glands [187].

Recurrent swellings of the salivary glands, predominantly of the parotid glands, often persist for years. They are mostly painless with the exception of slight tension pain which will be occasionally observed. The swelling is only very rarely, dependent on food intake, e.g., after simul-

---

[1] This paper is part of the habilitation thesis of *R. Chilla.*

taneous ingestion of certain antihypertensive drugs [44]. Chronic enlargement of the salivary glands, particularly of the parotid gland in its preauricular region, is not uncommon. Nearly always both sides are affected, although a unilateral predominance of the swelling was occasionally reported [21, 188] (fig. 1 and 2).

There is no predisposition as to sex, and the incidence has its peak between the 50th and 60th year of age [188]. The coincidence of sialadenosis with diseases of the endocrine glands, with malnutrition and with neurologic diseases is conspicuous [95]. The various types of sialadenosis have therefore been classified into three groups.

1. Hormonal Sialadenosis. Parotid swellings of the sialadenotic type have been described in connection with nearly all endocrine disorders although sialadenosis accompanying diabetes mellitus is the most common among the latter.

2. Dystrophic-Metabolic Sialadenosis. It is observed in protein deficiency [kwashiorkor and mangy: 75, 172], in the malnutrition of alcoholics [22] and in vitamin deficiency [beriberi, pellagra: 113, 169].

3. Neurogenic Sialadenosis. This type is found in dysfunction of the vegetative nervous system.

Secretory Mechanisms of the Parotid Gland

The occurrence of sialadenosis in combination with a multitude of endocrine diseases, nutritional deficiencies and neurologic disorders raises the question if all these diseases might be responsible for triggering a pathophysiologic mechanism damaging the salivary glands.

Histologic and electron microscopic examination of sialadenosis reveals a swelling of the glandular parenchyma due to hypertrophic acinar cells [63]. The number of zymogen granules in these cells is increased; structural changes of the granules can be observed by electron microscopy [63]. Since the zymogen granules are the main source of the protein components of glandular secretion, a disturbance of acinar protein secretion (proteodyschylia) has been discussed as one component of the clinical picture but also as the cause of sialadenosis [186]. We will therefore now describe the basic principles of the physiologic mechanisms leading to formation and secretion of parotid saliva.

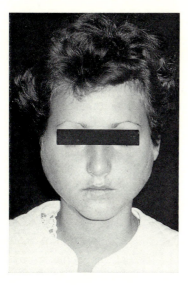

Fig. 1. 23-year-old woman with bilateral sialadenosis of the parotid glands of several years' standing. Note the characteristic 'hamster-like' facial expression (pouch cheeks).

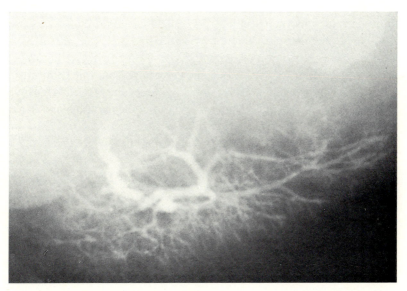

Fig. 2. Sialography of a sialadenosis of the right parotid gland. The multibranched duct system seen in this figure sometimes resembles the picture of a 'defoliated tree'.

Vegetative Innervation of the Parotid Gland

Although anatomy and histology of the parotid gland (serous acinar cells, myoepithelial cells, intercalated, striated, and secretory duct cells) were well known for decades, the contribution of the vegetative nervous system to glandular secretion remained a controversial matter. As early as 1851 *Ludwig* [129] had demonstrated that electric stimulation of a parasympathetic (chorda tympani) and also of a sympathetic nerve (cervical sympathetic trunk) induced saliva flow in the submandibular gland. The parotid gland, too, is innervated by both components of the autonomic nerve system [54]. Preganglionic parasympathetic fibers from the IXth cranial nerve travel to the otic ganglion; from there they arise as secreto-motor fibers and reach the parotid gland via the auriculotemporal nerve. Sympathetic fibers from the cervical ganglia accompany the blood vessels running to the parotid gland. Gangliocytes could not be found in the gland itself [61]. Once within the parotid gland, the postganglionic sympathetic and parasympathetic fibers reach the myoepithelial cells, the intercalated ducts and the acinar cells, coursing partly within the cytoplasm of the same Schwann cell scaffolding [80]. In man, only an epilemmal contact [9] of these cells with the terminal axons could be demonstrated so far [79], that is, the axon is outside the epithelial basement membrane. A hypolemmal contact, with the axons penetrating the epithelial basement membrane, was only found in some laboratory animals, especially in the rat [80].

Cholinergic and adrenergic terminal axons innervate the same acinar cell [91, 92]. The function of sympathetic nerve fibers in the human parotid gland was not clear for a long time, the more important role being attributed to its parasympathetic innervation [23]. According to *Rauch* [159], the postganglionic parasympathetic fibers prevail in the parotid gland. However, more recent investigations have shown that, quantitatively, the human parotid gland is furnished equally well with both sympathetic and parasympathetic nerve fibers [74].

Cholinergic, α- and β-adrenergic receptors are found at the acinar cell membranes of the parotid gland [182]. The β-receptors are of the 'β_1 type' [39, 56, 72]. The myoepithelial cells were reported to be equipped with α-adrenergic receptors [72, 213]. The role of cholinergic and adrenergic receptors in the acinar electrolyte and protein secretion was mainly studied in parotid tissue slices [20, 40] and in isolated acinar cells of laboratory animals, especially the rat, with more [133–135] or less success [15]. These studies yielded similar results, but of course their implications cannot be transferred to human beings without considerable reservations.

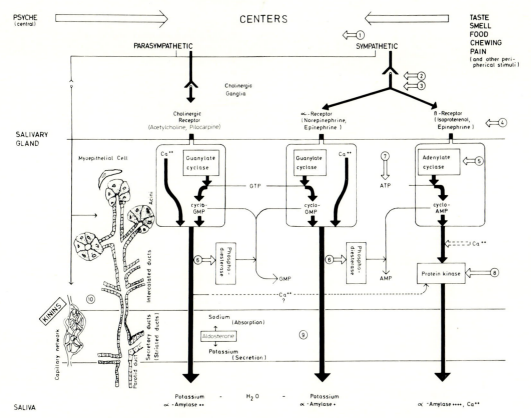

Fig. 3. Schematic diagram of the secretory mechanisms of the parotid gland. The adrenergic and cholinergic receptors of the acinar and also the myoepithelial cells are activated by various reflex arcs furnishing the gland with postganglionic parasympathetic and sympathetic nerve fibers. The numbers refer to the sites of action of the different pharmacologically active substances: 1 = clonidine, 2 = ganglioplegic substances, nicotine, 3 = guanethidine, reserpine, α-methyl-DOPA, 4 = sympathomimetics, parasympathomimetics, adrenergic and cholinergic receptor blockers, 5 = fluoride ions, 6 = caffeine, theophylline, 7 = 'metabolic poisons', e.g., dinitrophenol, oligomycin, 8 = tolbutamide, 9 = aldosterone antagonists.

Salivary Flow and Electrolyte Secretion

Via the 'gustatory-salivatory reflex' [61] and similar reflexes (fig. 3), the secretion of saliva from the parotid gland is increased (stimulated saliva) above the levels of resting secretion [95]. Besides afferent nerve pathways, vegetative centers and pre- as well as postganglionic vegetative fibers are also involved in these reflex arcs. Studies with microprobes have shown that saliva, while isotonic to plasma in the region of the acini and intercalated duct cells, becomes hypotonic to plasma in the region of the striated duct cells and in the more distal duct system [194].

The experimentally induced stimulation of the acinar α-adrenergic and of the cholinergic receptors leads, in the presence of Ca^{2+} ions, to the secretion of K^+ ions and water [17, 18, 40, 133, 134, 157]. An increased intracellular concentration of guanosine 3′,5′-monophosphate (cyclo-GMP) was observed at the same time, although this was not always accompanied by an increased acinar K^+ secretion [38, 40].

Saliva, initially isotonic to plasma, becomes hypotonic in the region of the striated duct cells which, histologically, resemble the distal tubules of the kidney. Readsorption of Na^+ and excretion of K^+ take place in this region under the influence of aldosterone [132].

Concerning saliva changes in the major secretory ducts, up to date studies have almost exclusively been available on the conditions in Wharton's duct [121, 153, 175]. Contraction of the myoepithelial cells results in a pressure increase in this duct system [72, 194].

Protein Secretion of the Parotid Gland

Under experimental conditions, more than 50% of the glandular protein can be secreted by the rat parotid gland [191], and 80–90% of this amount within the first 90 min after maximum stimulation. The acinar cells contain this 'exportable' protein mainly within the zymogen granules. These consist of densely packed protein molecules covered by a membrane [43, 167]. The main enzymes found in the zymogen granules of the rat parotid gland are α-amylase and also DNase, peroxidase, and RNase [112, 221]. The function of other proteins has not yet been elucidated [221]. Synthesis of these proteins, e.g. α-amylase, takes place in the rough endoplasmatic reticulum [86] and was also achieved in vitro [57]. The newly synthesized proteins aggregate and form the zymogen granules; it is presumed that the Golgi apparatus is responsible for transport functions in this process [61, 228]. The secretory granules undergo several maturation stages, their membrane fuses with the acinar cell membrane by exocytosis, and the content of the zymogen granules is then released into the acinar lumen. During the secretion process, several granules may merge into one, and very likely fragments of their membranes are used in the formation of new secretory granules [220]. 55% of acinar α-amylase is localized in the zymogen granules; the remainder exists in a free state in cytoplasmic fractions [181].

The release of zymogen granule content and thus secretion of amylase is mainly operated through the β-receptor mechanism, that is, via the sympathetic nerve system [12, 16, 182, 183]. Sympathomimetic agents such as epinephrine and especially isoproterenol induce a very strong amylase secretion in the rat and in man [71, 102, 125, 131, 204]. The mechanism of secretion has been elucidated in part (fig. 3). As in many other important metabolic and secretory processes, the cyclic adenosine 3′,5′-monophosphate (cyclo-AMP) plays here also a central role [19, 100, 190]. Sympathomimetics, under physiological conditions, mainly epinephrine and norepinephrine, activate the enzyme adenylate cyclase by stimulation of the β-receptors. Isoproterenol is the strongest activator of this enzyme which synthesizes cyclo-AMP from adenosine triphosphate (ATP). Experimental application of cyclo-AMP alone also induces amylase secretion [19, 55, 70, 189]. Ca^{2+} ions and a cyclo-AMP-dependent protein kinase are possibly involved in this process since the inhibition of this enzyme by the antidiabetic drug tolbutamide prevents amylase secretion despite high cyclo-AMP levels [100, 105, 190, 230].

Besides this experimentally well-established secretory mechanism, a direct activation of the protein kinase via a cholinergic receptor is discussed [143]. Here, too, Ca^{2+} ions are supposed to act as mediating substance [166]. The proposed process would explain the well-known amylase secretion by direct parasympathomimetic agents, e.g. pilocarpine [143]. Other investigators interpret the action of this drug by a mobilization of epinephrine (which would have to be stored in the glandular tissue) and therefore, in effect, also by the activation of adrenergic β-receptors [180]. However, very recent studies have shown that the exocytosis of amylase-containing zymogen granules can be a direct consequence of stimulation of cholinergic receptors [38, 137] but also of α-adrenergic receptors [229]. The simultaneous rise of the intracellular cyclo-GMP level [40, 229] was already mentioned.

In any case, amylase secretion via β-receptors is much stronger than that via cholinergic receptors, and stimulation of α-adrenergic receptors results in an even weaker enzyme secretion [123]. Cholinergic and α-adrenergic receptors were reported to cause mainly the excretion of older zymogen granules that extend towards the acinar lumen and, together with the β-receptor mechanism, to induce the fusion of secretory granules of different developmental stages [195]. Stimulation of β-receptors alone leads to exocytosis also of 'younger' granules. In this manner the acinar cell would be able to guarantee the release of secretable proteins dependent on intracellular storage time.

Influence of Hormones on Parotid Secretion

A great number of investigations has been carried out concerning the effects of hormones on parotid secretion and concerning the relationship between the parotid gland and the endocrine system. Parotin for instance, a proteohormone synthesized in the parotid gland, was reported to possess regulatory properties in protein synthesis and in calcification of cartilage [101, 149, 210], although such an endocrine function of salivary glands still lacks conclusive proof.

In experiments with rats it could be demonstrated that thyroxin increases the sensitivity toward epinephrine of the enzyme adenylate cyclase which is present in parotid acinar cells [146]. Prostaglandin E_1 is said to stimulate secretion not so much by influencing adenylate cyclase but rather by acting on the intracellular distribution of Ca^{2+} ions [124]. In man, synthetic calcitonine increases amylase secretion of the parotid gland but not of the pancreas [68].

Opinions differ concerning the effects of secretin and pancreozymin on parotid secretion. There are reports on investigations in which application of these substances had no influence on parotid secretion, especially of α-amylase [58, 68]; on the other hand, such influence was supposedly demonstrated by others [85, 144]. It is, however, known that some poly-peptides such as physalaemine and eldoisine stimulate the secretion of the salivary glands of the head [42, 215].

α-Amylase as a Secretory Product of the Parotid Gland

By quantity alone, α-amylase is a very important component of the zymogen granules and also the most important enzymatic secretion product of the parotid gland. Since furthermore the determination of amylolytic activity in serum, urine, and especially in saliva is of considerable diagnostic value, we will now deal with the properties of the parotid amylases in some detail.

α-Amylase (EC 3.2.1.1, α-1,4-glucan-4-glucanohydrolase) cleaves amylose, amylopectin, glycogen, and related poly- and oligosaccharides by hydrolyzing α-1,4-glucan links between two *D*-glucose units. The α-1,6-glucan links present in amylopectin and glycogen are not hydrolyzed by α-amylase. The cleavage products thus formed are the reducing substances maltose and limit dextrins of varying chain length [163]. Only very small amounts of glucose are formed under physiological conditions [152, 164], probably by hydrolysis of maltotriose.

The different α-amylases from animal and human sources that were studied so far, consist of a single polypeptide chain with a molecular weight of roughly between 50,000 and 60,000 daltons [111, 130, 145, 171]. The salivary amylases of human beings and of the rat and also the human pancreatic amylase contain one sulfhydryl group per enzyme molecule [206] while hog pancreatic amylase, binding two molecules maltotriose, contains two [128, 179, 211]. The enzyme has a pH optimum of about 7 [170, 208]. α-Amylases are calcium-metalloenzymes [98] and are inhibited by ethylene-diaminetetraacetate (EDTA) [140]. This property permits their differentiation from α-glucosidases [76, 78] which are frequently synthesized in the same salivary gland.

α-Amylase is activated by Cl⁻ ions [142]. Biogenic inhibitors were prepared from wheat extracts [66, 197] and are also produced by some *Streptomyces* species [115]. Some of these inhibitors differ in their effectivity on salivary and pancreatic amylases; this property has been used to differentiate between the two enzyme variants in human serum [67].

Preparation and purification of the α-amylases is facilitated by their strong affinity to substrate [127]. Since α-amylases from different organs exhibit different activities towards different varieties of starch, this behavior has also been used to distinguish between salivary and pancreatic amylases [88, 138, 207].

Isoamylases of Human Parotid Gland in Parotid Tissue,
Saliva and Serum

Human parotid amylase is no unimolecular enzyme. Electrophoretic separation procedures such as paper electrophoresis [69, 185], electrophoresis on cellulose acetate foil [11, 171], in agar gel [104] and in polyacrylamide gel [25, 33, 145, 160], as well as the application of electrofocusing, sometimes combined with electrophoresis in polyacrylamide gel [35, 165, 209, 219] revealed that α-amylase consists of a number of isoenzymes [139, 158]. These have slightly different molecular weights and differ mainly in their isoelectric points [110, 165]. *Kauffman* et al. [110] described for human parotid saliva a basic pattern of 5 isoamylases, 3 of which were glycoproteins (mol. wt. 62,000) while the other 2 (mol. wt. 56,000) did not contain any sugar moieties. Electrophoretic separation of the isoamylases in parotid saliva of more than 1,200 persons [141, 222] revealed that 99.3% of the members of the white race show a basic pattern comprising six isoamylases in the polyacrylamide system. This pattern is inherited as an autosomal dominant trait [103, 141]. The primary product of the amylase gene is altered, by 'post-translational' modifications involving glycosidation and

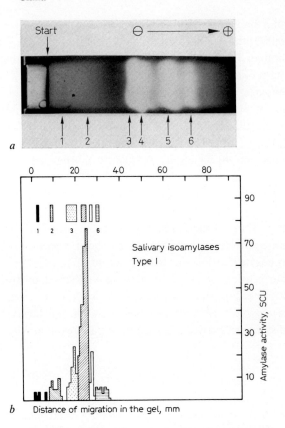

Fig. 4. Basic pattern of six isoamylases in parotid saliva. Top: Activity staining with Lugol's solution of the six isoamylases after electrophoresis in starch-containing poly-acrylamide gel. Bottom: Determination of amylase activity after elution of the isoenzymes from the gel. Electrophoretic conditions: 0.2 µg parotid saliva protein; 5% acrylamide, 0.25% bis-acrylamide; 0.1% starch; 2.5 h at 600 V, 60–80 mA, 0°C; buffer 125 *mM* tris-borate, pH 8.9.

deamidation, in such a way that the individual isoamylases are formed [106–108].

Our own investigations in which we used a vertical, starch-containing polyacrylamide slab gel, confirmed the basic pattern of six isoamylases (fig. 4) in human parotid saliva as well as in human parotid tissue [7, 46]. Up to six additional isoamylases, migrating faster towards the anode ('fast iso-amylases'), can be observed in parotid saliva [7]. These 'fast' isoamylases

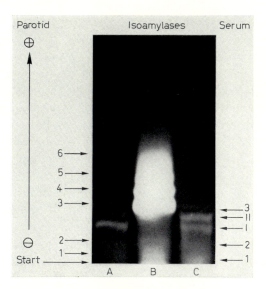

Fig. 5. Serum and parotid isoamylases in starch-containing polyacrylamide gel. Activity staining of the isoamylases with Lugol's solution. Electrophoretic conditions as in figure 4. A = Serum (10 μl), 1 day before parotidectomy; B = parotid gland extract (0.2 μg protein), basic pattern of six isoamylases (numbers 1–6); C = serum (10 μl), 2 days after parotidectomy; besides parotid isoamylases 1 and 2, two pancreatic isoamylases (I and II) and parotid isoamylase 3 are visible.

evolve from the isoenzymes of the basic pattern by deamidation of asparagin or of glutamin [111]; their number increases with age [7, 48] and in homozygous carriers of cystic fibrosis [52].

Besides for parotid gland and pancreas [200, 206, 212, 216], isoamylases have been described also for other human tissues such as submandibular gland [109, 119], mammary gland [118], ovary [202], lacrimal gland [87], liver [28], and lung [for references see 96]. Serum amylase (fig. 5) with a half-life of about 3 h [168] comprises isoamylases from pancreas and parotid gland [25, 120, 139, 150, 216] and is found regardless of involvement of the salivary glands. Other theories assuming liver as a source of the normal level of serum amylase [139, 148, 223, 224] have found less support.

The determination of amylase activity in serum (fig. 5) and urine, and differentiation between the individual isoamylases, has now gained considerable diagnostic importance [24, 83, 122, 170, 173] in the assessment of pancreatic and parotid diseases and in revealing macroamylasemia [26, 27].

Isoamylases of Rat Parotid Gland

Similar to man, the rat, experimental animal in this investigation, contains different numbers of isoamylases in its parotid gland, pancreas, and serum (fig. 6). Using the polyacrylamide electrophoresis system we found, as did other authors [160, 161] four isoamylases in the parotid gland. Two isoamylases of rat serum are identical to parotid isoenzymes with regard to their electrophoretic mobility (fig. 6) but differ clearly from the slow-moving pancreatic band found near the start (fig. 6). We also detected in rat serum one additional, more anodal, isoamylase whose electrophoretic mobility distinguishes it from all the other isoamylases observed in the investigated tissue extracts (fig. 6). The amylase isoenzymes of rat liver are also present in the parotid gland and in serum but their low activity suggests serum, and therefore originally the parotid gland, as their source. Our results are similar to those of *Skude* and *Mårdh* [201] and contradict at least the assumption that the amylolytic activity of rat serum has to be attributed solely to the liver amylases [81, 82, 89, 90].

The rat parotid gland which resembles the human parotid gland in its ultrastructure, its innervation pattern and its secretion products, served us as a model to induce nerve-mediated secretory disorders (see below). We studied their possible similarities to the clinical picture of sialadenosis in the attempt to gain a better understanding of the pathophysiology of sialadenosis.

Sialadenosis Caused by Disorders of Parotid Gland
Sympathetic Innervation

General

The histologic and electron microscopic examination of parotid tissue of patients suffering from a sialadenosis reveals as the cause of the paren-chymatous swelling the presence of enlarged acinar cells that are congested with zymogen granules. Some of these bodies show structural changes [63]. This congestion of secretory material in the acinar cells should be expected to correspond to an increased amylolytic activity in the acini. The origin of this secretory granule congestion remained, for the most part, unknown. Since the depletion of zymogen granules and thus secretion of amylase from the parotid gland, is mainly controlled by the sympathetic nervous system, we performed in vivo experiments affecting the sympathetic innervation of the rat parotid gland at various stages of the innervation pathway, and then

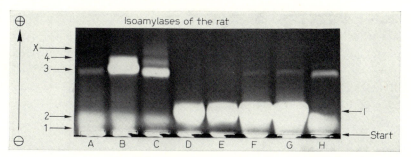

Fig. 6. Isoamylases of different tissues of the rat in starch-containing polyacrylamide gel. Activity staining with Lugol's solution. Electrophoretic conditions as in figures 4 and 5. Each 1 g of tissue was homogenized in 5 ml electrophoresis buffer. Prior to electrophoretic separation, extracts were diluted in buffer as stated below. A = *Gl. submandibularis* (dilution 1:50, 20 μl applied onto gel), four isoamylases as in parotid gland; B = *Gl. parotis* (1:1,000, 10 μl), four isoamylases; C = *serum* (1:10, 25 μl), four isoamylases as in parotid gland and additional isoamylase X; D = *pancreas* (1:1,000, 5 μl), one (iso)amylase I; E = *pancreas* (1:1,000, 10 μl), same as in D; F = *pancreas* (1:100, 10 μl), same as in D and isoamylase 3 (serum?); G = *pancreas* (1:50, 10 μl), same as in F; H = *liver* (1:10, 25 μl), distribution of isoamylases as in parotid gland and in serum (isoamylases 1–4). (F and G: Isoamylase I superimposing region of isoamylases 1 and 2.)

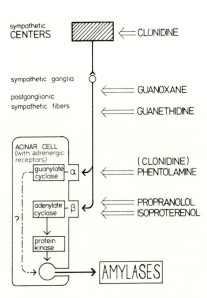

Fig. 7. Pathway of sympathetic innervation of the parotid acinar cell. The sites of action are shown of various pharmacons at different stages of the innervation pathway.

determined the amylase and isoamylase content of the gland (fig. 7). In this way we wanted to find out (1) possible similarities to the clinical picture of sialadenosis ('experimental sialadenosis') and (2) whether the side-effects of many antihypertensive drugs inhibiting the sympathetic nerve system, such as dryness of the mouth, initial parotid pain during mastication [29–31] and sialadenosis [188], could be attributed to disorders of acinar protein secretion.

Own Investigations

Experimental Animals and Preparation of Parotid Glands

Female rats (strain Sprague-Dawley NIH/HAN), weighing from 90 to 160 g, were purchased from 'Zentralinstitut für Versuchstiere' (Hannover, FRG) and used in our experiments. The animals were distributed 'randomly' (by lot procedure) among the control and experimental groups. All experimental animals received intraperitoneal injections of the various drugs while the controls were given the same volume of solvent alone [50]. The rats were kept under identical conditions (Altromin® standard diet, tap water ad libitum). After the specified times they were killed by ether inhalation, their left parotid glands were immediately removed, weighed and stored at $-70°C$ until extraction. We did not observe any appreciable decrease of isoamylase activity within 3–5 months of storage at this temperature.

The animals of the experimental groups were compared with those of the corresponding control groups by means of the distribution-free rank tests of *Wilcoxon* [226] and *Mann* and *Whitney* [136], with a preset significance level of $\alpha \, p \leq 0.01$ (error probability $p \leq 1\%$).

Determination of Protein and Amylase

We homogenized the glands, after thawing, in 125 mM Tris-borate buffer, pH 8.9 ('electrophoresis buffer') using 1 ml of buffer for 0.2 g of gland tissue, and determined the protein content of the extracts with the method of *Lowry* et al. [126], and the amylase activity with the assay of *Street* and *Close* [208].

This 'amyloclastic method' which makes use of the decreasing color intensity of the starch-iodine complex with increasing hydrolysis of starch by α-amylase, has been criticized mainly because unspecific destaining of this complex can occur, without hydrolysis of amylose, in the presence of albumin [154, 184, 227] or, according to more recent studies, of a lipoprotein [151]. Such unspecific action, however, affects the determination of amylase in serum more than that in tissue extracts of parotid gland.

Another type of amylase assays, the so-called 'saccharogenic methods', measures the liberation of reducing sugars by starch hydrolysis [147, 203]. A disadvantage of this method is its sensitivity to reducing compounds that are not amylose fragments. As opposed to the amyloclastic assay, the saccharogenic methods also measure to some extent α-glucosidase that frequently accompanies α-amylase in tissue extracts [77, 78].

Electrophoretic Separation and Determination of Isoamylase Activity

For the separation of the isoamylases present in the parotid extracts, we used the apparatus modified by *Stegemann* [196, 205] for vertical slab gel electrophoresis in 5% polyacrylamide. The addition of 0.1% starch alters the electrophoretic conditions in such a manner that the velocity of migration of the isoamylases is much stronger impeded by their high affinity to substrate than that of all other gland proteins and serum components. After electrophoresis for 2.5 h (in 125 mM Tris-borate buffer, pH 8.9, at 0°C, 600 V, 60–80 mA) only the isoamylases are found in the section of the gel near the start. They can be visualized by staining of the starch-containing gel with Lugol's solution after immersion in buffer containing chloride ions necessary for the activation of amylase. Following incubation, the isoamylases prevent formation of the starch-iodine complex due to their previous hydrolysis of starch and become visible as bright yellowish bands (fig. 6) before a blue background [3]. Unspecific destaining of gel portions by albumin is impossible as this serum protein has already migrated through the gel when the electrophoresis is terminated.

Isoamylase activities can be determined also quantitatively after elution from gel sections [3, 50, 51, 53]. All four isoamylases of rat parotid gland are seen as separate bands in the gel after staining (fig. 6) but isoamylases 1 and 2 and also isoamylases 3 and 4 lie too closely together to permit the separate determination of each individual isoenzyme. The activities of isoamylases 1 and 2 and of isoamylases 3 and 4 are therefore measured together.

Amylase, Protein and Isoamylase Content of Rat Parotid Gland after Inhibition and Stimulation of Its Sympathetic Innervation in vivo

Central Sympathetic Inhibition by Clonidine

Clonidine (2-[2,6-dichlorophenylamino]-2-imidazoline hydrochloride, Catapresan®) was synthesized in 1962 and intended to be used for detumescence of the nasal mucosa as were other imidazoline derivatives [84].

Shortly afterwards the antihypertensive effect of the compound was detected which led to its being predominantly used as an antihypertensive drug.

Like most hypotensive substances, clonidine blocks the sympathetic nervous system [97]. Contrary to the guanethidine derivatives, its main site of action is located in the central nervous system [99] and there mainly in the sympathetic cardiovascular regulation centers situated in the medulla oblongata [174] where it is said to directly stimulate α-adrenergic receptors [1].

While application of clonidine for 3 weeks leads to decreased amylolytic activities in the rat submandibular gland, histology and isoamylase pattern of the parotid gland do not differ from the controls [51]. A short-term application (1–3 days) of clonidine, however, decreases the acinar protein content (fig. 8) and the amylase activity shows a tendency to decline [4]. A brief initial, direct stimulation of peripheral α-adrenergic receptors described in addition to the central action of clonidine [116] could have caused exocytosis of zymogen granules and could thus explain the observed fall in enzyme activity [4].

Blockade of Postganglionic Sympathetic Fibers

Antihypertensive drugs such as guanethidine (Ismelin®) and related compounds (guanacline, Leron®; guanoxane, Envacar®) inhibit the transmission of impulses along the sympathetic postganglionic fibers [36, 37, 117]. *Kleine* [114] reported that primarily the release of epinephrine is prevented before the catecholamine store is slowly drained. The long-term application of guanethidine ([2-(octahydro-1'-azocinyl)-ethyl]-guanidine sulfate) and guanoxane (2-guanidinomethyl-[1,4]-benzodioxane) leads to the destruction of postganglionic sympathetic fibers in the rat [36, 37]. The effects of these substances are similar to those of 6-hydroxydopamine [213, 217.]

Application of guanethidine [50] and of guanoxane (fig. 9) [3] causes a massive acinar congestion of protein and amylase in the parotid gland of the rat. The activities of all four isoamylases reflect these changes. Despite undiminished drug levels, the retention of secretable gland protein slowly subsides during 3 weeks, and, in the case of guanethidine, has completely disappeared after an additional period of 2 weeks without treatment [50].

Inhibition of Adrenergic α- and β-Receptors

Propranolol (1-isopropylamino-3-[1-naphthyloxylpropane]-2-ol hydrochloride; propranolol hydrochloride, Dociton®) is a competitive antagonist of epinephrine at the adrenergic β-receptors which are mainly responsible for inducing exocytosis of the zymogen granules in rat parotid gland.

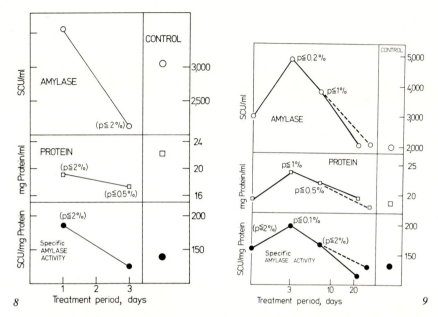

Fig. 8. Protein and amylase concentrations of rat parotid extracts after administration of *clonidine*. Glandular protein content is diminished, the amylase activity shows a tendency to decline. SCU = Street-Close units, p = error probability; level of significance at $p \leq 1\%$, higher values in brackets. The mean values of n animals of the different groups are given: control, n = 5; 1 day treated, n = 7; 3 days treated, n = 7. Experimental animals were given every 24 h i.p. injections of 0.075 mg clonidine.

Fig. 9. Protein and amylase concentrations of rat parotid extracts after application of *guanoxane*. The acinar protein and amylase content is distinctly increased during the first week of treatment. Regardless of continuation or termination (------) of drug administration, the values drop to the levels of the controls after 3 weeks. For SCU and p, see legend to figure 8. The mean values of n animals of the following groups are given: control, n = 10; 1 day treated, n = 7; 3 days treated, n = 7; 7 days treated, n = 7; 21 days treated, n = 7; 7 days treated and killed after an additional 2 weeks without treatment, n = 7. Experimental animals were given one daily dose of 7 mg guanoxane sulfate (i.p. injection).

Treatment of rats with propranolol increases the activity of amylase but not the concentration of protein (fig. 10) in parotid gland extracts [8]. The α-adrenergic receptors, causing depletion of 'older' zymogen granules adjacent to the acinar cell lumina [195], are not inhibited by propranolol, and the isoamylases present in the older granules might well have a lower enzymatic activity. This could explain our findings.

Inhibition of sympathetic α-adrenergic receptors by phentolamine (2-[N-*p*-tolyl-N-*m*-hydroxyphenylaminomethyl]-2-imidazolinemethane sulfo-

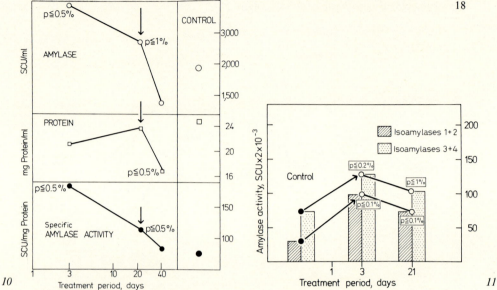

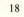

10

11

Fig. 10. Protein and amylase content of rat parotid extracts after sympathetic β-receptor block with *propranolol*. Only the amylase activity is increased after application of propranolol for 3 weeks. These changes are reversible within 3 more weeks following termination of treatment (↓). For SCU and p see legend to figure 8. The mean values of n animals of the following groups are given: control, n = 10; 3 days treated, n = 10; 21 days treated, n = 10; 21 days treated and killed after an additional 3 weeks without treatment, n = 10. Experimental animals received every 12 h one i.p. injection of 2 mg propranolol.

Fig. 11. Isoamylase activities of rat parotid gland after sympathetic α-receptor block with *phentolamine*. Activities of both groups of isoenzymes (isoamylases 1 + 2 and isoamylases 3 + 4) were determined after electrophoretic separation and elution from the polyacrylamide gel. Isoamylase activities are distinctly enhanced under the influence of α-receptor block. For SCU and p see legend to figure 8. The mean values of n animals of the different groups are given: control, n = 8; 3 days treated, n = 8; 21 days treated, n = 8. Experimental animals received every 24 h one i.p. injection of 1 mg phentolamine.

nate, Regitin®) enhances the activity of rat parotid isoamylases (fig. 11) without perceptible changes in the specific enzyme activities [45]. A disturbed discharge from the duct system of already secreted gland protein could explain this result because stimulation of α-receptors induces secretion of K^+ ions and water from the acinar cells, at least under experimental conditions [17, 18]. It was furthermore reported that contraction of the myoepithelial cells is effected by adrenergic α-receptors [72, 214]. On the other hand, the α-receptors are probably also active to some extent in protein secretion from the gland [123, 195].

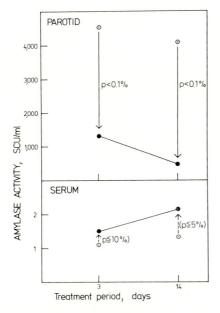

Fig. 12. Activity of α-amylase in rat parotid extracts and serum after administration of *isoproterenol* (IPR). While the amylase activities are clearly reduced in parotid extracts, they show a tendency to increase in serum. For SCU and p see legend to figure 8. ● = Experimental group, 20 mg IPR/day, n = 8; ⊙ = control group, n = 8.

Stimulation of Adrenergic Receptors

By stimulation of the sympathetic adrenergic β-receptors which is accompanied by activation of the enzyme adenylate cyclase, isoproterenol (1-[3,4-dihydroxyphenyl]-2-isopropylamino ethanol; isoprenaline [IPR]; isoprenaline sulfate, Aludrin®) causes a massive secretion of amylase from the parotid gland [14, 41, 231]. IPR induces in vivo chronic enlargement of the parotid gland that manifests itself histologically as an increase in volume of the acinar cells which contain more secretory granules [198]. Besides this hypertrophy, repeated, unphysiologic secretory stimuli exerted by prolonged IPR treatment also induce hyperplasia of salivary glands [13, 14, 61, 193]. Enlargement of salivary glands was also observed in asthma patients who had frequently used aerosols containing sympathomimetics [34]. In animal experiments, the IPR-induced hypertrophic and hyperplastic parotid gland was employed as an 'experimental model of sialadenosis' [6, 10, 192, 193].

IPR treatment reduces the activity of amylase in parotid gland extracts despite the histologically confirmed increase in number of secretory granules

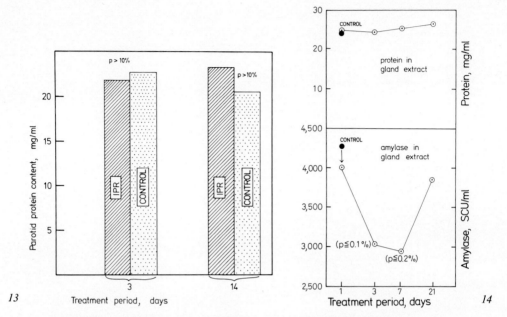

13   Treatment period, days   Treatment period, days   14

Fig. 13. Protein concentration of rat parotid extracts after administration of *iso-proterenol* (IPR). There is no difference between the protein concentrations of parotid extracts from experimental and control animals. p = Error probability, level of significance at p≦1%. Mean values are given for experimental and control groups (each group, n = 8). Experimental animals were given one daily i.p. injection of 20 mg IPR.

Fig. 14. Protein and amylase concentrations of rat parotid extracts after application of *amitriptyline*. Similar to the parotid gland of IPR-treated rats, the amylase activity is reduced in the extracts following administration of amitriptyline while the protein content remains unchanged. Despite continued drug application, the amylase activity reaches the level of the controls after 3 weeks. For SCU and p see legend to figure 8. The mean values of n animals of the following groups are given: control, n = 8; 1 day treated, n = 8; 3 days treated, n = 8; 7 days treated, n = 8; 21 days treated, n = 8. Experimental animals received every 12 h one i.p. injection of 1.5 mg amitriptyline.

in the acinar cells (fig. 12) while the protein content does not change (fig. 13). At the same time, the values of serum amylase activity show a tendency to increase (fig. 12). This might be due to increased permeation of salivary isoamylases into serum following damage to the acinar cells which was observed by *Simson* [199] after application of IPR to rats.

Amylase activity and protein content of rat parotid gland behave in a similar fashion after application of amitriptyline (5-[3′-dimethylaminopropylidene]-10,11-dihydro-5H-dibenzo[a,d]-cycloheptene; Laroxyl®) for 1 week. While the protein content of the gland remains constant, its amylase activity drops (fig. 14) [47]. Analogous results were obtained for the iso-amylase activities [47]. The 'amino-potentiating effect' of amitryptyline [156] intensifying the action of norepinephrine is assumed to be due to inhibited uptake of catecholamines into the storage sites. Activation of adrenergic receptors at the acinar cells, increased by the described effect, could have caused the amitriptyline-induced decrease of acinar amylase activity [47].

Discussion

Interference with the sympathetic innervation of the parotid gland at different levels along its course results in very similar changes of protein content and concentration of α-amylase and its isoenzyme pattern in the parenchyma of the gland. Principally, two different forms of reaction of the parotid gland can be distinguished; they are characterized by either an increase or by a decrease of acinar protein and amylase content. Since these changes can be traced back to disorders of protein secretion from the gland (proteodyschylia), the two forms of gland reaction to disturbance of its sympathetic innervation can be defined as follows [47]:

(1) *Inhibitory proteodyschylia* due to inhibition of physiologic protein secretion, accompanied by congestion of amylase in the acinar cells.

(2) *Stimulatory proteodyschylia* due to unphysiologic rise of protein secretion with concomitant decline in acinar amylase activity.

In contrast to the effects of natural aging processes [53] and cytostatic agents [5] on the rat parotid gland, the ratio between the individual iso-amylase activities remains more or less unchanged in both types of proteo-dyschylia. According to our definition, the disorders of protein secretion caused by inhibition or stimulation of the sympathetic innervation of the gland can be classified into two types of parotid gland reaction:

(1) Blockade of the postganglionic sympathetic fibers by guanoxane and guanethidine as well as inhibition of the α- and β-adrenergic receptors by phentolamine and propranolol lead to an 'inhibitory proteodyschylia'. In all these instances, the protein and amylase content of the gland is more or less enhanced.

(2) The direct or indirect activation of adrenergic receptors by isopro-terenol and probably also by amitriptyline and clonidine causes a 'stimula-tory proteodyschylia'. This type of reaction is characterized by a diminished protein and amylase content of the parotid gland.

Besides morphologic studies, there were so far only very few investigations on the effects of sympathetic stimulation or inhibition on the 'exportable' protein of the parotid gland in vivo. *Wilborn* and *Schneyer* [225] observed a congestion of zymogen granules in the gland cells 2 weeks after surgical sympathectomy. The electron microscopic picture of acinar cells containing densely packed secretory granules caused these authors to speak of 'dark cells'. Despite this accumulation of amylase-containing zymogen granules [86, 181, 228], the amylolytic activity of the rat parotid gland remained unaltered after elimination of the sympathetic nervous system [176]. This was explained by the occurrence of 'light acinar cells' in sympathectomized parotid glands. As opposed to the 'dark cells', the 'light cells' contain fewer secretory granules but exhibit all morphologic signs of an active protein metabolism. The simultaneous presence of 'dark' and 'light' cells in parotid tissue extracts is assumed to be responsible for the unchanged amylolytic activity of sympathectomized parotid glands.

These results were confirmed particularly by sympathetic inhibition for 3 weeks produced by guanoxane [3]. But also after application of guanethidine [50] and propranolol [8] the amylase concentration in the gland again declines after 3 weeks although it does not reach the still lower level of the untreated controls. An investigation within the first week of treatment yields principally different results. Following 'pharmacological sympathectomy' by guanoxane (fig. 9) and guanethidine as well as β-receptor inhibition by propranolol (fig. 10), we found a distinct increase of amylase activity in the parotid extracts during the first week [3, 8, 50].

There are several ways to explain *Schneyer* and *Hall's* [176] and our findings of the unchanged or again diminished glandular amylase activity 2 or 3 weeks after sympathectomy. Enzyme synthesis, which under physiological conditions is controlled in the parotid gland by the parasympathetic nervous system [176–178, 225] could be reduced in its response, but this explanation is contradicted by the electron microscopic finding of zymogen granule congestion. On the other hand, amylase might lose activity after prolonged storage in the acinar cell; and finally, automatic secretion processes [73] and also increased amylase secretion via cholinergic receptors might develop in the sympathectomized parotid gland.

As could be expected from investigations of parotid tissue slices, in vivo stimulation of β-receptors leads to a decrease of glandular amylase content [14, 41, 162]. On the other hand, the unphysiologically strong stimulation exerted by IPR activates DNA [13] and protein synthesis [177, 178] in the acinar cell.

The morphologic similarity of the parotid gland of IPR- and guanacline-treated rats to swelling of the human salivary glands of the head in sialadenosis has been known for some time [60, 62]. The parotid gland of the IPR-treated rat was used as an 'experimental model of sialadenosis' [6, 10] since the studies of *Selye* et al. [192, 193]. Similar to sialadenosis, IPR causes a swelling of the rat parotid gland that is not due to inflammatory infiltrations but to enlargement of the acinar cells, as revealed by histologic examination. The cells contain electron-optically less dense secretory granules [2, 198] and can therefore be compared with the 'light' cells [162]. According to our investigations, such cells contain significantly less secretable protein. Since the total number of zymogen granules is not reduced, their protein content must be lower due to their lower electron-optical density.

The side-effects of some antihypertensive substances, such as 'dryness of the mouth' and 'initial parotid pain' during mastication [for references see 44], but especially the development of a 'neurogenic sialadenosis' following therapy with guanacline [32, 62, 65, 155], initiated ultrastructural studies of the parotid gland of guanacline-treated rats [188]. The glands showed a parenchymatous swelling caused by enlarged acinar cells. Such changes meet the requirements of the term 'sialadenosis' according to the definition given by *Seifert* [186]. As another model of 'experimental sialadenosis', the parotid gland of guanacline-treated rats, however, mainly shows the 'dark type of acinar cells' [60]. They are closely packed with protein-rich zymogen granules.

Our studies with guanoxane and guanethidine (substances that are chemically related to guanacline and that also inhibit the transmission of impulses in the region of the postganglionic sympathetic fibers) revealed a retention of secretable protein within the parenchyma of the rat parotid gland. Application of these compounds therefore induces an 'inhibitory proteodyschylia' comparable with sympathetic α- and β-receptor inhibition. The parotid gland of IPR-treated rats is characterized by opposite changes; it shows 'light acinar cells' containing zymogen granules of lower electron-optical density, a decrease of secretable protein and therefore, 'stimulatory proteodyschylia'.

Based on their ultrastructural studies of the parotid glands of sialadenosis patients, *Donath* and *Seifert* [63] distinguished between three different types of sialadenosis:

(1) A dark granular type (dark acinar cells, densely packed, containing protein-rich secretory granules; no signs of increased protein synthesis in the gland cells).

(2) A light granular type (light acinar cells, containing secretory granules of low optical density; the acinar cells exhibit the morphologic signs of an increased protein synthesis).

(3) A mixed granular type (simultaneous presence of 'light' and 'dark' acinar cells).

These types of human sialadenosis can be experimentally induced in the rat by application of isoproterenol (light granular type) or guanacline (dark and mixed granular type).

The quantitative determination of the amount of secretable gland protein, especially of α-amylase, under the influence of experimentally induced changes of the sympathetic innervation of the parotid gland, has rendered it possible to assign to the morphologic types of sialadenosis the more functional terms of 'inhibitory' and 'stimulatory' proteodyschylia. 'Inhibitory proteodyschylia', characterized by retention of secretable protein, corresponds to the 'dark granular type' of sialadenosis with congestion of protein-rich zymogen granules. It can be experimentally produced by guanacline, guanoxane and guanethidine, or by inhibition of sympathetic α- and β-adrenergic receptors, e.g., by phentolamine and propranolol, respectively. 'Stimulatory proteodyschylia' (experimentally induced mainly by isoproterenol but also by amitriptyline and clonidine), characterized by decreased glandular amylase concentration, corresponds to the 'light granular type' with protein-deficient zymogen granules and the signs of enhanced protein synthesis caused by excessive stimulation.

The simultaneous action of inhibitory and stimulatory effects on glandular protein secretion and synthesis has to be postulated for the 'mixed granular type' of sialadenosis. Accepting the hypothesis of *Seifert* and *Donath* [188] that sialadenosis is the consequence of a peripheral vegetative neuropathy, simultaneous inhibition and stimulation of acinar protein secretion would seem possible: The neurogenic transmitter, released by destruction of peripheral sympathetic nerve structures, could lead to stimulation of protein secretion and synthesis by triggering a process of denervation secretion [73]. This 'stimulatory proteodyschylia' would then cause the 'light granular type of sialadenosis'. Following longer lasting denervation of the acinar cells one would have to expect the 'dark granular type of sialadenosis' resulting from the 'inhibitory proteodyschylia'. Denervation and re-innervation processes simultaneously taking place in different acinar cells could produce the morphologic signs of the 'mixed granular type of sialadenosis', with inhibition and stimulation of protein secretion existing side by side.

A pathogenetic pattern of sialadenosis as proposed above would explain the wide variation in the results of sialochemical as well as sialometric determinations in sialadenosis patients [49]. Besides aptyalism we also observed hypersalivation [for definition see 159] but could never find the reduced amylase content in sialadenotic saliva described by *Seifert* [187]. Depending on the presence of 'inhibitory' or 'stimulatory' proteodyschylia, different results will have to be expected. The diagnosis of sialadenosis with the aid of sialochemistry will therefore remain very difficult in the future.

Sialadenosis, when interpreted as a peripheral vegetative neuropathy [188], would explain the frequent connection of the disease with endocrine disorders and malnutrition. Neuropathia diabetica is known to accompany diabetes mellitus, and other neuropathies are not rare in alcoholics and in avitaminosis such as beriberi and pellagra. It is therefore not surprising that all therapeutic attempts have so far more or less failed although healing or improvement of the basic disease has been successful in the abolishment of the concomitant neuropathy to a certain extent. The sufficient stabilization of diabetes or the ingestion of proteins and vitamins in endocrine and metabolic sialadenoses is rather important in this connection. However, it is just the endocrine and neurogenic sialadenoses that frequently defy therapy [159].

Surgical removal of salivary glands which requires absolute competence in facial nerve surgery may be indicated as 'ultima ratio' in the, albeit rare, painful cases of sialadenosis. Whether or not parotidectomy can be replaced by operative ligation of the secretory ducts [59, 64, 93, 94, 218] cannot yet be decided with certainty.

Sialadenosis as the result of antihypertensive medication vanishes after discontinuation of drug application [for references see 44]. Following treatment with guanacline, however, there have been cases in which complaints persisted even after termination of the antihypertensive therapy [32]. This phenomenon was interpreted by irreversible destruction of vegetative nerve fibers by the action of the antihypertensive drug [36, 37]. The results of our investigations on the effects of clonidine, guanoxane and guanethidine have demonstrated that other antihypertensive substances, too, can at least experimentally induce sialadenosis-like changes in the parotid gland.

An answer to the question how far pharmacologic blockade of adrenergic and cholinergic receptors of the acinar cells is suitable for the therapy of sialadenosis, demands further clinical and experimental studies. Progress in the elucidation of its pathogenesis has raised hopes for new possibilities in the successful therapy of human sialadenosis.

Summary

Sialadenosis is a noninflammatory disease of the salivary glands of the head. It is observed in connection with endocrine disorders, malnutrition and neurologic diseases. The parotid glands are predominantly affected by a parenchymatous swelling. Based on morphologic and biochemical investigations it can be assumed that disorders of the gland's acinar protein secretion are responsible for sialadenosis. Changes in secretory behavior are caused by either excessive stimulation ('stimulatory proteodyschylia') or by inhibition of secretion ('inhibitory proteodyschylia'). The origin of these secretory disorders is very likely to be found in the vegetative nerve system.

The pathophysiology of sialadenosis can therefore only be understood after elucidation of the physiologic mechanisms of salivary gland secretion. Research in the field of biophysical and biochemical principles underlying parotid secretion has made considerable progress in recent years. A comprehensive review of this new evidence is necessary for the understanding of experimental studies on the pathogenesis of sialadenosis.

References

1 Andén, N.E.: Effects of amphetamine and some other drugs on central catecholamine mechanisms; in Costa, Garattini, Int. Symp. Amphetamines and Related Compounds (Raven Press, New York 1970).

2 Ansel, D.G.: Rat salivary glands after long-term isoproterenol administration. Archs. Otolar. *100:* 256–261 (1974).

3 Arglebe, C.; Chilla, R.: Über ein biochemisches Modell neurogener Sialosen. Z. Lar. Rhinol. *54:* 542–550 (1975).

4 Arglebe, C.; Chilla, R.: Early effects of clonidine (Catapresan®) on rat salivary glands. Archs. Oto-Rhino-Lar. *212:* 133–136 (1976).

5 Arglebe, C.; Chilla, R.: Spontane und künstlich erzeugte Enzymveränderungen in der Rattenohrspeicheldrüse. Ein experimentelles Alterungsmodell? HNO *25:* 51–54 (1977).

6 Arglebe, C.; Bremer, K.; Chilla, R.: Hyperamylasaemia in isoprenaline-induced experimental sialadenosis in the rat. Archs oral Biol. *23:* 997–999 (1978).

7 Arglebe, C.; Chilla, R.; Opaitz, M.: Age-dependent distribution of isoamylases in human parotid saliva. Clin. Otolaryngol. *1:* 249–256 (1976).

8 Arglebe, C.; Eysholdt, U.; Chilla, R.: Pharmacological inhibition of salivary glands: a possible therapy for sialosis and sialoadenitis. Effect of experimentally induced β-receptor block on the rat parotid gland. ORL *38:* 218–229 (1976).

9 Arnstein, C.: Zur Morphologie der sekretorischen Nervenendapparate. Anat. Anz. *10:* 410–419 (1895).

10 Arold, R.; Schätzle, W.: Die 'experimentelle Sialadenose' und ihre Beeinflussung durch β-Rezeptoren-Blocker. Arch. klin. exp. Ohr.-Nas.-KehlkHeilk. *203:* 274–288 (1973).

11 Aw, S.E.: Separation of urinary isoamylases on cellulose acetate. Nature, Lond. *209:* 298–300 (1966).

12 Babad, H.; Ben-Zvi, R.; Bdolah, A.; Schramm, M.: The mechanisms of enzyme secretion by the cell. 4. Effects of inducers, substrates, and inhibitors on amylase secretion by rat parotid slices. Eur. J. Biochem. *1:* 96–101 (1967).

13 Barka, T.: Stimulation of DNA synthesis by isoproterenol in the salivary gland. Expl. Cell Res. *39:* 355–364 (1965).

14 Barka, T.; Burke, G.T.: Secretory behaviour of hypertrophic and hyperplastic salivary gland. Histochem. J. *9:* 453–466 (1977).

15 Barka, T.; Noen, H. van der: Dissociation of rat parotid gland. Lab. Invest. *32:* 373–381 (1975).

16 Batzri, S.; Selinger, Z.: Enzyme secretion mediated by the epinephrine β-receptor in rat parotid slices. Factors governing efficiency of the process. J. biol. Chem. *248:* 356–360 (1973).

17 Batzri, S.; Selinger, Z.; Schramm, M.; Robinovitch, M.R.: Potassium release mediated by the epinephrine α-receptor in rat parotid slices. Properties and relation to enzyme secretion. J. biol. Chem. *248:* 361–368 (1973).

18 Batzri, S.; Amsterdam, A.; Selinger, Z.; Ohad, I.; Schramm, M.: Epinephrine-induced vacuole formation in parotid gland cells and its independence of the secretory process. Proc. natn. Acad. Sci. USA *68:* 121–123 (1971).

19 Bdolah, A.; Schramm, M.: The function of 3′:5′ cyclic AMP in enzyme secretion. Biochem. biophys. Res. Commun. *18:* 452–454 (1965).

20 Bdolah, A.; Ben-Zvi, R.; Schramm, M.: The mechanisms of enzyme secretion by the cell. 2. Secretion of amylase and other proteins by slices of rat parotid gland. Archs Biochem. Biophys. *104:* 58–66 (1964).

21 Becker, W.: Die Klinik der Erkrankungen der grossen Kopfspeicheldrüsen. Z. Lar. Rhinol. Otol. *37:* 205–240 (1958).

22 Becker, W.; Gosepath, P.: Zum Thema Lebercirrhose und Parotisfunktion. Z. Lar. Rhinol. Otol. *41:* 603–607 (1962).

23 Berger, A.S.V.; Emmelin, N.G.: Physiology of the salivary glands (Arnold, London 1960).

24 Berk, J.E.; Fridhandler, L.: Pursuit of the elusive: adventure in quest of a specific test for pancreatic amylase. Mount Sinai J. Med. *43:* 321–337 (1976).

25 Berk, J.E.; Hayashi, S.; Searcy, R.L.; Hightower, N.: Differentiation of parotid and pancreatic amylase in human serum. Am. J. dig. Dis. *11:* 695–701 (1966).

26 Berk, J.E.; Kizu, H.; Wilding, P.; Searcy, R.L.: Macroamylasemia: a newly recognized cause for elevated serum amylase activity. New Engl. J. Med. *277:* 941–946 (1967).

27 Berk, J.E.; Kizu, H.; Take, S.; Fridhandler, L.: Macroamylasemia: serum and urine amylase characteristics. Am. J. Gastroent., N.Y. *53:* 223–229 (1970).

28 Bhutta, I.H.; Rahman, M.A.: Serum amylase activity in liver disease. Clin. Chem. *17:* 1147–1149 (1971).

29 Bock, K.D.: Fehler und Gefahren bei der Hochdruckbehandlung. Dt. med. Wschr. *88:* 836–847 (1963).

30 Bock, K.D.: Vermeidbare und unvermeidbare Komplikationen der Langzeittherapie mit Antihypertonika. Therapiewoche *18:* 1102–1108 (1968).

31 Bock, K.D.: Gefahren der modernen antihypertensiven Therapie. Z. Allgemeinmed. *46:* 1287–1290 (1970).

32 Bock, K.D.; Huep, W.W.: Irreversibler Parotisschmerz nach Verabreichung von Guanaclin. Dt. med. Wschr. *96:* 1649–1650 (1971).

33 Boettcher, B.; Lande, F.A. de la: Electrophoresis of human salivary amylase in gel slabs. Analyt. Biochem. *28:* 510–514 (1969).

34 Borsanyi, S.J.; Blanchard, C.L.: Asymptomatic parotid swelling and isoproterenol. Laryngoscope 72: 1777–1783 (1962).

35 Burdett, P.E.; Kipps, A.E.; Whitehead, P.H.: A rapid technique for the detection of amylase isoenzymes using an enzyme sensitive 'test-paper'. Analyt. Biochem. 72: 315–319 (1976).

36 Burnstock, G.; Doyle, A.E.; Gannon, B.J.; Gerkens, J.F.; Iwayama, T.; Mashford, M.L.: Prolonged hypotension and ultrastructural changes in sympathetic neurones following guanacline treatment. Eur. J. Pharmacol. 13: 175–187 (1971).

37 Burnstock, G.; Evans, B.; Gannon, B.J.; Heath, J.W.; James, V.: A new method of destroying adrenergic nerves in adult animals using guanethidine. Br. J. Pharmacol. 43: 295–301 (1971).

38 Butcher, F.R.; McBridge, P.A.; Rudich, L.: Cholinergic regulation of cyclic nucleotide levels, amylase release, and K^+-efflux from rat parotid glands. Mol. cell. Endocrinol. 5: 243–254 (1976).

39 Butcher, F.R.; Goldman, J.A.; Nemerovski, M.: Effect of adrenergic agents on α-amylase release and adenosine 3′:5′-monophosphate accumulation in rat parotid tissue slices. Biochim. biophys. Acta 392: 82–94 (1975).

40 Butcher, F.R.; Rudich, L.; Emler, C.; Nemerovski, M.: Adrenergic regulation of cyclic nucleotide levels, amylase release, and potassium efflux in rat parotid gland. Molec. Pharmacol. 12: 862–870 (1976).

41 Byrt, P.: Secretion and synthesis of amylase in the rat parotid gland after isoprenaline. Nature, Lond. 212: 1212–1215 (1966).

42 Cantalamessa, F.; Caro, G. de; Perfumi, M.: Effects of chronic administration of eldoisin or physalaemin on the rat salivary glands. Pharmacol. Res. Commun. 7: 259–271 (1975).

43 Castle, J.D.; Jamieson, J.D.; Palade, G.E.: Secretion granules of the rabbit parotid gland. J. Cell Biol. 64: 182–210 (1975).

44 Chilla, R.; Arglebe, C.: Pharmakotherapie der Hypertonie und ihre Bedeutung für die Funktion der Kopfspeicheldrüsen. Münch. med. Wschr. 117: 1425–1428 (1975).

45 Chilla, R.; Arglebe, C.: Effects of α- and β-adrenergic receptor blockade on the isoamylases of rat parotid gland. Archs Oto-Rhino-Lar. 220: 187–192 (1978).

46 Chilla, R.; Bobke, H.; Arglebe, C.: Postoperative Hyperamylasämie. Bestimmung der Serumisoamylasen nach chirurgischen Eingriffen an der Ohrspeicheldrüse. Medsche Klin. 73: 626–632 (1978).

47 Chilla, R.; Hoffmann, G.; Arglebe, C.: Die 'stimulatorische Proteodyschylie' in der Amitriptylin (Laroxyl®)-behandelten Rattenparotis. Tierexperimentelle Untersuchungen über die Auswirkung einer antidepressiven Pharmakotherapie auf die Ohrspeicheldrüsen. Archs Oto-Rhino-Lar. 217: 61–67 (1977).

48 Chilla, R.; Kropp, T.; Arglebe, C.: Amylaseaktivität und Isoamylasenmuster im Parotisspeichel des Menschen. Z. Lar. Rhinol. 56: 912–918 (1977).

49 Chilla, R.; Opaitz, M.; Arglebe, C.: Flussrate, Amylase- und Proteingehalt des Parotisspeichels bei Sialadenose. Z. Lar. Rhinol. 57: 274–279 (1978).

50 Chilla, R.; Rieger, R.; Arglebe, C.: Die Sialadenose des therapierten Hypertonikers. I. Experimentelle Untersuchungen über die Auswirkungen von Guanethidin (Ismelin®) auf die Ohrspeicheldrüsen der Ratte. Archs Oto-Rhino-Lar. 211: 185–192 (1975).

51 Chilla, R.; Arold, R.; Flucke, K.-H.; Arglebe, C.: The effect of clonidine treatment on the salivary glands of the rat. Results of biochemical and histological investigations. Archs Oto-Rhino-Lar. *209:* 47–57 (1975).

52 Chilla, R.; Doering, K.-M.; Lubahn, H.; Arglebe, C.: Über das Auftreten 'schneller Isoamylasen' im Mukoviszidosespeichel. Archs Oto-Rhino-Lar. *214:* 367–369 (1977).

53 Chilla, R.; Niemann, H.; Arglebe, C.; Domagk, G.F.: Age-dependent changes in the α-isoamylase pattern of human and rat parotid glands. ORL *36:* 373–382 (1974).

54 Clara, M.: Das Nervensystem des Menschen (Barth, Leipzig 1959).

55 Cope, G.H.; Williams, M.A.: Quantitative analyses of the constituent membranes of the parotid acinar cells and of the changes evident after induced exocytosis. Z. Zellforsch. mikrosk. Anat. *145:* 311–330 (1973).

56 Corbett, A.D.; Main, B.E.; Muir, T.C.; Templeton, D.: The receptors involved in catecholamine mediated growth and secretion in rat parotid gland. Br. J. Pharmacol. *58:* 281P–282P (1976).

57 Cwinkel, B.; Avner, R.; Czosnek, H.H.; Hochberg, A.A.; Groot, N. de: The synthesis of α-amylase by rough and in vitro reconstituted rough endoplasmic reticulum derived from rat parotid gland. Mol. Biol. Rep. *2:* 455–463 (1976).

58 Descos, F.; Andre, F.; Lambert, R.; Andre, C.: Influence of secretin on salivary mucous secretion in man. Digestion *9:* 199–204 (1973).

59 Diamant, H.: Ligation of the parotid duct in chronic recurrent parotitis. Acta otolar. *49:* 375–380 (1958).

60 Donath, K.: Ultrastrukturelle Acinusveränderungen der Rattenparotis unter der Einwirkung von Antihypertensiva (Guanacline). Archs Oto-Rhino-Lar. *206:* 77–90 (1973).

61 Donath, K.: Die Sialadenose der Parotis. Ultrastrukturelle, klinische und experimentelle Befunde zur Sekretionspathologie (Fischer, Stuttgart 1976).

62 Donath, K.; Burkhardt, A.: Experimentelle Parotisveränderungen nach chemisch induzierter Sympathicusdegeneration. Verh. dt. Ges. Path. *57:* 449 (1973).

63 Donath, K.; Seifert, G.: Ultrastructural studies of the parotid gland in sialadenosis. Virchows Arch. Abt. A Path. Anat. *365:* 119–135 (1975).

64 Donath, K.; Hirsch-Hoffmann, H.U.; Seifert, G.: Zur Pathogenese der Parotisatrophie nach experimenteller Gangunterbindung. Ultrastrukturelle Befunde am Drüsenparenchym der Rattenparotis. Virchows Arch. Abt. A Path. Anat. *359:* 34–48 (1973).

65 Donath, K.; Seifert, G.; Pirsig, W.: Sympathicusveränderungen in der Parotis bei Guanacline-Therapie. Virchows Arch. Abt. A Path. Anat. *360:* 195–207 (1973).

66 O'Donnell, M.D.; McGeeney, K.F.: Purification and properties of an α-amylase inhibitor from wheat. Biochim. biophys. Acta *422:* 159–169 (1976).

67 O'Donnell, M.D.; Fitzgerald, O.; McGeeney, K.F.: A new method for detecting pancreatic and salivary gland malfunction. Ir. J. med. Sci. *145:* 267–268 (1976).

68 Drack, G.T.; Koelz, H.R.; Blum, A.L.: Human calcitonin stimulates salivary amylase output in man. Gut *17:* 620–623 (1976).

69 Dreiling, D.A.; Janowitz, H.D.; Josephberg, L.J.: Serum isoamylases. An electrophoretic study of the blood amylase and the patterns observed in pancreatic disease. Ann. intern. Med. *58:* 235–244 (1963).

70 Durham, J.P.; Butcher, F.R.: The effect of catecholamine analogues upon amylase

secretion from the mouse parotid gland in vivo: relationship to changes in cyclic AMP and cyclic GMP levels. FEBS Lett. *47:* 218–221 (1974).

71 Durham, J.P.; Galanti, N.: The effect of isoproterenol upon the activity and intracellular distribution of pyrimidine nucleoside kinases in the mouse parotid gland. J. biol. Chem. *249:* 1806–1813 (1974).

72 Emmelin, N.: Control of salivary glands; in Emmelin, Zotterman, Oral physiology. Proc. Int. Symp. Wenner-Green Center, Stockholm 1971 (Pergamon Press, New York 1971).

73 Emmelin, N.; Trendelenburg, U.: Degeneration activity after parasympathetic or sympathetic denervation. A. Rev. Physiol. *66:* 147–211 (1972).

74 Eneroth, C.-M.; Hökfelt, T.; Norberg, K.-A.: The role of parasympathetic and sympathetic innervation for the secretion of human parotid and submandibular gland. Acta oto-lar. *68:* 369–375 (1969).

75 Fontoynont, M.: Le mangy. Presse méd. *19:* 455–459 (1911).

76 Franzini, C.; Bonini, P.A.: Alpha-glucosidases in human urine. Clinica chim. Acta *17:* 505–510 (1967).

77 Franzini, C.; Bonini, P.A.: Lack of α-amylase in horse serum. Experientia *25:* 597–598 (1969).

78 Franzini, C.; Bonini, P.A.; Sola, M.L.: α-Amylases and α-glucosidases in pig serum. Enzymologia *36:* 117–131 (1969).

79 Garrett, J.R.: The innervation of normal human submandibular and parotid salivary glands. Archs oral Biol. *12:* 1417–1436 (1967).

80 Garrett, J.R.: Recent advances in physiology of salivary glands. Br. med. Bull. *31:* 152–155 (1975).

81 McGeachin, R.L.; Potter, B.A.: Electrophoretic behaviour of rat serum amylase. Nature, Lond. *198:* 751 (1961).

82 McGeachin, R.L.; Gleason, J.R.; Adams, M.R.: Amylase distribution in extrapancreatic, extrasalivary tissues. Archs Biochem. Biophys. *75:* 403–411 (1958).

83 Goldberg, D.M.; Spooner, R.J.: Amylase, isoamylase, and macroamylase. Digestion *13:5* 6–75 (1975).

84 Graubner, W.; Wolf, M.: Kritische Betrachtungen zum Wirkungsmechanismus des 2-(2,6-Dichlorphenylamino)-2-imidazolin-hydrochlorids. Arzneimittel-Forsch. *16:* 1055–1058 (1966).

85 Grimmel, K.; Rossbach, G.; Kasper, H.: Amylase activity of parotid saliva in acute and chronic pancreatitis. Acta hepato-gastroenterol. *23:* 334–344 (1976).

86 Gromet-Elhanan, Z.; Winnick, T.: Microsomes as sites of α-amylase synthesis in the rat parotid gland. Biochim. biophys. Acta *69:* 85–96 (1963).

87 Haeringen, N.J. van; Ensink, F.; Glasius, E.: Amylase in human tears fluid: origin and characteristics, compared with salivary and urinary amylases. Expl. Eye Res. *21:* 395–403 (1975).

88 Hall, F.F.; Ratliff, C.R.; Hayakawa, T.; Culp, T.W.; Hightower, N.C.: Substrate differentiation of human pancreatic and salivary alpha-amylases. Am. J. dig. Dis. *15:* 1031–1038 (1970).

89 Hammerton, K.; Messer, M.: Electrophoretic studies on mammalian α-amylases. Proc. Aust. biochem. Soc. *3:* 15 (1970).

90 Hammerton, K.; Messer, M.: The origin of serum amylase. Electrophoretic studies of the isoamylases of the serum, liver, and other tissues of adult and infant rats. Biochim. biophys. Acta *244:* 441–451 (1971).

91 Hand, A.R.: Nerve-acinar cell relationships in the rat parotid gland. J. Cell Biol. *47:* 540–543 (1970).

92 Hand, A.R.: Adrenergic and cholinergic nerve terminals in the rat parotid gland. Electron microscopic observations on permanganate-fixed glands. Anat. Rec. *173:* 131–140 (1972).

93 Harrison, J.D.; Garrett, J.R.: Histological effects of ductal ligation of salivary glands of the cat. J. Path. Bact. *118:* 245–254 (1976).

94 Harrison, J.D.; Garrett, J.R.: The effects of ductal ligation on the parenchyma of salivary glands of cat studied by enzyme histochemical methods. Histochem. J. *8:* 35–44 (1976).

95 Haubrich, J.: Klinik der nichttumorbedingten Erkrankungen der Speicheldrüsen. Archs Oto-Rhino-Lar. *213:* 1–59 (1976).

96 Heffernon, J.J.; Smith, W.R.; Berk, J.E.; Fridhandler, L.; Glauser, F.L.; Montgomery, K.A.: Hyperamylasemia in heroin addicts. Am. J. Gastroent., N.Y. *66:* 17–22 (1976).

97 Hoefke, W.; Kobinger, W.: Pharmakologische Wirkungen des 2-(2,6-Dichlorphenylamino)-2-imidazolin-hydrochlorids, einer neuen antihypertensiven Substanz. Arzneimittel-Forsch. *16:* 1038–1050 (1966).

98 Hsiu, J.; Fischer, E.H.; Stein, E.A.: Alpha-amylases as calcium-metallo-enzymes. II. Calcium and the catalytic activity. Biochemistry *3:* 61–66 (1964).

99 Hukahara, T., Jr.; Otsuka, Y.; Takeda, R.; Sakai, F.: Die zentralen Wirkungen des 2-(2,6-Dichlorphenylamino)-2-imidazolin-hydrochlorids. Arzneimittel-Forsch. *18:* 1147–1153 (1968).

100 Ishida, H.; Miki, N.; Yoshida, H.: Role of Ca^{2+} in the secretion of amylase from the rat parotid gland. Jap. J. Pharmacol. *21:* 227–238 (1971).

101 Ito, Y.; Mizutani, A.: Studies on the salivary gland hormones. XIII. Purification of parotin. Jap. Pharmacol. *72:* 239–245 (1952).

102 Johnson, D.A.; Sreebny, M.S.; Sreebny, L.M.: Effect of isoproterenol on synthesis and secretion in the rat parotid gland. Lab. Invest. *28:* 263–269 (1973).

103 Kamaryt, J.; Laxová, R.: Amylase heterogeneity. Some genetic and clinical aspects. Humangenetik *1:* 579–586 (1965).

104 Kamarýt, J.; Laxová, R.: Amylase heterogeneity variants in man. Humangenetik *3:* 41–45 (1966).

105 Kanamori, T.; Hayakawa, T.; Nagatsu, T.: Adenosine 3′:5′-monophosphate-dependent protein kinase and amylase secretion from rat parotid gland. Biochem. biophys. Res. Commun. *57:* 394–398 (1974).

106 Karn, R.C.; Rosenblum, B.B.; Ward, J.C.; Merritt, A.D.: Genetic and post-translational mechanisms determining human amylase isozyme heterogeneity; in Markert, Isozymes. IV. Genetics and evolution, pp. 745–761 (Adademic Press, New York 1975).

107 Karn, R.C.; Shulkin, J.D.; Merritt, A.D.; Newell, R.C.: Evidence for post-transcriptional modification of human salivary amylase (Amy₁) isozymes. Biochem. Genet. *10:* 341–350 (1973).

108 Karn, R.C.; Rosenblum, B.B.; Ward, J.C.; Merritt, A.D.; Shulkin, J.D.: Immunological relationships and posttranslational modifications of human salivary amylase (Amy₁) and pancreatic amylase (Amy₂) isozymes. Biochem. Genet. *12:* 485–499 (1974).

109 Kauffman, D.L.; Watanabe, S.; Evans, J.R.; Keller, P.J.: The existence of glycosy-lated and non-glycosylated forms of human submandibular amylase. Archs oral Biol. *18:* 1105–1111 (1973).

110 Kauffman, D.L.; Zager, N.I.; Cohen, E.; Keller, P.J.: The isoenzymes of human parotid amylase. Archs Biochem. Biophys. *137:* 325–339 (1970).

111 Keller, P.J.; Kauffman, D.L.; Allan, B.J.; Williams, B.L.: Further studies on the structural differences between the isoenzymes of human parotid α-amylase. Biochemistry *10:* 4867–4874 (1971).

112 Keller, P.J.; Robinovitch, M.; Iversen, J.; Kauffman, D.L.: The protein composition of rat parotid saliva and secretory granules. Biochim. biophys. Acta *379:* 562–570 (1975).

113 Kenawy, M.R.: Endemic enlargement of parotid gland in Egypt. Trans. R. Soc. trop. Med. Hyg. *31:* 339–350 (1937).

114 Kleine, U.: Über den Wirkungsmechanismus von Guanethidin. Ärztl. Forsch. *17:* 498–501 (1963).

115 Koba, Y.; Najima, M.; Ueda, S.: Further purification of amylase inhibitor produced by *Streptomyces* spec. Agric. Biol. Chem. *40:* 1167–1173 (1976).

116 Kobinger, W.: Pharmacological basis of the cardio-vascular actions of clonidine; in Onesti, Kim, Moyer, Hypertension: mechanisms and management (Grune & Stratton, New York 1973).

117 Kroneberg, G.; Schümann, H.J.; Eckardt, A.: Untersuchungen zum Wirkungs-mechanismus des Guanethidins. Naunyn-Schmiedebergs Arch. exp. Path. Pharmak. *243:* 16–25 (1962).

118 Kuttner, M.; Somogyi, M.: Diastase in milk. Proc. Soc. exp. Biol. Med. *32:* 564–566 (1934).

119 Lamberts, B.L.; Meyer, T.S.; Osborne, R.M.: A comparative study of human parotid and submaxillary amylase. Archs oral Biol. *16:* 517–526 (1971).

120 Lande, F.A. de la; Boettcher, B.: Electrophoretic examination of human serum amylase isoenzymes. Enzymologia *37:* 335–342 (1969).

121 Laugesen, L.P.; Nielsen, J.O.D.; Poulsen, J.H.: Partial dissociation between salivary secretion and active potassium transport in the perfused cat submandibular gland. Pflüger's Arch. *364:* 167–173 (1976).

122 Lehrner, L.M.; Ward, J.C.; Karn, R.C.; Ehrlich, C.E.; Merritt, A.D.: An evaluation of the usefulness of amylase isoenzyme differentiation in patients with hyper-amylasemia. Am. J. clin. Path. *66:* 576–587 (1976).

123 Leslie, B.A.; Putney, J.W.; Sherman, J.M.: α-Adrenergic, β-adrenergic and cholin-ergic mechanisms for amylase secretion by rat parotid gland in vitro. J. Physiol., Lond. *260:* 351–370 (1976).

124 Lillie, J.H.: An effect of prostaglandin E_1 on the acinar cell of the rat parotid gland. J. Ultrastruct. Res. *49:* 50–59 (1974).

125 Lindsay, R.H.; Ueha, T.; Hulsey, B.S.; Hanson, R.W.: Relationship of chemically initiated enzyme secretion to metabolism in rat parotid in vitro. Am. J. Physiol. *221:* 80–85 (1971).

126 Lowry, O.H.; Rosebrough, N.J.; Farr, A.L.; Randall, R.J.: Protein measurement with the Folin phenol reagent. J. biol. Chem. *193:* 265–275 (1951).

127 Loyter, A.; Schramm, M.: The glycogen-amylase complex as a means of obtaining highly purified α-amylase. Biochim. biophys. Acta *65:* 200–206 (1962).

128 Loyter, A.; Schramm, M.: Multimolecular complexes of α-amylase with glycogen limit dextrin. Number of binding sites of the enzyme and size of the complexes. J. biol. Chem. *241:* 2611–2617 (1966).

129 Ludwig, C.: Neue Versuche über Beihilfe der Nerven zur Speichelabsonderung. Z. rat. Med. *1:* 255–277 (1851).

130 Malacinski, G.M.; Rutter, W.J.: Multiple molecular forms of α-amylase from the rabbit. Biochemistry *8:* 4382–4390 (1969).

131 Mandel, I.D.; Katz, R.: The effect of pharmacologic agents on the salivary secretion and composition. 2. Isoproterenol, alpha- and beta-adrenergic blockers. J. oral Ther. Pharm. *4:* 260–269 (1968).

132 Mangos, J.A.; McSherry, N.R.: Micropuncture study of sodium and potassium excretion in rat parotid saliva: role of aldosterone. Proc. Soc. exp. Biol. Med. *132:* 797–801 (1969).

133 Mangos, J.A.; McSherry, N.R.; Barber, T.: Dispersed parotid acinar cells. III. Characterization of cholinergic receptors. Am. J. Physiol. *229:* 566–569 (1975).

134 Mangos, J.A.; McSherry, N.R.; Barber, T.; Arvanitakis, S.N.; Wagner, V.: Dispersed parotid acinar cells. II. Characterization of adrenergic receptors. Am. J. Physiol. *229:* 560–565 (1975).

135 Mangos, J.A.; McSherry, N.R.; Butcher, F.; Irwin, K.; Barber, T.: Dispersed rat parotid acinar cells. I. Morphological and functional characterization. Am. J. Physiol. *229:* 553–559 (1975).

136 Mann, H.B.; Whitney, D.R.: On a test of whether one of two random variables is stochastically larger than the other. Ann. math. Statist. *18:* 50–60 (1947).

137 Maurs, C.; Herman, G.; Busson, S.; Ovtracht, L.; Rossignol, B.: Regulation of protein secretion and metabolism in rat salivary glands. J. Microscopy *20:* 187–196 (1974).

138 Meites, S.; Rogols, S.: Serum amylases, isoenzymes, and pancreatitis. I. Effect of substrate variation. Clin. Chem. *14:* 1176–1184 (1968).

139 Meites, S.; Rogols, S.: Amylase isoenzymes. CRC crit. Rev. clin. Lab. Sci. *2:* 103–138 (1971).

140 Mermall, H.L.; Hanhila, M.O.; Reeres, W.M.: Effects of cations on the activation of salivary amylase. I. Na^+, K^+, Ca^{2+} and Mg^{2+}. J. dent. Res. *52:* 1148 (1973).

141 Merritt, A.D.; Rivas, M.L.; Bixler, D.; Newell, R.: Salivary and pancreatic amylase: electrophoretic characterizations and genetic studies. Am. J. hum. Genet. *25:* 510–522 (1973).

142 Meur, S.K.; De, K.B.: Anionic activation of human salivary amylase. Experientia *32:* 1133–1135 (1976).

143 Monnard, P.; Schorderet, M.: Cyclic adenosine $3':5'$-monophosphate concentration in rabbit parotid slices following stimulation by secretagogues. Eur. J. Pharmacol. *23:* 306–310 (1973).

144 Mulcahy, H.; Fitzgerald, O.; McGeeney, K.F.: Secretin and pancreozymin effect on salivary amylase concentration in man. Gut *13:* 850 (1972).

145 Muus, J.; Vnenchak, J.M.: Isoenzymes of salivary amylase. Nature, Lond. *204:* 283–285 (1964).

146 Nelson, T.E.; Stouffer, J.E.: Thyroxine modulation of epinephrine stimulated secretion of rat parotid α-amylase. Biochem. biophys. Res. Commun. *48:* 480–485 (1972).

147 Noelting, G.; Bernfeld, P.: Sur les enzymes amylolytiques. III. La β-amylase: dosage d'activité et contrôle de l'absence d'α-amylase. Helv. chim. Acta *31:* 286–290 (1948).

148 Nothman, M.M.; Callow, A.D.: Investigations on the origin of amylase in serum and urine. Gastroenterology *60:* 82–89 (1971).

149 Ogata, A.; Ito, Y.; Nozaki, N.: On the parotid gland hormone. Med. Biol. *5:* 253–259 (1944).

150 Otsuki, M.; Saeki, S.; Yuu, H.; Maeda, M.; Baba, S.: Electrophoretic pattern of amylase isoenzymes in serum and urine of normal persons. Clin. Chem. *22:* 439–444 (1976).

151 Pasternack, A.; Stenman, U.H.: False rise of starch-iodine determined amylase values caused by heparin treatment during haemodialysis. Clinica chim. Acta *65:* 213–221 (1975).

152 Pazur, J.H.: Enzymes in synthesis and hydrolysis of starch; in Whistler, Paschall, Starch: chemistry and technology, vol. I (Academic Press, New York 1965).

153 Peterson, O.H.: The effect of dinitrophenol on secretory potentials, secretion and potassium accumulation in the perfused cat submandibular gland. Acta physiol. scand. *80:* 117–121 (1970).

154 Pimstone, N.R.: A study of the starch iodine complex: a modified colorimetric micro-determination of amylase in biological fluids. Clin. Chem. *10:* 891–906 (1964).

155 Pirsig, W.; Proescher, H.J.; Donath, K.: Zur Ultrastruktur geschädigter Nerven in der Parotis bei Guanacline-therapierten Hypertonikern: Morphologische Substrate zum Parotisschmerz. Arch. klin. exp. Ohr.-Nas.-KehlkHeilk. *205:* 103–109 (1973).

156 Pöldinger, W.: Kompendium der Psychopharmakatherapie (Hoffmann-La Roche, Grenzach 1971).

157 Putney, J.W.: Biphasic modulation of potassium release in rat parotid gland by carbachol and phenylephrine. J. Pharmac. exp. Ther. *198:* 375–384 (1976).

158 Rajasingham, R.; Bell, J.L.; Baron, D.N.: A comparative study of the isoenzymes of mammalian α-amylase. Enzyme *12:* 180–186 (1971).

159 Rauch, S.: Die Speicheldrüsen des Menschen. Anatomie, Physiologie und klinische Pathologie (Thieme, Stuttgart 1959).

160 Robinovitch, M.R.; Sreebny, L.M.: Separation of rat parotid isoamylases by preparative polyacrylamide gel electrophoresis. Archs oral Biol. *15:* 1381–1384 (1970).

161 Robinovitch, M.R.; Sreebny, L.M.: On the nature of the molecular heterogeneity of rat parotid amylase. Archs oral Biol. *17:* 595–600 (1972).

162 Robinovitch, M.R.; Keller, P.J.; Johnson, D.A.; Iversen, J.M.; Kauffman, D.L.: Changes in rat parotid salivary proteins induced by chronic isoproterenol administration. J. dent. Res. *56:* 290–303 (1977).

163 Robyt, J.F.; French, D.: Multiple attack hypothesis of α-amylase action: action of porcine pancreatic, human salivary, and *Aspergillus oryzae* α-amylases. Archs. Biochem. Biophys. *122:* 8–16 (1967).

164 Robyt, J.F.; Whelan, W.J.: The α-amylases; in Radley, Starch and its derivatives, pp. 430–476 (Chapman & Hall, London 1968).

165 Rosenmund, H.; Kaczmarek, M.J.: Isolation and characterization of isoenzymes of human salivary and pancreatic α-amylase. Clinica chim. Acta *71:* 185–189 (1976).

166 Rossignol, B.; Herman, G.; Keryer, G.: Inhibition by colchicine of carbamylcholine induced glycoprotein secretion by the submaxillary gland. A possible mechanism of cholinergic induced protein secretion. FEBS Lett. *21:* 189–194 (1972).

167 Rothman, S.S.; Burwen, S.; Liebow, C.: The zymogen granule: intragranular organization and its functional significance; in Ceccarelli, Clementi, Meldolesi, Advances in cytopharmacology, vol. 2 (Raven Press, New York 1974).

168 Ryan, J.; Appert, H.: Circulatory turnover of pancreatic amylase. Proc. Soc. exp. Biol. Med. *149:* 921–925 (1975).

169 Salomon, T.: Enlarged parotids and pellagra. J. trop. Med. Hyg. *61:* 253–259 (1958).

170 Salt, W.B.; Schenker, S.: Amylase – its clinical significance: a review of the literature. Medicine *55:* 269–289 (1976).

171 Sanders, T.G.; Rutter, W.J.: Molecular properties of rat pancreatic and parotid α-amylase. Biochemistry *11:* 130–136 (1972).

172 Sandstead, H.R.; Koehn, C.J.; Sessions, S.M.: Enlargement of the parotid gland in malnutrition. Am. J. clin. Nutr. *3:* 198–214 (1955).

173 Schiwara, H.-W.: Nachweis der Isoamylasen mit Amylopectin Azur als Substrat. Z. klin. Chem. klin. Biochem. *11:* 319–320 (1973).

174 Schmitt, H.; Schmidt, H.: Localization of the hypotensive effect of 2-(2,6-dichloro-phenylamino)-2-imidazoline hydrochloride (St 155, catapresan). Eur. J. Pharmacol. *6:* 8–12 (1969).

175 Schneyer, L.H.: Secretion of potassium by perfused excretory duct of rat sub-maxillary gland. Am. J. Physiol. *217:* 1324–1329 (1969).

176 Schneyer, C.A.; Hall, H.D.: Function of the rat parotid gland after sympathectomy and total postganglionectomy. Am. J. Physiol. *211:* 943–949 (1966).

177 Schneyer, C.A.; Hall, H.D.: Parasympathetic regulation of mitosis induced in rat parotid by dietary change. Am. J. Physiol. *229:* 1614–1617 (1975).

178 Schneyer, C.A.; Hall, H.D.: Neurally mediated increase in mitosis and DNA of rat parotid with increase in bulk of diet. Am. J. Physiol. *230:* 911–915 (1976).

179 Schramm, M.: Unmasking of sulfhydryl groups in pancreatic α-amylase. Biochemistry *3:* 1231–1234 (1964).

180 Schramm, M.: Amylase secretion in rat parotid slices by apparent activation of endogenous catecholamine. Biochim. biophys. Acta *165:* 546–549 (1968).

181 Schramm, M.; Danon, D.: The mechanisms of enzyme secretion by the cell. 1. Storage of amylase in the zymogen granules of the rat parotid gland. Biochim. biophys. Acta *50:* 102–112 (1961).

182 Schramm, M.; Selinger, Z.: The function of α- and β-adrenergic receptors and a cholinergic receptor in the secretory cell of the rat parotid gland; in Ceccarelli, Clementi, Meldolesi, Advances in cytopharmacology, vol. 2 (Raven Press, New York 1974).

183 Schramm, M.; Ben-Zvi, R.; Bdolah, A.: Epinephrine-activated amylase secretion in parotid clices and leakage of the enzyme in the cold. Biochem. biophys. Res. Commun. *18:* 446–451 (1965).

184 Searcy, R.L.; Hayashi, S.; Hardy, E.M.; Berk, J.E.: The interaction of human serum protein fractions with the starch iodine complex. Clinica chim. Acta *12:* 631–638 (1965).

185 Searcy, R.L.; Ujihara, I.; Hayashi, S.; Berk, J.E.: An intrinsic disparity between amyloclastic and saccharogenic estimations of human serum isoamylase activities. Clinica chim. Acta *9:* 505–508 (1964).

186 Seifert, G.: Die Sekretionsstörungen (Dyschylien) der Speicheldrüsen; in Cohrs, Giese, Meessen, Ergebnisse der allgemeinen Pathologie und pathologischen Anatomie, vol. 44, pp. 103–188 (Springer, Berlin 1964).

187 Seifert, G.: Klinische Pathologie der Sialadenitis und Sialadenose. HNO *19:* 1–9 (1971).

188 Seifert, G; Donath, K.: Die Sialadenose der Parotis. Dt. med. Wschr. *100:* 1545–1548 (1975).

189 Selinger, Z.; Naim, E.: The effect of calcium on amylase secretion by rat parotid slices. Biochim. biophys. Acta *203:* 335–337 (1970).

190 Selinger, Z.; Schramm, M.: Control of reactions related to enzyme secretion in rat parotid gland. Ann. N.Y. Acad. Sci. *185:* 395–402 (1971).

191 Selinger, Z.; Sharoni, Y.; Schramm, M.: Modification of the secretory granule during secretion in the rat parotid gland; in Ceccarelli, Clementi, Meldolesi, Advances in cytopharmacology, vol. 2 (Raven Press, New York 1974).

192 Selye, H.; Cantin, M.; Veilleux, R.: Abnormal growth and sclerosis of the salivary glands induced by chronic treatment with isoproterenol. Growth *25:* 243–248 (1961).

193 Selye, H.; Veilleux, R.; Cantin, M.: Excessive stimulation of salivary gland growth by isoproterenol. Science *133:* 44–45 (1961).

194 Shannon, I.L.; Suddick, R.P.; Dowd, F.J.: Saliva: composition and secretion (Karger, Basel 1974).

195 Sharoni, Y.; Eimerl, S.; Schramm, M.: Secretion of old versus new exportable protein in rat parotid slices. Control by neurotransmitters. J. Cell Biol. *71:* 107–122 (1976).

196 Siepmann, R.; Stegemann, H.: Enzym-Elektrophorese in Einschlusspolymerisaten des Acrylamids. A. Amylasen, Phosphorylasen. Z. Naturf. *22b:* 949–955 (1967).

197 Silano, V.; Furia, M.; Gianfreda, L.; Macri, A.; Palescandolo, R.; Rab, A.; Scardi, V.; Stella, E.; Valfre, F.: Inhibition of amylases from different origins by albumins from the wheat kernel. Biochim. biophys. Acta *391:* 170–178 (1975).

198 Simson, J.V.A.: Alterations in salivary glands of rats following isoproterenol administration as revealed by electron microscopy. Anat. Rec. *157:* 321–322 (1967).

199 Simson, J.V.A.: Evidence of cell damage in rat salivary glands after isoproterenol. Anat. Rec. *173:* 437–452 (1972).

200 Skude, G.; Ihse, I.: Salivary amylase in duodenal aspirates. Scand. J. Gastroent. *11:* 17–20 (1976).

201 Skude, G.; Mårdh, P.-A.: Isoamylases in blood, urine, and tissue homogenates from some experimental mammals. Scand. J. Gastroent. *11:* 21–26 (1976).

202 Skude, G.; Mårdh, P.-A.; Westrom, L.: Amylases of genital tract. 1. Isoamylases of genital tract tissue homogenates and peritoneal fluid. Am. J. Obstet. Gynec. *126:* 652–656 (1976).

203 Somogyi, M.: Micromethods for estimation of diastase. J. biol. Chem. *125:* 399–414 (1938).

204 Speirs, R.L.; Herring, J.; Cooper, W.D.; Hardy, C.C.; Hind, C.R.K.: The influence of sympathetic activity and isoprenaline on the secretion of amylase from the human parotid gland. Archs oral Biol. *19:* 747–752 (1974).

205 Stegemann, H.: Apparatur zur thermokonstanten Elektrophorese und Focussierung und ihre Zusatzteile. Z. analyt. Chem. *261:* 388–391 (1972).

206 Stiefel, D.J.; Keller, P.J.: Preparation and some properties of human pancreatic amylase including a comparison with parotid amylase. Biochim. biophys. Acta *302:* 345–361 (1973).

207 Stiefel, D.J.; Keller, P.J.: Comparison of human pancreatic and parotid amylase on different substrates. Clin. Chem. *21:* 343–346 (1975).

208 Street, H.V.; Close, J.R.: Determination of amylase activity in biological fluids. Clinica chim. Acta *1:* 256–268 (1956).

209 Takeuchi, T.; Matsushima, T.; Sugimura, T.: Separation of human α-amylase isozymes by electrofocusing and their immunological properties. Clinica chim. Acta *60:* 207–213 (1975).

210 Takizawa, N.: A pathological research on the internal secretion of the salivary glands. Acta path. jap. *4:* 229–266 (1954).

211 Telegdi, M.; Fabian, F.; El-Sewedy, S.M.; Straub, B.F.: Microheterogeneity in porcine pancreatic amylase preparations due to disulfide-sulfhydryl exchange. Biochim. biophys. Acta *429:* 860–869 (1976).

212 Thaysen, E.H.; Müllertz, S.; Worning, H.; Bang, H.O.: Amylase concentration of duodenal aspirates after stimulation of the pancreas by a standard meal. Gastroenterology *46:* 23–31 (1964).

213 Thoenen, H.; Tranzer, J.P.: The pharmacology of 6-hydroxydopamine. A. Rev. Pharmacol. *13:* 169–180 (1973).

214 Thulin, A.: Influence of autonomic nerves and drugs on myoepithelial cells in parotid glands of cat. Acta physiol. scand. *93:* 477–482 (1975).

215 Thulin, A.: Secretory and motor effects in the submaxillary gland of the rat of some polypeptides and autonomics drugs. Acta physiol. scand. *97:* 343–348 (1976).

216 Townes, P.L.; Moore, W.D.; White, M.R.: Amylase polymorphism: studies of sera and duodenal aspirates in normal individuals and in cystic fibrosis. Am. J. hum. Genet. *28:* 378–389 (1976).

217 Tranzer, J.P.; Thoenen, H.: An electron microscopic study of selective, acute degeneration of sympathetic nerve terminals after administration of 6-hydroxydopamine. Experientia *24:* 155–156 (1968).

218 Vogt, K.: Die Ligatur des Ductus parotideus. Pathophysiologie – Indikation – Erfolgskontrolle. Mschr. Ohrenheilk. Lar.-Rhinol. *108:* 324–329 (1974).

219 Wadström, T.; Nord, C.-E.; Kjellgren, M.: A rapid method for separation and detection of human salivary amylase isoenzymes by isoelectric focusing in polyacrylamide gel. Scand. J. dent. Res. *84:* 234–239 (1976).

220 Wallach, D.; Kirshner, N.; Schramm, M.: Non-parallel transport of membrane proteins and content proteins during assembly of the secretory granule in rat parotid gland. Biochim. biophys. Acta *375:* 87–105 (1975).

221 Wallach, D.; Tessler, R.; Schramm, M.: The proteins of the content of the secretory granules of the rat parotid gland. Biochim. biophys. Acta *382:* 552–564 (1975).

222 Ward, J.C.; Merritt, A.D.; Bixler, D.: Human salivary amylase: genetics of electrophoretic variants. Am. J. hum. Genet. *23:* 403–409 (1971).

223 Warshaw, A.L.: Studies on isoenzymes of human amylase: evidence for a circulating amylase not of pancreatic or salivary origin. J. surg. Res. *16:* 360–365 (1974).

224 Warshaw, A.L.; Bellini, C.A.; Lee, K.-H.: Electrophoretic identification of an isoenzyme of amylase which increases in serum in liver disease. Gastroenterology *70:* 572–576 (1976).

225 Wilborn, W.H.; Schneyer, C.A.: Effect of postganglionic sympathectomy on the ultrastructure of the rat parotid gland. Z. Zellforsch. mikrosk. Anat. *130:* 471–480 (1972).

226 Wilcoxon, F.: Probability tables for individual comparisons by ranking methods. Biometrics *3:* 119–122 (1947).

227 Wilding, P.: The electrophoretic nature of human amylase and the effect of protein on the starch-iodine reaction. Clinica chim. Acta *12:* 97–104 (1965).

228 Williams, M.A.; Cope, G.H.: A system for the study of zymogen granule genesis in rabbit parotid gland tissue in vitro. J. Anat. *116:* 431–444 (1973).

229 Wojcik, J.D.; Grand, R.J.; Kimberg, D.V.: Amylase secretion by rabbit parotid gland. Role of cyclic AMP and cyclic GMP. Biochim. biophys. Acta *411:* 250–262 (1975).

230 Wray, L.; Harris, A.W.: Adenosine 3′:5′-monophosphate dependent protein kinase in adipose tissue: inhibition by tolbutamide. Biochem. biophys. Res. Commun. *53:* 291–294 (1973).

231 Zengo, A.N.; Mandel, I.D.; Solomon, A.; Block, P.: Chemistry of rat saliva following isoproterenol administration. J. oral Ther. Pharm. *4:* 359–363 (1968).

Priv.-Doz. Dr. Reinhard Chilla,
Universitäts-Hals-Nasen-Ohren-Klinik, Geiststrasse 5/10, D–3400 Göttingen (FRG)

Adv. Oto-Rhino-Laryng., vol. 26, pp. 39–48 (Karger, Basel 1981)

Etiology and Pathogenesis of the Inflammatory Diseases of the Cephalic Salivary Glands

J. Haubrich

HNO-Klinik, Städtische Krankenanstalten, Krefeld, BRD

Introduction

As shown by the extensive literature published on the subject over the years, the tumorous diseases of the salivary glands are sufficiently well known, but many questions concerning inflammatory changes, especially of the parotid gland, remain unsolved and this hampers specific diagnosis and effective therapy. The difficulties arise from the circumstance that such diseases cannot be diagnosed and treated by the otorhinolaryngologist alone but require co-operation with the internist, the immunologist, the dermatologist, and the pathologist.

On the basis of increasingly differentiated pathoanatomical investigations of a considerably broadened scope of clinical and laboratory methods and of more and more detailed physiological and biochemical studies, the complex matter of the inflammatory diseases of the cephalic salivary glands could be more profoundly elucidated. In his monograph *Rauch* [23] was the first to give a detailed description and classification of these diseases. The pathoanatomical studies of *Seifert* and his colleagues [26–33] provided decisive impulses for the study of their etiology and pathogenesis.

This group of diseases comprises inflammations of the cephalic salivary glands with different etiologies and pathogenetic principles. For some of them the isolated study of individual diseased glands must be preferred to a more generalized view that takes into account the complex pathological processes. It is the aim of the present study to characterize certain clinical pictures from the group of inflammatory diseases of the salivary glands whose classification can be derived from etiological and pathogenetic concepts (table I).

Table I. Classification of the inflammatory diseases of the salivary glands according to etiological and pathogenetic aspects [after ref. 3, 27, 28]

Bacterial sialadenitis
Acute parotitis
Chronic-recurrent parotitis
Tuberculous and luetic sialadenitis

Viral sialadenitis
Parotitis epidemica
Cytomegaly
Coxsackie virus infection

Mycotic sialadenitis
Actinomycosis

Irradiation-induced sialadenitis
Parotitis induced by ionizing radiation

Electrolyte sialadenitis
Parotitis due to metabolic disorder of salivary electrolytes
Final stage: sialolithiasis

Immunosialadenitis
Allergic sialadenitis (e. g., food allergy)
Chronic-myoepithelial sialadenitis (Sjögren syndrome)
Chronic epithelioid-cellular sialadenitis (sarcoidosis, Heerfordt syndrome, febris uveoparotidea)

Special form
Chronic-sclerosing sialadenitis of the submandibular gland (Küttner tumor);
etiology as yet unknown

Acute Sialadenitis

Acute sialadenitis is encountered most frequently in the region of the parotid glands. Ascending infections with streptococci A and *Staphylococcus aureus* are responsible in the majority of cases. Decrease or cessation of salivary flow is of great importance for the pathogenesis of acute parotitis. Salivary secretions, when produced in sufficient amounts, obviously exhibit an effective defense mechanism which is evident also by the low incidence of acute parotitis in the presence of extended inflammatory or tumorous alterations in the oral cavity. Deficient salivary composition, for instance in connection with wasting diseases or desiccating intestinal infections, plays only a secondary role in the pathogenesis of the inflammatory process.

Postoperative Parotitis

A special form of parotitis is the inflammatory change that can occur uni- or bilaterally after laparotomies or other big operations (postoperative parotitis). As far as etiology and pathogenesis are concerned not all questions are answered yet. It is remarkable that the submandibular gland is not involved in the pathological process, possibly due to the high mucin content of its secretion. The disease is not decisively influenced even by high doses of antibiotics. Morphological, functional and neurovegetative connections between parotid gland and the pancreas could indicate certain pathogenetic analogies: An increased permeability of membranes causes hypoxemic tissue damage which leads to involvement of secretory parenchyma and thus to exudation of parotid secretion into the neighboring tissue. Consequently, therapy is attempted by stellate ganglion block aimed at interruption of the neurovegetative dysregulation. Inclusion into the therapy of Trasylol® is supposed to inhibit the autodigestive processes by inactivation of trypsin.

Chronic-Recurrent Parotitis

The etiology of this disease, with a higher incidence in juvenile than adult age, is still largely unknown. The juvenile form is characterized by the observation that the disease very often heals spontaneously around puberty. If chronic-recurrent parotitis occurs in adults, intermittent attacks recur during various periods of time until atrophy of the glandular parenchyma and eventually gradual cessation of salivary flow develop after the disease has persisted for a long time. Abolished salivary flow then favors ascending bacterial infections.

Carious teeth or chronic-recurrent tonsillitis are supposed to be causative factors in the etiology of the disease. *Becker* et al. [2] discussed a primary parotid malformation favoring the development of an inflammatory process.

Viral Sialadenitis

Parotitis epidemica, cytomegaly and coxsackie infection are of importance among the virus-induced forms of parotitis.

Parotitis epidemica is a viral general disease involving the salivary, especially the parotid, glands. Parotitis is nearly always a symptom of the pathological process even though it may not be clinically prominent. (Pathoanatomical changes do always exist!) The infectious agents are neurogenic viruses which are also involved in the diseases accompanying parotitis epidemica (damage to the statoacoustic and abducent nerves).

Cytomegaly, caused by the salivary gland virus, may be found as fetal disease (sialadenalous fetopathy) or as generalized disease of early infancy. Premature infants or newborns with severe dyspepsia are predominantly affected. Infection is in most cases diaplacentally but airborne and smear infections are also possible. *Miklos* [20] focused attention on the not rare coincidence of cytomegaly and interstitial pneumonia. Cytomegaly may also develop following organ transplantations and immunosuppressive therapy, and was further observed in the course of acute leukosis.

Infection with coxsackie virus causes a disease very similar to parotitis epidemica, often combined with angina and gingivitis. The virus is excreted via pharyngeal mucosa and intestine.

Irradiation-Induced Sialadenitis

The development of irradiation-induced sialadenitis depends on the following factors: type, dose and fractionation of irradiation. It is furthermore decisive whether the glands are located in the center or at the margin of the field of irradiation. Last but not least the individually very different sensitivity to irradiation of the secretory glandular parenchyma plays a role in this connection. *Seifert and Donath* [28] have conducted thorough investigations on the development of this type of sialadenitis. Transient hyposialism and a change in viscosity of saliva and hence, dryness of the mouth, are encountered after 1,000–1,500 rad. This phase is initiated by irradiation-induced enzyme dysregulation and reduced blood circulation in the glandular parenchyma. Owing to its high rate of protein turnover and the very sensitive ergastoplasm of its serous acini the parotid gland is particularly affected. The following stages of irradiation sialadenitis can be distinguished:

1. Focal dose below 1,000 rad: transient reduction of salivary flow.
2. Focal dose from 1,000 to 1,500 rad: clinically clearly demonstrable dryness of the mouth due to hyposialism.
3. Focal dose from 4,000 to 5,000 rad: frequently irreversible damage to the glandular parenchyma followed by tissue atrophy and irradiation-induced fibrosis.

Treatment with high-energy radiation results above all in damage to nuclear and intracytoplasmatic cell organelle membranes, leading to the observed morphological changes of the gland with concomitant reduction of salivary flow and alteration of salivary viscosity.

Electrolyte Sialadenitis

This form of sialadenitis is a secretory disorder caused by changed salivary electrolyte composition. *Seifert* and *Donath* [28] gave a detailed description of the morphological substrate of the disease and characterized it by the term 'dyschylia'. In more than 25% of parotid glands subjected to pathoanatomical investigation, intracanalicular sphero- and microliths were found. This percentage is even higher (40%) in patients with additional diabetes mellitus and liver cirrhosis [25]. The course of the disease can be described as follows: In a first stage the changed electrolyte composition of the saliva leads to changed salivary viscosity. Owing to its increased viscosity the secretory product is congested in the terminal excretory ducts. The salivary obstructions thus produced are followed by changes presenting themselves as epithelial metaplasia, duct proliferations and interstitial inflammations. These changes eventually increase the primary damage by sialolith formation in the larger excretory ducts. The pathogenetic chain therefore stretches from a primary secretory disorder to the formation of sialoliths. The significance of the shift in salivary electrolyte composition for the induction of inflammatory changes of the glandular parenchyma can also be demonstrated in experimental iodide sialadenitis.

Chronic-Sclerosing Sialadenitis (Küttner Tumor)

Chronic-sclerosing sialadenitis of the submandibular gland (Küttner tumor) constitutes a special form of inflammatory changes. Morphologically, chronic inflammation with destruction of acini, interstitial lymphocytic reaction and connective tissue transformation are found, the latter sometimes leading to a clinical picture resembling cirrhosis [17, 26, 29]. So far little is known about the etiology of the disease. According to *Seifert* [26], duct alterations with enlargement of the lumen and also formation of diverticula and secretory disorders are of decisive importance. Dilations and ramifications of the duct system always favor congestion of secretory products so that in many cases inspissation of secretion is the final result. *Bhaskar* [6] experimentally ligated the excretory duct of the submandibular gland and was able to produce similar changes as in chronic-sclerosing sialadenitis. Identical changes were experimentally induced by application of iodide [33] and by injection of sclerosing solutions [22]. *Waterhouse* and *Doniach* [35] directed attention to the not uncommon coincidence of lympho-cytic infiltrations in the submandibular gland with rheumatoid arthritis and lymphocytic thyroiditis. From the different experimental results it can be concluded that a disorder of the immunological system is a triggering factor in the development of chronic-sclerosing sialadenitis.

Immunosialadenitis

This clinical picture is defined by inflammatory changes of the salivary glands which are induced by antigen-antibody reactions. The inflammation is unspecific and often disappears after elimination of the allergen. For a better understanding the following facts have to be taken into consideration: The salivary glands are involved in the defense system in several ways. Among the unspecific factors are the lysozymes which are formed in specializ-ed basal cells of the striated ducts [15] and the neuraminic acid-containing mucins which form at the epithelial surface a protective coat against offend-ing viruses or bacteria. A special secretory immunological system is formed by immunoglobulin A (IgA) and immunoconglutinin present in the salivary glands [11, 16, 21, 24]. Since under normal conditions no plasma cells can be demonstrated in the stroma of salivary glands, so far no safe conclusions can be drawn regarding the site of IgA synthesis. The secretory component is synthesized in the epithelial cells of the proximal duct system and possibly is excreted into the glandular lumen together with IgA. A process of this kind would permit specific antibody reaction against certain antigens.

Clinically important is the acute immunosialadenitis that can be induced by drugs or food allergens. The unspecific inflammatory changes disappear after elimination of the allergen.

Chronic-Myoepithelial Sialadenitis (Sjögren Syndrome)

Chronic-myoepithelial sialadenitis is counted among the group of allergenic diseases with immunopathological reactions [12]. According to *Seifert* and *Geiler* [31, 32] the parotitis is characterized by the following morphological trias: atrophy of the glandular parenchyma, interstitial lymphocytic infiltrations and myoepithelial proliferations. The hypothesis regarding the etiology of the disease is supported by experimental studies in which sialadenitis was produced by injection of immunoglobulins against extracts from rat salivary glands [10, 14, 18]. In the parenchyma of the gland tissue necroses are found directly neighboring antibody complexes. Investigations employing immunofluorescence further indicated the involvement of immunopathological processes. In the serum of patients with chronic-myoepithelial sialadenitis antibodies were found that were directed against components of salivary duct epithelia [5, 19]. Moreover, coincidenec of Sjögren syndrome, struma Hashimoto, lupus erythematodes disseminatus and antinuclear factors could be demonstrated [1, 4, 9, 27, 34]. *Bertram* [4] conducted extensive comparative studies of Sjögren syndrome and auto-aggressive diseases with the following result: In the serum of Sjögren patients antibodies against the cytoplasm of excretory duct epithelia were found in 75% of cases (control group 7.4%). The same antibodies occurred in 27% of cases in lupus erythematodes disseminatus and in 12.5% of cases in struma Hashimoto. In 71% of patients with Sjögren syndrome a positive LE phenomenon, that is, antinuclear factors, could be demonstrated. These results are of great importance as they support the hypothesis of autoimmunization in Sjögren syndrome.

Epithelioid-Cellular Sialadenitis (Sarcoidosis, Heerfordt Syndrome)

Epithelioid-cellular sialadenitis is morphologically characterized by the occurrence of epithelioid-cellular granuloma in the glandular parenchyma and/or in the intra- and periglandular lymph nodes, respectively. There is no conformity of opinion regarding etiology of the disease, but some authors suggested that an allergic-hyperergic pathological process is involved. As judged from the morphological findings, the clinical picture is that of a specifically localized form of sarcoidosis.

Development of Malignant Lymphomas in the Course of Immunosialadenitis

Lastly the observation must be noted that in the course of an immunosialadenitis, especially in its chronic-myoepithelial form, tumors of the lymphoma type of various degrees of malignancy may develop [7, 8, 13]. This can be explained by the fact that, besides immunoglobulin synthesis, the cells of the immunological system possess the ability for malignant transformation. Immunoplastic lymphomas develop in the majority of cases. Therefore the sudden enlargement of a parotid gland in the course of a chronic-myoepithelial sialadenitis is highly suspicious with respect to the development of a malignant process.

Conclusions

The complexity of the inflammatory pathological processes in the salivary glands, especially in the parotid gland, requires subtle diagnostic techniques. A multitude of clinical, pathological and anatomical as well as laboratory investigation methods are now available. This permits to make a safe diagnosis in most cases. However, many questions concerning etiology and pathogenesis of the inflammatory diseases of the cephalic salivary glands remain unanswered. This impedes a specifically directed therapy which will have to be the aim of further clinical and theoretical research.

References

1   Bark, C.J.; Perzik, S.C.: Mikulicz's disease, sialoangiectasis and autoimmunity based upon a study of parotid lesions. Am. J. clin. Path. *49:* 683 (1968).
2   Becker, W.; Matzker, J.; Ruckes, J.: Zur Morphologie der 'diffusen, kugelförmigen Gangektasien' in der Glandula parotis. Lar. Rhinol. Otol. *39:* 479 (1960).
3   Becker, W.; Haubrich, J.; Seifert, G.: Krankheiten der Kopfspeicheldrüsen; in Berendes, Link, Zöllner, Hals-Nasen-Ohrenheilkunde in Praxis und Klinik, vol. 3, pp. 12.1–12.55 (Thieme, Stuttgart 1978).
4   Bertram, U.: Xerostomia, clinical aspects, pathology and pathogenesis. Acta odont. scand. *25:* suppl. 49, p. 1 (1967).
5   Bertram, U.; Halberg, P.: A specific antibody against the epithelium of the salivary ducts in sera from patients with Sjögren syndrome. Acta allerg. *19:* 458 (1964).
6   Bhaskar, S.N.: Regeneration of rabbit submaxillary gland following obstructive adenitis. J. dent. Res. *40:* 744 (1961).
7   Bloch, K.J.; Buchanan, W.W.; Wohl, M.J.; Bunim, J.J.: Sjögren's syndrome. A clinical, pathological and serological study of sixty-two cases. Medicine, Baltimore *44:* 187 (1965).
8   Bolognini, G.; Riva, G.: Lymphoproliferative Erkrankungen und Paraproteinämien beim Sjögren-Syndrom. Schweiz. med. Wschr. *105:* 1493 (1975).
9   Bunim, J.J.: A broader spectrum of Sjögren's syndrome and its pathogenetic implications. Ann. rheum. Dis. *20:* 1 (1961).
10 Cheung, C.W.: Experimental sialoadenitis in guinea-pigs. J. Path. Bact. *88:* 592 (1964).

11 Eichner, H.; Münzel, M.; Bretzel, G.; Hochstrasser, K.: Vergleichende Untersuchungen der Proteinfraktionen von menschlichem Parotissekret mittels ein- und zweidimensionaler Immunelektrophorese, Immunodiffusion und Diskelektrophorese. Lar. Rhinol. Otol. *54:* 105 (1975).

12 Ericson, S.; Sundmark, E.: Studies on the sicca syndrome in patients with rheumatoid arthritis. Acta rheum. scand. *16:* 60 (1970).

13 Gravanis, M.B.; Giansanti, J.S.: Malignant histopathologic counterpart of the benign lymphoepithelial lesion. Cancer, Philad. *26:* 1332 (1970).

14 Haferkamp, O.: Ein tierexperimenteller Beitrag zur Immunpathologie der Speicheldrüsen. Virchows Arch. Abt. A Path. Anat. *335:* 298 (1962).

15 Kraus, F.W.; Mestecky, J.: Immunohistochemical localization of amylase, lysozyme and immunoglobulin in the human parotid gland. Archs oral Biol. *16:* 781 (1971).

16 Lachmann, P.J.; Thomson, R.A.: Immunoconglutinins in human saliva – a group of unusual IgA antibodies. Immunology *18:* 157 (1970).

17 Lentrodt, J.: Beitrag zur Kenntnis der Küttnerschen Tumoren. Dt. Zahnärztebl. *18:* 125 (1964).

18 McCabe, B.F.: The evidence for an auto-immune mechanism in Mikulicz's disease. Laryngoscope *71:* 396 (1961).

19 McSveen, R.N.M.; Goudie, R.B.; Anderson, J.R.; Armstrong, E.M.; Murray, M.A.; Mason, D.K.; Jasani, M.K.; Boyle, J.A.; Buchanan, W.W.; Williamson, J.: Occurrence of antibody to salivary duct epithelium in Sjögren's disease, rheumatoid arthritis and other arthrites. A clinical and laboratory study. Ann. rheum. Dis. *26:* 402 (1967).

20 Miklos, C.: Cytomegalie. Zentbl. allg. Path. path. Anat. *101:* 496 (1960).

21 Proescher, H.J.: Immunglobuline im Parotisspeichel gesunder Erwachsener. Arch. klin. exp. Ohr.-Nas.-KehlkHeilk. *205:* 113 (1973).

22 Rabin, M.A.; Murane, T.W.; Doku, H.C.: Histologic response of rat submandibular glands to the intraglandular administration of a sclerosing solution. Oral Surg. *29:* 635 (1970).

23 Rauch, S.: Die Speicheldrüsen des Menschen (Thieme, Stuttgart 1959).

24 Ruhwinkel, B.; Münzel, M.: Der Immunglobulingehalt des menschlichen Parotissekretes. Lar. Rhinol. Otol. *54:* 361 (1975).

25 Seemann, N.: Pathohistologische Untersuchungen zur Häufigkeit der Sialolithiasis und Sialadenitis der Parotis. HNO, Berl. *17:* 3 (1969).

26 Seifert, G.: Mundhöhle, Mundspeicheldrüsen, Tonsillen und Rachen; in Doerr, Uehlinger, Spezielle pathologische Anatomie, vol. 1, pp. 1–415 (Springer, Berlin 1966).

27 Seifert, G.: Klinische Pathologie der Sialadenitis und Sialadenose. HNO, Berl. *19:* 1 (1971).

28 Seifert, G.; Donath, K.: Die Morphologie der Speicheldrüsenerkrankungen. Arch. Ohr.-Nas.-KehlkHeilk. *213:* 111, 371 (1976).

29 Seifert, G.; Donath, K.: Zur Pathogenese des Küttner-Tumors der Submandibularis. Analyse von 349 Fällen mit chronischer Sialadenitis der Submandibularis. HNO, Berl. *25:* 81 (1977).

30 Seifert, G.; Geier, W.: Zur Pathologie der Strahlen-Sialadenitis. Lar. Rhinol. Otol. *50:* 376 (1971).

31 Seifert, G.; Geiler, G.: Speicheldrüsen und Rheumatismus. Dt. med. Wschr. *82:* 1415 (1957).

32   Seifert, G.; Geiler, G.: Vergleichende Untersuchungen der Kopfspeichel- und
     Tränendrüsen zur Pathogenese des Sjögren-Syndroms und der Mikulicz-Krankheit.
     Virchows Arch. path. Anat. Physiol. *330:* 402 (1957).
33   Seifert, G.; Junge-Hülsing, G.: Untersuchungen zur Jod-Sialadenitis und Jod-131-
     Aktivität der Speicheldrüsen. Z. Path. *74:* 485 (1965).
34   Walser, A.; Juankovic, M.; Baur, M.: Sjögren-Syndrom und Struma lymphomatcsі
     Hashimoto. Schweiz. med. Wschr. *95:* 763 (1965).
35   Waterhouse, J.P.; Doniach, I.: Post-mortem prevalence of foci lymphocytic adenitis
     of the submandibular salivary gland. J. Path. Bact. *91:* 53 (1966).

Prof. J.Haubrich, MD, HNO-Klinik, Städtische Krankenanstalten
D-4150 Krefeld (FRG)

Adv. Oto-Rhino-Laryng., vol. 26, pp. 49–96 (Karger, Basel 1981)

Cytological Diagnosis of Sialadenosis, Sialadenitis, and Parotid Cysts by Fine-Needle Aspiration Biopsy[1]

Manfred Droese

Department of Pathology, University of Göttingen, Göttingen, FRG

Introduction

The principal symptom of pathological changes of the major and minor cephalic salivary glands is the swelling of the diseased gland. Differential diagnosis of swellings encompasses a wide spectrum of nontumorous diseases as well as benign and malignant tumors. Although anamnesis, clinical examination and technical methods of investigation yield informations pointing to a certain direction, morphological investigation is decisive for the diagnosis.

While swellings of the minor salivary glands and of the sublingual and submandibular glands are usually histologically examined after total extirpation or exploratory excision, often combined with frozen sections [16], exploratory excisions from parotid swellings are rejected by many authors [9, 36, 44] and only sometimes supported in a few special cases [6, 42, 45, 78]. The rejection is based mainly on the following three points: (1) exploratory excision involves the danger of injuring the facial nerve; (2) exploratory excisions which must spare the facial nerve are often performed too superficially and not extensively enough; wrong conclusions can be drawn from a nonrepresentative sample; (3) tumor tissue may be disseminated into healthy neighboring tissue by destruction of the tumor capsule, endangering the success of radical surgical intervention which may become necessary.

Not only exploratory excisions alone but also exploratory biopsies with thick needles carry the risk of tumor cell propagation and nonrepresentative tissue sampling. They are therefore not advocated [42].

---

[1] This paper is part of the habilitation thesis of *M. Droese.*

Today, two different diagnostic concepts are generally applied to swellings of the parotid gland. The majority of clinicians omit preoperative morphological investigations, deciding on the indication of operation on the basis of the results of clinical examination alone, and performing extensive surgery in combination with the technique of frozen sections [16, 45]. This procedure is termed 'grand biopsy' [16] and will therapeutically suffice in many cases. It can be extended at any time to radical surgery should the result of intraoperative histological examination make this inevitable. However, critics of this method maintain that operative measures are not indicated for a big number of nonneoplastic diseases [36, 42].

Fine-needle biopsy with cytological evaluation of the punctates constitutes the diagnostic alternative to grand biopsy [36, 42]. In this way many patients with nontumorous diseases of the parotid gland are spared surgical intervention.

Under the aspects of tumor cell propagation and damage to the facial nerve, fine-needle biopsy is without risk [36]. Although it cannot be denied that even with this technique nonrepresentative material may be aspirated, the mistake rate will not be higher than that of exploratory excision or of biopsy with a thick needle, the reason being that a thin needle is able to penetrate into deeper layers of tissue without danger, and fan- or cone-shaped needle manipulation will explore an area of tissue whose dimension corresponds very well to that of a sample obtained by excision [40, 80].

Fine-needle aspiration biopsies of salivary gland swellings were for the first time performed in 1953, at Radiumhemmet, Karolinska Hospital, in Stockholm [33, 36, 50]. Most authors of later publications from other Scandinavian centers [7, 46, 49, 56], France [1, 11, 13–15, 17], the USSR [47, 54, 55], the United States [39], United Kingdom [77], and Germany [27, 28, 42] reported on small series or single cases, mostly without comparison with the results of histological investigation. As evident from extent and documentation of results, only few publications permit critical assessment of the method [27, 28, 33, 49, 50, 56].

Reproducible diagnostic criteria are the most important prerequisite for a broad application of aspiration biopsy cytology in the diagnosis of swellings of the salivary glands. Initiatory studies dealing with the establishment of such criteria come from the Stockholm group and concern the most frequent tumor types [31, 32, 34, 35, 81].

Important aspects of salivary gland cytology are still untouched by research. Thus a detailed investigation of salivary gland inflammations and

Table I. Localization of 574 swellings of the salivary glands of 572[1] patients

Localization	n	%
Parotid gland	511[1]	89.0
Submandibular gland	44	7.7
Minor salivary glands	16	2.8
Sublingual gland	2	0.3
Ectopic salivary gland tissue	1	0.2

[1] 2 patients had a bilateral parotid tumor.

cysts is missing so far, and furthermore it remains an open question whether or not sialadenosis can be diagnosed by means of aspiration cytology.

It is the aim of the present study to establish, on the basis of extensive biopsy material and by application of morphometry, satisfactory cytological criteria for the diagnosis of sialadenosis, the different forms of sialadenitis, and of cysts of the salivary glands.

Patients and Methods

Patients

From 1975 to 1978, a total number of 572 patients with swellings of the salivary glands were examined by aspiration cytology. More than one biopsy was taken from 97 patients (before operation or in the course of follow-up for recurrences) so that altogether 694 fine-needle biopsies were evaluated. 326 patients (56.9%) including 2 with bilateral parotid tumor underwent surgery.

The largest number of biopsies were taken from swellings of the parotid gland. The submandibular gland, the minor salivary glands of the oral cavity, the sublingual gland and ectopic salivary gland tissue are following with decreasing order of frequency (table I).

Cytological Technique

The equipment for obtaining the fine-needle biopsies consisted of a pistol grip, a 20-ml disposable syringe and a disposable needle No. 17 (fig. 1). The punctation technique corresponded to the method introduced by *Franzén* et al. [40]. In most cases the swelling was punctured twice from different directions. The individual phases of biopsy taking are schematically depicted in figure 2.

The aspirated tissue samples were spread on microscopic slides, air-dried and stained according to May-Grünwald-Giemsa (MGG).

Analysis of Cellular Pattern

In order to obtain reproducible cytodiagnostic criteria the cytological preparations of the various pathological entities were analyzed observing the following aspects: type, differentiation and arrangement of cells; shape, structure and staining of noncellular

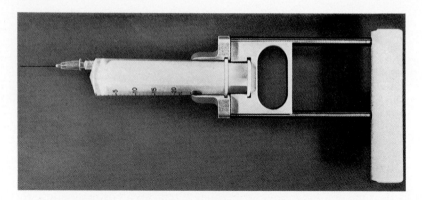

Fig. 1. Equipment for taking fine-needle biopsies.

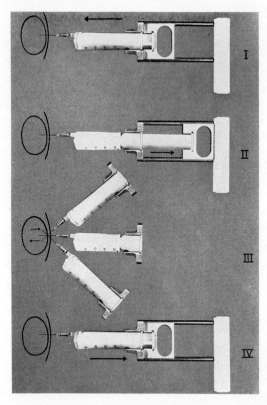

Fig. 2. The four stages of taking fine-needle biopsy samples (schematic representation). Stage I: puncture of the lesion. Stage II: creation of negative pressure. Stage III: fan-like deployment of the needle during aspiration. Stage IV: equalization of pressure and withdrawal of the needle. Modified after *Zajicek* [80].

elements. Some of these characteristics were semiquantitatively evaluated. The combinations of features found for the different pathological entities were correlated to the corresponding histological findings. In the sialadenitis group, cases without histological examination were also included in the analysis when clinical investigation had shown the typical symptoms of the respective form of inflammation.

All histological preparations were subjected to reinvestigation; the cases of sialadenitis were reclassified following the schedule of *Seifert* and *Donath* [68].

Morphometric Studies

Morphometric studies for sialadenosis were carried out with fine-needle biopsies and compared with the corresponding histological specimens. Measurements were performed with an ocular micrometer attached to a Zeiss photomicroscope. The cytological specimens were scanned by tracing a meander line on the slide, and in each punctate the biggest diameter of at least 12 clearly definable acini was determined. Three fields of vision, with as little admixture of fat, connective tissue and blood vessels as possible, were selected in the histological sections and the biggest diameters of at least 12 acini measured in each field of vision (eyepiece × 12.5, lens × 25).

An analysis of variance was computed for the group of normal cases as well as for the group of sialadenoses. The linear regression between the mean acinar diameters in the cytological and the corresponding histological preparations of the normal cases was also calculated, the cytological measurements being regarded as independent variables and the histological data as dependent variables. The frequency distributions of the values measured in the two groups of sialadenoses and controls were graphically represented as histograms and the statistical parameters computed for both distributions.

Sialadenosis

Sialadenosis belongs to the differential diagnostic spectrum of bilateral and, less frequently, unilateral parotid swellings. The term 'sialadenosis' was coined by *Rauch* [59] and was introduced, in modified form, into the nomenclature of the WHO [76]. The most precise definition of this pathologic entity was given by *Seifert* [63]: 'Sialadenoses are noninflammatory, parenchymatous diseases of the salivary glands, caused by metabolic and secretory disorders of the glandular parenchyma and in most cases accompanied by a recurrent, painless bilateral swelling of the salivary glands, especially the parotid.'

Due to the increased occurrence of sialadenosis in endocrinopathies, metabolic disorders and neurogenic diseases, the following clinical forms are distinguished: endocrine, dystrophic-metabolic and neurogenic sialadenosis [67]. There is no evident sex disposition; the highest incidence occurs between the 4th and 7th decade of life [25].

Morphologically characteristic of sialadenosis are increased acinar diameters. The mean acinar diameter lies between 35 and 52 µm with a maximum extending up to 100 µm [24]. In an earlier investigation, a mean acinar diameter of 40 µm was reported for sialadenosis and of 30 µm for parotid control tissue [21].

The cytoplasm of the swollen acinar cells is either granular, alveolate translucent or contains a mixture of these two forms (fig. 5). Ultrastructurally the secretory granules of different optical densities correspond to the light-microscopical cytoplasmic structure.

The myoepithelial cells in the region of the acini and the proximal duct system reveal regressive changes. The interstitial gland tissue contains no inflammatory infiltrations [67]. Ultrastructurally demonstrable degeneration phenomena at the vegetative terminal axons in human sialadenosis and analogous experimental findings after chemical sympathicolysis or denutrition favor the pathogenetical hypothesis of a primary alteration of the vegetative nervous system. Etiologically the sialadenoses are attributed to a neurohormonally induced neuropathy of the vegetative nervous system [22–24, 67]. The bilateral occurrence and the tendency of recurrence of the process are in good agreement with this interpretation [25].

Chronic-recurrent, bilateral and painless swellings of the salivary glands (especially of the parotid) a known endocrine, metabolic or neurogenic basic disease or antihypertensive therapy [2, 20], as well as the absence of general or local symptoms of a sialadenitis justify the clinical diagnosis of a sialadenosis [42]. Sialographic and scintigraphic characteristics supply additional diagnostic parameters [12, 53, 67]. The analysis of saliva is less revealing as the results show a wide range of variation [42, 67].

The clinical diagnosis of sialadenosis is difficult in the initial phase, if the swelling predominates on one side, and if a syntropy with a typical basic disease cannot be established anamnestically. In such cases the histopathological (morphometric) investigation, which requires an exploratory excision, gains decisive value.

In order to avoid the risk of an exploratory excision and to minimize the amount of diagnostic work involved we have tried to make a morphometric diagnosis of sialadenosis based on cytological samples.

Patients

We performed a comparative morphometric investigation of the cytological and histological preparations from 6 samples of normal parotid tissue in order to find out whether the mean acinar diameter in the cytological punctate differs from that in the histological preparation.

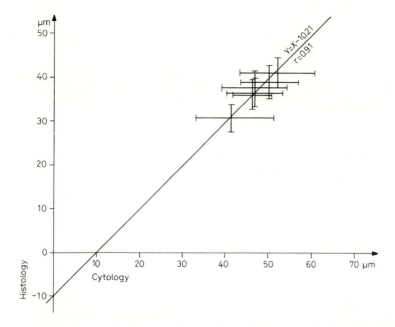

Fig. 3. Linear regression between the mean acinar diameters determined by morphometry in cytological and corresponding histological preparations from six normal parotid glands.

Without knowledge of the clinical diagnoses we then selected, in order of admission, for morphometric examination 41 cases with cell-rich parotid biopsies that had been previously diagnosed as normal tissue. Following clinical diagnosis, these cases included 10 sialadenoses and 18 cases with no pathological findings in the parotid gland. No safe diagnosis was possible in 13 instances. The group of sialadenoses comprised 4 endocrine and 2 metabolic forms, and 4 cases without syntropic basic disease. The group of controls was formed by those cases in which biopsies had been performed for the exclusion of tumor recurrences or of lymph node metastases in the region of the salivary glands.

Results

Morphometry

The linear regression plot of the mean acinar diameters, determined in cytological and corresponding histological preparations of six normal parotid glands, shows a very high correlation ($r = 0.96$) between the cytological and the histological data. The straight line of regression follows the equation $y = x - 10.21$ µm. It must be noted, however, that the mean values of both variables are scattered over a wide range (fig. 3).

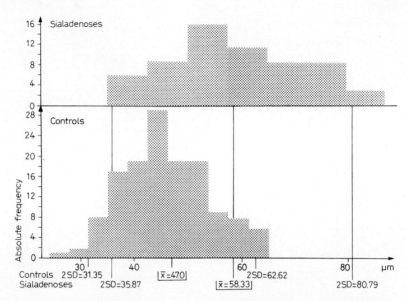

Fig. 4. Histograms of the frequency distributions of acinar diameters determined by morphometry in cytological preparations from 10 sialadenoses and 18 controls. 2 SD range of the arithmetic mean $(\bar{x})$ of the acinar diameters of both groups.

The analysis of variance of the cytological and histological data reveals a confidence level of 99.79% ($F = 4.24$, $n_1 = 5$, $n_2 = 69$) and of 95.3% ($F = 2.39$, $n_1 = 5$, $n_2 = 65$), respectively, for the hypothesis that the diameters of the acini are different in each patient.

The distribution of the cytological data is highly symmetrical in the sialadenosis and control groups (fig. 4). The slope of the distribution is <0.5 in both groups. The arithmetic mean of the acinar diameters is 58.33 μm for the sialadenoses and 47.0 μm for the controls. The range of 2 SD encompasses 36–81 μm for the sialadenoses and 31–62 μm for the controls. In both groups, 95% of the cases lie within these ranges. It is not advisable to make a quantitative comparison between the means of both distributions, coupled with a level of significance (e.g. by means of a t test), because the analysis of variance yields a confidence level of far over 90% for the statement that there exists no common mean value for both groups.

Cytomorphology

As far as number, composition and placement of the cells are concerned, the salivary gland biopsies of patients with sialadenosis do not differ from those of the controls. The punctates predominantly contain aspirated whole acini, free acinar cells and a few clusters of epithelial duct cells and lipocytes. The majority of aspirated acini are arranged in large aggregates associated with duct fragments or lipocyte clusters. The picture of a rudimentary lobulated structure is sometimes observed (fig. 5a).

Only a few acini show distinct cell boundaries so that the hypertrophy of the individual acinar cells is not clearly recognizable and measurable. Some acini are enveloped by a metachromatically staining basal membrane. The histologically discerned forms of cytoplasmic differentiation (granular, alveolar, mixed) can be demonstrated cytologically in both groups (fig. 5b).

In the sialadenosis group the biopsies nearly always contain single extremely big acini. Furthermore, a high vulnerability of the cytoplasm is evident.

Discussion

The increase of the acinar diameters is the decisive criterion for the histomorphological diagnosis of sialadenosis [21, 24, 67]. The technique of morphometric investigation is, in our opinion, transferable to fine-needle biopsies, since part of the acini are aspirated in toto.

Using the histological method, approximate diagnostic values of acinar diameters are given for sialadenosis of 50–70 μm while for control tissue these values are reported to range from 30 to 40 μm [24, 67].

New ranges for acinar diameters of both groups (sialadenosis and control) had to be determined for the cytological diagnostic technique since this alters the relative sizes. Cells in the air-dried punctate smear are generally bigger than in the mounted section. Two factors are mainly responsible for this phenomenon. Firstly, isolated cells that are no longer subject to pressure exerted by neighboring cells can expand on the microscopic slide, and secondly, the cells are not exposed to formol mounting which, by dehydration, results in a shrinking of cells.

By comparative measurements of the acinar diameters in cytological and histological specimens of normal parotid glands we could demonstrate the size relations for acini, depending on the choice of method. The cytological mean acinar diameters are bigger than the corresponding histological values by 10 μm (fig. 3). In the samples derived from sialadenosis the mean acinar diameter measured in cytological preparations is 58 μm, and in control samples 47 μm (fig. 4). The difference of 11 μm corresponds to the difference of 10 μm calculated from the mean acinar diameters found with

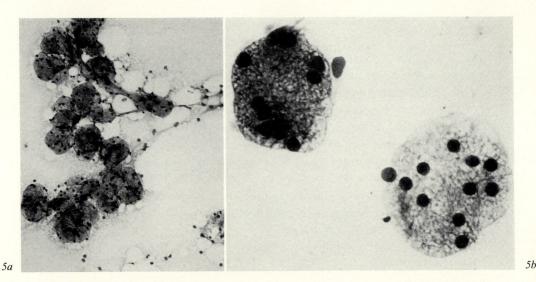

5a   5b

the histological method where values of 40 μm (sialadenosis) and 30 μm (control) were determined for the acini [21].

The arithmetic mean of the acinar diameters of sialadenosis lies within the 2 SD range of the arithmetic mean of the acinar diameters of the controls (fig. 4). In the cytological evaluation of fine-needle biopsies it can therefore be assumed that only mean acinar diameters of 62 μm and more (with an error probability of 5%) may be considered as a morphological criterion of sialadenosis.

On the basis of the reported findings it seems justified to include biopsy cytology in the diagnosis of sialadenosis. Particularly in clinically doubtful cases the cytological method could supply important diagnostic aid.

Sialadenitis

According to their etiology the following inflammations of the salivary glands are distinguished: bacterial sialadenitis, viral sialadenitis, immuno-sialadenitis, electrolyte sialadenitis and chronic sialadenitis of the sub-mandibular gland, the so-called Küttner tumor [65, 69].

The position of aspiration cytology in the diagnosis of inflammations of the salivary glands has up to now not been evaluated. Some cytological reports mention only in passing the different forms of sialadenitis under the aspect of tumor diagnosis [17, 46, 49, 56, 77].

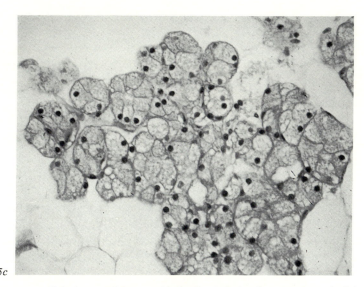

5c

Fig. 5. Sialadenosis of the parotid gland. *a* Lobulated arrangement of acini with granular cytoplasm, surrounded by lipocytes. MGG × 110. *b* 2 acini with a maximum diameter of 56 μm (left) and 66 μm (right). Granular and alveolar cytoplasmic structure. MGG × 490. *c* Gland lobule with predominantly alveolar cytoplasmic structure of the acinar cells. Lipomatosis. HE × 275.

Cytomorphologic descriptions and attempts to define the diagnostic criteria of the various forms of inflammation are so far only tentative [7, 80]. In the present study we have tried to close this gap. The following forms of inflammation were included in the investigation: acute purulent sialadenitis (18 cases), chronic-recurrent parotitis (26 cases), irradiation-induced sialadenitis (1 case), epithelioid-cellular sialadenitis (3 cases), myoepithelial sialadenitis (20 cases) and chronic sialadenitis of the submandibular gland (5 cases).

Acute Purulent Sialadenitis

Acute purulent sialadenitis of the salivary glands is mostly a secondary disease in the course of severe general diseases. It is usually induced by retrograde canalicular infection of the salivary glands with streptococci and staphylococci.

Table II. Cells and noncellular elements in biopsies from 18 patients with acute purulent sialadenitis

Cells and noncellular elements	Frequency of occurrence	Cells and noncellular elements	Frequency of occurrence
Neutrophilic granulocytes	18	Duct epithelia	8
Lymphocytes	5	Cell debris	15
Macrophages	13	Protein precipitates	16
Fibroblasts	4	Stroma particles	3
Acinar epithelia	7	Capillary fragments	4

The extended salivary ducts contain aggregated leukocytes. Focal destructions of the duct epithelium prepare the invasion of the glandular parenchyma by the inflammation with a resulting purulent histolysis. The parotid gland is most frequently affected. This form of inflammation has its highest incidence in the 6th decade of life [64, 65, 69].

Patients

The clinical diagnosis of an acute purulent sialadenitis was made in 18 cases. Following antibiotic therapy a regression of the symptoms of inflammation was observed in all instances. 4 cases were histologically examined with a resulting diagnosis of purulent sialadenitis concomitant with granulating tissue reaction. In 13 instances the inflammation was located in the parotid and in 5 cases in the submandibular gland.

Results

The cytological diagnosis of acute purulent sialadenitis was made in all 18 cases. The biopsies are cell-rich and contain predominantly neutrophilic granulocytes (table II). The background of the cytologic preparation is nearly without exception filled with cell debris and granular or filamentous protein precipitate (fig. 6a). More than half of the punctates contain numerous macrophages with phagocytosis of cell detritus. Acinar and duct epithelia showing regressive changes can be demonstrated in less than half of the biopsies. Fibroblasts, metachromatic stroma particles or fragments of capillaries can be recognized in a few cases (fig. 6b).

Discussion

The cytologic picture of acute purulent sialadenitis is determined by the actual stage of inflammation. The acute stage is characterized by a combination of neutrophilic granulocytes with cell debris and/or protein precipitates. The topical assignation of the inflammatory process is only successful

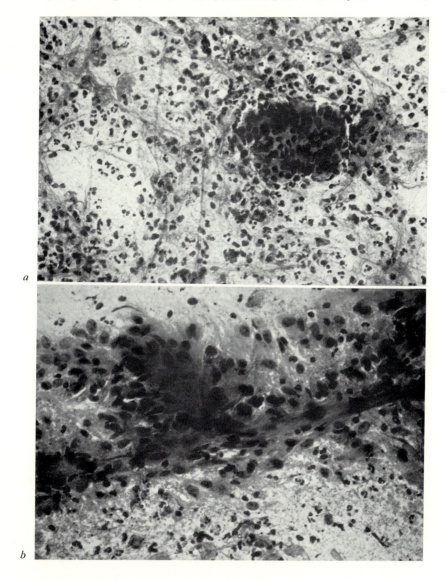

Fig. 6. Acute purulent parotitis. *a* Filamentous eosinophilic protein precipitate, neutrophilic granulocytes, histiocytes and one aggregate of duct epithelia. MGG. × 290. *b* Capillary fragments, fibroblasts and cell debris. Granulation reaction. MGG. × 470.

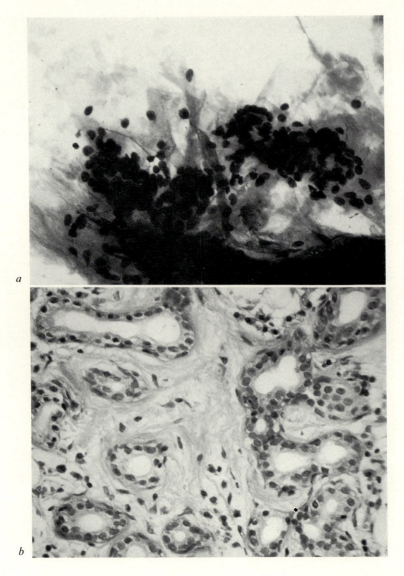

Fig. 7. Chronic-recurrent parotitis. *a* Aggregates of duct epithelia and membranous stroma particles. MGG. × 290. *b* Periductal fibrosis and lymphocytic infiltration. HE × 290.

Table III. Preoperative cytological diagnosis in 9 patients with histologically verified chronic-recurrent parotitis

Cytological diagnosis	Histological diagnosis chronic-recurrent parotitis
Chronic-recurrent parotitis	2
Parotid cyst	2
Benign epithelial parotid tumor with cyst formation	2
Suspicion of highly differentiated mucoepidermoid tumor	1
Cell material not evaluable	2

if one can demonstrate salivary gland epithelia. These exhibit the signs of toxic damage.

After repairing processes have started, one finds elements of the granulating tissue reaction which include fibroblasts, stroma particles and fragments of capillaries. Duct regeneration products, occurring in the punctate as duct epithelia in a tubular formation, are an exception.

Chronic-Recurrent Parotitis

Chronic-recurrent parotitis is mainly caused by streptococci and staphylococci. This form of inflammation is in its further course characterized by disorders of secretion and by immunologic factors. It occurs uni- or bilaterally, mainly in children and in the 4th and 5th decade of life with a predilection of women [64, 65, 71].

The histologic picture shows the following symptoms: duct dilation, microlith formation, periductal lymphocytic infiltrations with formation of lymph follicles, destruction of the secretory acinar tissue, duct proliferations, metaplasia of the duct epithelium, interstitial fibrosis and lipomatosis [64, 69].

Patients
The clinical diagnosis of chronic-recurrent parotitis was made in 26 patients and confirmed in 9 cases by histological examination.

Results
Out of 9 histologically verified cases of chronic-recurrent parotitis, only 2 were correctly classified by cytological investigation. In 3 cases the diagnosis of cystic epithelial tumor was made, and in 2 instances parotid

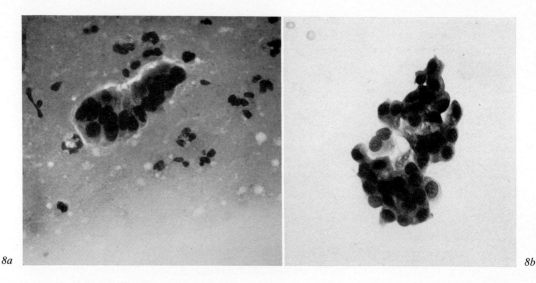

cysts were assumed. 2 biopsies did not contain any evaluable cell material (table III). In the group only examined by cytology the following diagnoses were given: 13 cases of chronic-recurrent parotitis, 3 cases of purulent parotitis with granulation reaction, and 1 parotid cyst.

In the group studied by cytology and histology, the specimen background is filled with diffuse eosinophilic protein precipitates or with basophilic mucus (fig. 8a). Some biopsies further contain metachromatic stroma particles (fig. 7a), cholesterol crystals or cell debris. Neutrophilic granulocytes, histiocytes and lymphocytes are found in 6 punctates, and exclusively eosinophilic granulocytes in 1 case. There is not one biopsy where the inflammatory cells are domineering. The predominant component is formed by aggregates or tubular formations of duct epithelia (fig. 7a). In a few punctates mucusforming cylindrical epithelia (fig. 8a, b) or metaplastic squamous epithelia can be recognized.

14 biopsies of the only cytologically examined group are identical in their composition to that of the punctates of the first group. In a few cases plasma cells, germinal center cells, fibroblasts, lipocytes and needle-shaped crystals are also found. Some of the punctates contain a small number of acinar cells with degenerative changes. In 3 biopsies the cellular picture corresponds to that of an acute purulent parotitis with granulation reaction (table IV).

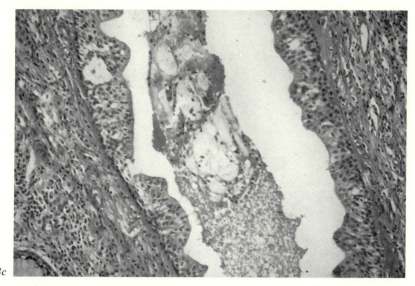

8c

Fig. 8. Chronic-recurrent parotitis. *a* Precipitated mucus, neutrophilic granulocytes and palisade-like arrangement of cylindrical epithelia. MGG. × 285. *b* Papilliform arrangement of duct epithelia. MGG. × 285. *c* Ectatic salivary duct filled with secretory product. Pseudopapillary proliferation of epithelia and leukocytic infiltrations. HE × 115.

Discussion

The cytological picture of chronic-recurrent parotitis is characterized mainly by two features: small or moderate numbers of neutrophilic and eosinophilic granulocytes; lymphocytes and histiocytes in varying numbers as well as varying amounts of duct epithelia, arranged in aggregates or tubular formations. Whereas punctates from normal parotid glands contain largely acinar epithelia but only a few duct epithelia, an inversion of this quantitative ratio is to be observed in chronic-recurrent parotitis due to destruction of acinar tissue and duct proliferation. The acinar cells can even be missing altogether.

The precipitation of protein throughout the specimen warrants the assumption of a tissue alteration with duct dilation or cyst formation. Microliths, signifying dyschylia, were not found.

Metaplastic duct epithelia are prominent in the punctate as goblet cells with basophilic mucus or as squamous epithelia. While the cytological symptoms of duct ectasis or cyst formation can be nearly always demonstrated, the metaplasia of epithelium is more or less a rare phenomenon.

Table IV. Cells and noncellular elements in biopsies of chronic-recurrent parotitis

Cells and noncellular elements	Cytological/histological examination	Cytological examination
Neutrophilic granulocytes	5	15
Eosinophilic granulocytes	1	
Lymphocytes	3	13
Plasma cells		2
Germinal center cells		4
Histiocytes	5	11
Fibroblasts		2
Lipocytes		4
Mucus-forming cylindrical epithelia	3	1
Metaplastic squamous epithelia	1	1
Duct epithelia	5	14
Acinar epithelia		9
Protein precipitates	6	16
Mucus	3	1
Cell debris	3	13
Cholesterol crystals	1	
Needle-shaped crystals		2
Stroma particles	1	6
Capillary fragments		3

9 cases examined by cytology and histology and 17 cases only examined by cytology.

Also, the cytological characteristics of an interstitial fibrosis or lipomatosis such as fibroblasts, stroma particles and lipocytes, can only be found in some biopsies.

There is one remarkable case of prominent eosinophilia indicating that the morphological aspect of chronic-recurrent parotitis is not only determined by bacterial infection but secondarily also by immunological processes. In 4 cases germinal center cells point to the same direction. These cells indicate formation of lymph follicles [71]. Focal purulent histolytic transformations of tissue result in cellular pictures that cannot be differentiated from an acute purulent parotitis.

Although the equivalent of different histomorphologic aspects of this form of inflammation are not decisive in the cytological diagnosis, they may be responsible for a false diagnosis with operative consequences if they occur in the punctate exclusively or predominantly. The combination of cyst formation and duct proliferation caused the wrong diagnosis of a cystic epithelial tumor. A cyst with goblet cell metaplasia gave rise to the false diagnosis of mucoepidermoid tumor. A comparable diagnostic situation exists with the adenolymphomas.

Irradiation-Induced Sialadenitis

This type of sialadenitis can be induced by tumor irradiation. Damaged membranes of epithelial and endothelial cells play a leading role in the pathogenesis of this form of inflammation [73]. The severity of irradiation-induced changes depends on the radiation dose [66]. An acute and a chronic form of irradiation-induced sialadenitis are distinguished.

The effect of irradiation first becomes manifest in the acinar cells by swelling, vacuolization and degranulation of the cytoplasm, followed by acinar cell necroses. The acute type of this sialadenitis is further characterized by interstitial edema and by interstitial cell infiltrations. The damage to the blood vessels becomes histologically evident as a wall sclerosis with partial obliteration of the lumen [65, 66]. The chronic irradiation-induced sialadenitis is marked by parenchymatous atrophy, duct ectasis, metaplasia and proliferations of the duct epithelium. Pronounced epithelial dysplasia is occasionally encountered [65, 66].

Case Report

We had the opportunity to study the cytological and histological specimens of a case of chronic irradiation-induced sialadenitis. 10 months prior to taking the biopsy, a 73-year-old man had been treated by irradiation because of a non-Hodgkin lymphoma of the immunoblastic type in the tonsillar area. Only after knowledge of the case history the cytological diagnosis of irradiation-induced sialadenitis was given while previously a malignant tumor had been suspected.

The cell-deficient punctate smears contain few aggregates of duct epithelia with irregular arrangement of the nuclei. In some places the duct epithelia are forming tubular structures (fig. 9a). Part of the nuclei are pyknotic while others show small or large vacuoles. A slight nuclear polymorphism is notable in all cellular aggregates. Furthermore, fibroblasts, metachromatic stroma particles and lipocytes can be demonstrated (fig. 9b).

The surgical specimen is characterized by lipomatosis of the gland, interstitial fibrosis, diffuse round-cell infiltrations and duct proliferations with dysplastic and regressively changed nuclei (fig. 9c).

Discussion

As in other forms of chronic sialadenitis the duct epithelia are prominent in cytology. The lipomatous and fibrous transformation of the body of the

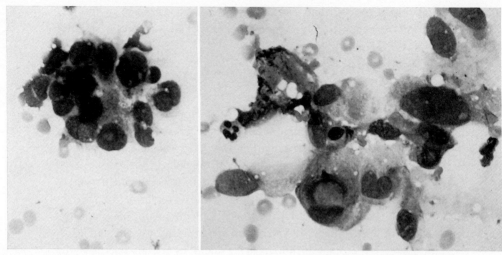

9a   9b

gland manifests itself cytologically by a small number of lipocytes, fibroblasts and stroma particles as well as by the complete absence of acinar
cells. The cells from dysplastic duct regeneration products can, as in the
described case, pretend the presence of a tumor.

Merely the numerous nuclear vacuoles can be regarded as symptoms
of the effect of irradiation. However, these changes are not to be interpreted
as specific for damage by irradiation. Analogous cellular changes were also
observed in follicle epithelia after treatment of the thyroid gland with
radioactive iodine [26].

Irradiation-induced sialadenitis, as a rule, cannot be diagnosed by the
cytologist without knowledge of the anamnesis since the combination of
epithelial damage and vascular lesion, guiding the histologist in his diagnosis, is impossible to demonstrate by cytological examination alone.

Epithelioid-Cellular Sialadenitis

Epithelioid-cellular sialadenitis is one component of Boeck's disease
[64] and a constituent of Heerfordt's syndrome, a special form of manifestation of this disease. In 1–4% of all cases of sarcoidosis, epithelioid-
cellular sialadenitis is to be expected [57]. The Hamburg Salivary Gland
Register lists 17 cases observed within 10 years [68]. Women in their 3rd
and 4th decade of life are predominantly affected [69]. The parotid gland is
involved in most cases but also the minor salivary glands are attacked [74].

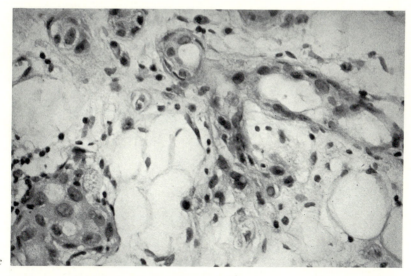

9c

Fig. 9. Irradiation-induced parotitis. *a* Tubular formation of duct epithelia with dysplastic nuclei. MGG. × 470. *b* Fibroblasts and metachromatic stroma material. MGG. × 520. *c* Interstitial fibrosis and lipomatosis, duct dysplasia and lymphocytic infiltration. HE × 285.

The histological picture is characterized by miliary granulomas first developing pericanalicularly. The granulomas are formed by epithelioid cells, giant cells of the Langhans type and lymphocytes. In contrast to tuberculosis one finds no caseous but, if at all, fibrinoid necroses. The granulomas have a tendency towards hyalinization. The inflammatory process preferentially destroys the acini of the gland. Duct obstructions with secretory congestion and microlith formation are secondary phenomena [64, 65].

Patients

Among the patients examined we find 3 with a histologically ascertained epithelioid-cellular parotitis.

Results

In all 3 cases the cytological diagnosis of epithelioid-cellular sialadenitis was made. The 3 biopsies are cell-rich and identical in their cell composition. Epithelioid-cell complexes are prominent (fig. 10a). The preparations contain lymphocytes in small to moderate numbers. Giant cells of the Langhans type can in no case be demonstrated. Duct epithelia as a component of the glandular parenchyma occur in aggregates and in tubular arrangement.

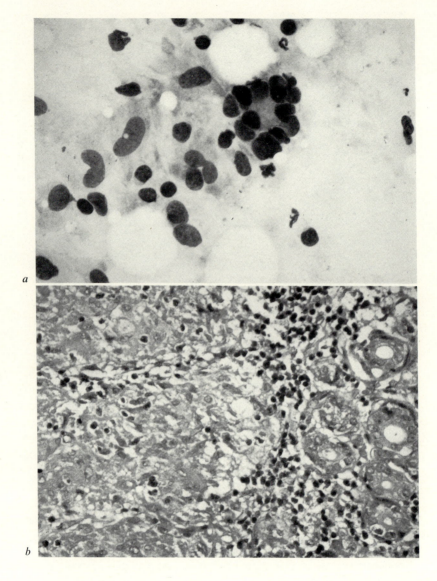

Fig. 10. Epithelioid-cellular parotitis. *a* Tubular formation of duct epithelia, epithelioid cells and lymphocytes. MGG. × 470. *b* Epithelioid cell granuloma surrounded by lymphocytes and salivary ducts. HE × 290.

Cell detritus and small stroma particles can be seen in some places in the specimen background. Histology shows complete destruction of the acinar tissue in all 3 cases (fig. 10b). Giant cell formations and fibrinoid necroses are not visible.

Discussion

The cytological diagnosis of an epithelioid-cellular sialadenitis can be made without difficulty if the punctate contains epithelioid cells and duct epithelia. As in other forms of chronic sialadenitis one finds, besides aggregates of duct epithelia, small stroma particles and cell debris. An absence of duct epithelia in the biopsy from the parotid gland makes a para- or intraglandular lymph node sarcoidosis likely. As far as differential diagnosis is concerned, we have finally to mention the very rare tuberculosis of the salivary glands [64] and the para- or intraglandular lymph node tuberculosis which is more frequent. While the caseating form of tuberculosis can be recognized according to the experience from lung and lymph node cytology, the productive form of tuberculosis cannot be distinguished from Boeck's granulomatosis.

Myoepithelial Sialadenitis

Myoepithelial sialadenitis [4, 62] is interpreted as autoimmunological disease of the salivary glands, on the basis of an autoantigen antibody reaction against salivary duct epithelia [19, 69]. In the Anglo-Saxon literature the synonym 'benign lymphoepithelial lesion' is standard usage [38, 41, 75].

From the histological point of view, myoepithelial sialadenitis is marked by three features: interstitial lymphoplasmatic-cellular infiltrations with lymph follicle formation, myoepithelial cell islets [8, 19, 52, 65] and destruction of the secretory parenchyma of the gland. The duct system of the gland is partially preserved, and duct ectases, cysts, secretory plaques and microliths are formed as a result of disorders of secretion.

The myoepithelial cell islets originate from the intercalated ducts and pass several stages of development [19]. In an early stage they contain epithelia from intercalated ducts and myoepithelia, are surrounded by a basal membrane and possess a residual lumen. The lumen disappears in the further course of development and the epithelia are obliterated. The cell islets increase in size due to proliferation of the myoepithelia and extended lymphohistiocytic infiltration. The basal membrane is dissolved and the cell islets eventually become subject to hyalinic transformation. The development of myoepithelial cell islets is regarded as pathognomonic [18, 52, 71].

The pathological process affects the parotid and the minor salivary glands. Myoepithelial sialadenitis preferentially occurs in women with the peak of incidence in the 6th and 7th decades of life [69].

On the average, a 10-year standing of myoepithelial sialadenitis can give rise to the development of a malignant lymphoma [3, 5, 10, 43]. The hypothesis was therefore put forward that long-term stimulation of immunologically active cells can lead to neoplastic transformation after previous myoepithelial sialadenitis [43]. Immunoglobulin-producing non-Hodgkin lymphomas of the lymphoplasmacytoid and immunoblastic types are mostly observed.

Patients

The patients are divided into two groups. The first group comprises 11 cases with a histologically verified diagnosis of myoepithelial sialadenitis. Although 3 more cases were histologically examined, the biopsies only yielded inadequate tissue (adipose tissue or normal salivary gland tissue). These 3 cases are therefore dealt with in the second group which was only cytologically examined. This group contains 9 cases. In agreement with the clinical picture the cytological diagnosis (or suspicion) of myoepithelial sialadenitis was made in all cases.

Results

After cytological examination, the disease was suspected in only 2 of altogether 11 cases of histologically verified myoepithelial sialadenitis. Chronic sialadenitis without further classification was determined in 3 cases. The remaining 6 biopsies were falsely interpreted as lymphadenitis, cyst or adenolymphoma (table V).

The specimen background is filled with precipitated protein or cell debris in the majority of the cytologically and histologically studied cases (table VI). Diffuse protein precipitates can be demonstrated mainly in 5 cases which histologically present extended duct ectases and multiple small cysts. Part of the cysts contain concrements and are lined with metaplastic squamous epithelium. Cyst fluid was aspirated twice during fine-needle biopsy. Lymphocytes, mostly present in big numbers, are a constant finding. Germinal center cells are relatively frequent but plasma cells and histiocytes are rather rare. Xanthoma cells and neutrophilic granulocytes in the punctate are an exception and can also histologically only be seen in a few ectatic ducts or periductally.

Epithelia are demonstrable in all but 2 biopsies. They appear as small and large aggregates characterized by pronounced overlapping of nuclei

Table V. Preoperative cytological diagnoses in 11 patients with histologically verified myoepithelial sialadenitis

Cytological diagnosis	Histological diagnosis myoepithelial sialadenitis
Suspicion of myoepithelial sialadenitis	2
Chronic sialadenitis	3
Lymphadenitis	3
Cyst	2
Suspicion of adenolymphoma	1

Hyalinic material can be histologically demonstrated in myoepithelial cell islets in 3 cases. It appears in one biopsy as plaque-like metachromatically staining particles. The punctates of the only cytologically examined cases yield identical cytologic pictures.

Table VI. Cells and noncellular elements in biopsies of myoepithelial sialadenitis

Cells and noncellular elements	Frequency of occurrence	
	cytological/histological examination	cytological examination
Protein precipitates	10	6
Cell debris	9	6
Cholesterol crystals		1
Hyalinic plaque	1	
Duct epithelia/myoepithelia	9	9
Acinar epithelia	1	1
Metaplastic squamous epithelia	2	
Lymphocytes	11	9
Plasma cells	2	1
Germinal center cells	8	5
Histiocytes	2	2
Xanthoma cells	3	
Neutrophilic granulocytes	3	

11 cases examined by cytology and histology and 9 cases only examined by cytology.

(fig. 11a) or in tubular formations (fig. 12a). In all cases pronounced regressive cellular changes are observed and naked nuclei often form lumps of large aggregates. Occasionally the cytoplasm is oxyphilic (fig. 12b). These cells are very similar to the oxyphilic epithelia in biopsies from adenolymphomas.

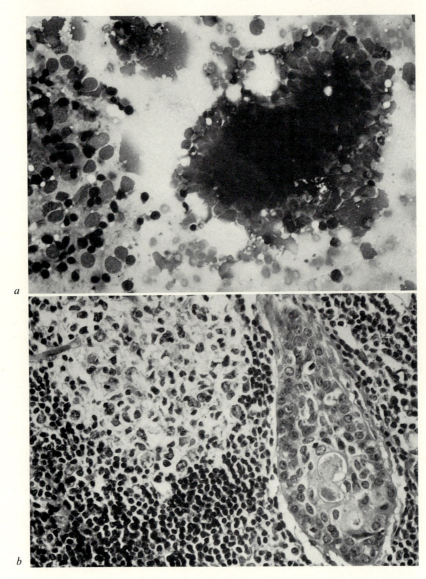

Fig. 11. Myoepithelial parotitis. *a* Epithelial aggregation consisting of several layers, surrounded by cell debris: equivalent of a myoepithelial islet. Lymphocytes and centroblasts: equivalent of a lymph follicle. MGG. × 290. *b* Myoepithelial islet surrounded by diffuse lymphocytic infiltration with lymph follicle. HE × 290.

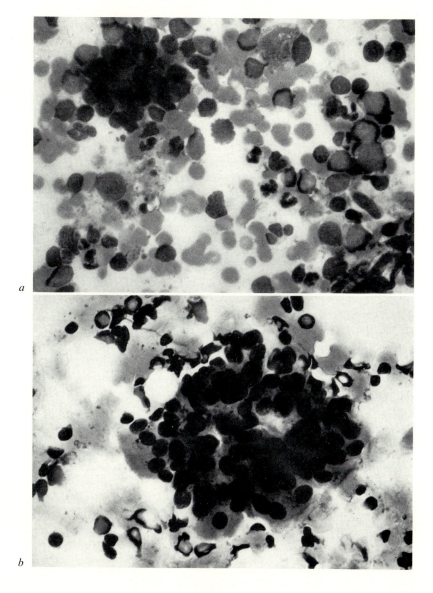

Fig. 12. Myoepithelial parotitis. *a* Tubular formation of duct epithelia surrounded by cells of a lymph follicle. Differential diagnosis: chronic-recurrent parotitis. MGG. × 470. *b* Epithelia with oxyphilic cytoplasm surrounded by lymphocytes. Differential diagnosis: adenolymphoma. MGG. × 470.

Discussion

A small number of acinar epithelia or their complete absence indicates the destruction of the secretory parenchyma of the gland. The pathognomonic myoepithelial cell islets cannot be identified with certainty in the punctate. Cytologically equivalent to these islets are aggregates of cells that cannot unequivocally be distinguished from aggregates of duct epithelia (fig. 11a). Conspicuous are alone the dense packing of nuclei and a high vulnerability of the cells. Spreading of the punctate strongly alters the shape of the nuclei in the marginal portions of the cell aggregates, and nuclear filaments forming matted clusters can always be demonstrated. Hyalinic plaques, when present, indicate myoepithelial cell islets.

The cytological diagnosis of myoepithelial sialadenitis is therefore based on three criteria: numerous lymphocytes, vulnerable epithelia in conglomerates and aggregates of cell debris.

Other cytological elements such as protein precipitates and microliths, indicating duct ectases and cysts, as well as metaplastic squamous epithelia, are only of little diagnostic value since they also occur in other chronic forms of sialadenitis.

On the basis of the above-mentioned criteria the diagnosis of myoepithelial sialadenitis can be made retrospectively in 8 of the 11 histologically verified cases. False positive diagnoses are possible if only lymphocytes or cyst fluid are aspirated [56]. Cases with strong hyalin formation in the myoepithelial islets and with development of gland sclerosis can hardly be diagnosed by cytology for lack of aspirated cell material. By differential diagnosis myoepithelial sialadenitis can be distinguished from adenolymphoma [18, 56]. In our own experience confusion with adenolymphoma is possible if the epithelia exhibit oxyphilic cytoplasm and if duct ectases or cysts are encountered at biopsy.

Since myoepithelial sialadenitis can give rise to the development of malignant lymphomas the differential diagnosis between these two transformations is of great clinical importance. Whereas non-Hodgkin lymphomas of the immunoblastic type can be reliably defined by cytology, lymphoplasmacytoid lymphomas cannot safely be differentiated from myoepithelial sialadenitis [46, 80]. A number of investigators have erroneously interpreted Hodgkin as well as non-Hodgkin lymphomas as myoepithelial sialadenitis [49], an experience we had to make ourselves recently. A patient was operated, based on the cytologic differential diagnosis discussed above, and histological examination revealed the presence of a non-Hodgkin lymphoma of low-grade malignancy. The punctate in this case contained neoplastic lymphocytes and preexisting duct epithelia in tubular formations and aggregates.

Chronic Sialadenitis of the Submandibular Gland

The clinical picture of chronic sialadenitis of the submandibular gland was first described by *Küttner* [48] after whom this disease is therefore also named Küttner's tumor [58]. Its development encompasses four stages: focal sialadenitis (stage 1), diffuse lymphocytic sialadenitis with fibrosis of the salivary gland (stage 2), chronic-sclerosing sialadenitis with sclerosis of the salivary gland (stage 3) and chronic-progressive sialadenitis with cirrhosis of the salivary gland (stage 4) [70]. In particular the stages 3 and 4 of this form of inflammation are accompanied by a tumor-like induration of the gland.

This disease is more frequent in men, with a peak of incidence between the 4th and 6th decades of life. Three etiological factors are supposed to be responsible for the development of Küttner's tumor: an obstructive secretory disorder and an immunologic reaction of the duct system [63, 69, 70]. The initial factor is a disorder of salivary electrolytes (dyschylia) leading, due to increasing viscosity of the saliva and obstruction by mucus, to sialolithiasis which is found in 40–50% of cases [69]. The dyschylia eventually induces an obstructive electrolyte sialadenitis [63, 69, 70]. Dyschylia and electrolyte sialadenitis correspond to stage 1 of chronic sialadenitis of the submandibular gland. Stages 2 and 3 are characterized by duct alterations (metaplasia, dysplasia and duct regeneration products), destructions of parenchyma and ascending infections, all of which trigger an immunpathologic reaction of the duct system. These in turn produce the final stage of the inflammatory process, stage 4 [70].

Patients
We have among our patients 5 cases of chronic sialadenitis of the submandibular gland, 2 of whom had also a sialolithiasis. 2 patients were operated. The histological examination of the specimens taken during operation yielded the diagnosis of chronic sialadenitis of the submandibular gland in the stages 1 and 2.

Results
The cytologic diagnosis of chronic sialadenitis of the submandibular gland was made in 4 cases, and the tentative diagnosis of highly differentiated mucoepidermoid tumor was given in 1 case.

Table VII. Cells and noncellular elements in biopsies of chronic sialadenitis of the submandibular gland

Cells and noncellular elements	Frequency of occurrence		cytological examination
	cytological/histological examination		
	stage 1	stage 2	
Protein precipitates	1		1
Mucus	1		
Cell debris		1	2
Stroma particles		1	2
Duct epithelia	1	1	3
Mucus-forming epithelia	1		1
Acinar epithelia	1		1
Neutrophilic granulocytes	1	1	1
Lymphocytes	1	1	3
Germinal center cells	1	1	2

2 cases examined by cytology and histology and 3 cases only examined by cytology.

The components of all 5 biopsies are numerous aggregates of duct epithelia or duct epithelia in tubular formation, as well as lymphocytes in small or moderate numbers (table VII). Neutrophilic granulocytes can be demonstrated in 3 cases, and additional germinal center cells in 4 cases. In stage 1 of this chronic sialadenitis the cellular aspect is predominantly marked by mucusforming epithelia, basophilic mucus and eosinophilic protein precipitates (fig. 13a, b). In stage 2 of the disease the punctate contains small metachromatic stroma particles and cell detritus (fig. 14a). The same elements are present in the specimens of 2 only cytologically examined cases which would make them stage 1 or 2. Acinar epithelia are found in small numbers in 2 biopsies.

Discussion

It is remarkable that chronic sialadenitis of the submandibular gland makes up 50% of all inflammations of the salivary glands in the Hamburg Salivary Gland Register [70] while among our own patients it was found in only 2 out of 36 histologically verified cases of sialadenitis.

Since stage 1 of Küttner's tumor is a focal sialadenitis, the diagnostic possibilities of punctate cytology are probably very much restricted. The

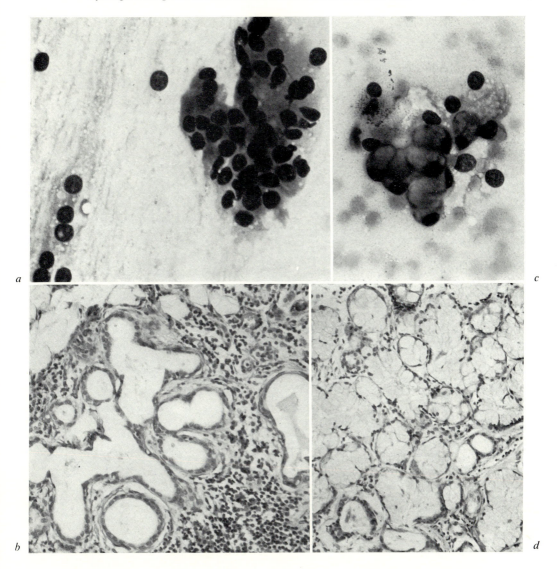

Fig. 13. Chronic sialadenitis of the submandibular gland (stage 1). *a* In the background, basophilic mucus and a papilliform aggregation of duct epithelia. MGG. × 460. *b* Mucus-containing goblet cells. Differential diagnosis: highly differentiated mucoepidermoid tumor. MGG. × 460. *c* Ectatic ducts and lymphocytic infiltration. HE × 150. *d* Mucus-filled acini, HE × 150.

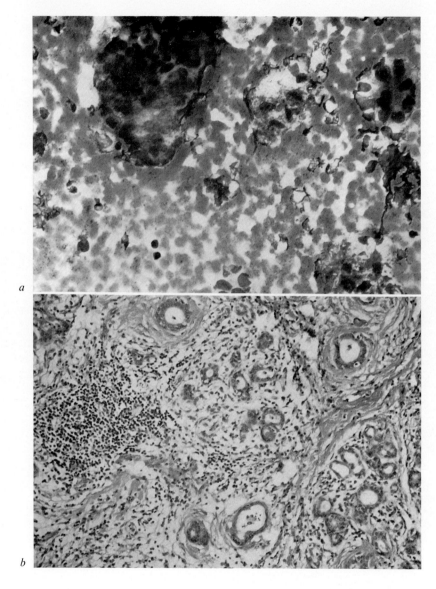

Fig. 14. Chronic sialadenitis of the submandibular gland (stage 2). *a* Aggregates of duct epithelia, partially with tubular structure (top right) and ruptured metachromatic stroma particles. MGG. × 290. *b* Periductal fibrosis and lymphocytic infiltration. HE × 117.

focal lymphocytic infiltrations are, if at all, encountered only accidentally. This assumption is corroborated by our experience in the cytologic diagnosis of the focal lymphocytic thyreoiditis [29]. The stiuation, however, is different if the morphologic phenomena of the secretory disorder are dominating, since mucoid dyschylia, microlith formation and duct ectases are represented by perceptible corresponding cytological phenomena: mucus, secretory plaque and diffuse protein precipitates. But the danger of a pronounced mucoid dyschylia imitating a highly differentiated mucoepidermoid tumor ought not to be oberlooked.

The diagnosis by punctate cytology is more promising in stage 2 when the process of inflammation is spreading in a diffuse manner. Destruction of the secretory parenchyma of the gland results, as in other forms of chronic sialadenitis, in a preponderance of duct epithelia (fig. 14a). Duct regeneration products are forming tubular configurations in the punctate. Canalicular bacterial infections are represented by focal accumulations of neutrophilic granulocytes. Small stroma particles are an indication of periductal fibroses. Metaplasia of squamous epithelial and goblet cells is also involved in the formation of the cellular picture. Analogous pictures are observed in punctates of chronic-recurrent parotitis and myoepithelial parotitis.

We did not investigate inflammations of the stages 3 and 4. It must be expected that punctate cytology is considerably reduced in its diagnostic value in cases of pronounced sclerosis and cirrhosis of the salivary glands. As in irradiation-induced sialadenitis, confusion with a carcinoma has to be avoided whenever pronounced duct dysplasia has been demonstrated.

Conclusions

Inflammations of the salivary glands are characterized by three features: primary inflammatory reaction of the interstitial vascularized connective tissue and alterations of the acini of the gland and of the salivary duct system. The three functional systems involved display a limited number of morphologic reactions. Their combination is determined by the etiological nature of the noxious event and by various pathogenetic factors [69].

The morphologic reaction of the three functional systems can be demonstrated, with certain reservations, in the cytologic punctate. We will first discuss the reactions of the interstitial vascularized connective tissue. The composition of the cellular infiltrations can be unequivocally identified and forms the basis of a cytological classification of the inflammations of the salivary glands. The cytological method is restricted by the following factors: in parotid biopsies the lymphoplasmatic cellular infiltrations of the immunologic forms of sialadenitis can only be distinguished from the lymphocytic cells of intra- and paraglandular lymph nodes if inflammation-induced reactions of the salivary duct system and the glandular acini exist side by side at the same time. Protein precipitates may correspond to an interstitial edema as well as to a duct ectasis. Stroma particles point to fibrosis but do not indicate grade and location.

The various inflammatory noxae induce toxic damage to the cell organelles, dissolution of membranes or atrophy due to pressure, and thereby finally lead to destruction of the acini of the gland [69]. This unidirectional reaction manifests itself in the cytological punctate as a reduction in numbers or as total lack of acinar cells.

The reactions of the salivary duct system, namely epithelial metaplasia and dysplasia as well as duct regeneration products, can be identified in the biopsy. Differential diagnosis, however, is limited by the fact that myoepithelial cell islets of immunosialadenitis cannot be distinguished from unspecific duct regeneration products with certainty. As was already mentioned, protein precipitates may be considered as an indication of a duct ectasis but are ambivalent. In contrast to these reservations microliths are to be regarded as unequivocal signs of a disorder of secretion.

The diagnostic problems involved in punctate cytology are finally augmented by identical pathogenetic factors becoming effective in the different forms of chronic sialadenitis. Chronic-recurrent parotitis, primarily induced by bacteria, is influenced in its course more and more by secretory disorders and by immunological processes, and myoepithelial parotitis and irradiation-induced sialadenitis are shaped by dyschylia [71].

In summing up, the following statements can be made:

The purulent histolysis present in acute purulent sialadenitis is definitely reflected by cytologic phenomena. The combination of inflammatory cells and predominance of epithelia of the salivary duct system forms the major diagnostic criterion of a chronic sialadenitis. With the exception of its epithelioid-cellular form which has a specific cytological substrate, the cytological classification of chronic parotitis is only possible to a limited extent. The diagnosis of chronic sialadenitis of the submandibular gland is supported by the topography. Epithelial metaplasia and dysplasia, when occurring in the punctate in a dominant proportion, can give rise to the false positive diagnosis of a tumor.

Parotid Cysts

Of the cysts that are forming in the major and minor salivary glands, the cytologist mainly concerns himself with the parotid cysts. The dysgenetic cysts of the submandibular and sublingual glands, the so-called Merkel's ducts [61] or the ranula, as well as the relatively frequent retention cysts of the minor salivary glands are rarities in aspiration-cytological diagnostics.

An incidence of 2–6% is given for parotid cysts in the operation material of several investigators [30, 60, 72, 79]. Acquired and congenital cysts are being distinguished, the latter comprise dermoid and branchial cysts. Acquired cysts are retention cysts developing by obstruction of the salivary duct system, caused by scarry structures in sialadenitis, and by sialoliths, inspissated mucus, trauma of different origins, parasites, and tumors [60, 79].

Parotid cysts are found in all age groups. In contrast to infancy and childhood where cysts are usually benign, in adult age they often constitute only one component of a benign or malignant tumor. Owing to this circumstance, diagnosis and treatment of parotid cysts is problematic.

The retention cysts contain a clear serous or turbid, creamy or viscid fluid. They are lined by mono- or multiple-layered epithelium exhibiting the forms of differentiation typical for ductal epithelium: cubical and cylindrical epithelia, mucus-forming cells, squamous epithelia and oncocytes. The cysts are enclosed by a collagenous connective tissue capsule. Chronic-inflammatory infiltrations or granulomatous reactions can be demonstrated in neighboring tissue [60, 79]. Neoplastic retention cysts are mostly observed in adenolymphoma, mucoepidermoid tumors, pleomorphic adenoma and adenoid-cystic carcinoma. Part of the neoplastic cysts, however, are extravasations or pseudocysts due to necrosis [79].

The branchial cysts are derived from the first branchial cleft [64] and are localized in the outer lobe of the gland. They contain fluid, crumbly masses and keratinous material; their walls are formed by mono- or multiple-layered squamous epithelium and a collagenous connective tissue capsule. According to *Work* [79], cysts without cutaneous appendages are termed type I, and those with cutaneous appendages and cartilagenous residues, type II. Branchial cysts are embedded in lymphatic tissue in which lymph follicles may be present [60, 64, 79]. On account of this characteristic, terms such as 'benign cystic lymph nodes' or 'benign lymphoepithelial cyst' were also proposed for branchial cysts [8]. These authors hold that such cysts develop from salivary ducts trapped during embryogenesis in lymph nodes.

Patients

Fine-needle biopsy of 520 clinically diagnosed parotid swellings resulted in the aspiration of cyst fluid in 40 cases (7.7%). The maximum volume was 20 ml. Cysts were present in all age groups with a predilection of the 7th decade of life. 27 patients were operated. No surgical intervention was attempted in 13 cases due to reasons of age or poor general condition of the patients, or following normalization of palpatory findings after emptying of the cyst.

Results

6 retention cysts (of inflammatory, traumatic, or unknown genesis), 2 branchial cysts and 3 epidermal inclusion cysts were cytologically classified as nonneoplastic cysts. 3 retention cysts were incorrectly interpreted. Adenolymphoma was diagnosed in 1 case and in 2 cases the tentative diagnosis of mucoepidermoid tumor was made (table VIII).

13 cyst biopsies were taken from tumors, and 7 monomorphic adenomas' 2 pleomorphic adenomas, 3 benign mesenchymatous tumors and 1 malignant tumor (diagnosed as metastasis of a squamous epithelial carcinoma in a periglandular lymph node) were histologically determined. Cytologically, only 4 adenolymphomas were correctly classified. In the remaining cases the cyst was not interpreted as component of a tumor (table IX).

From the 13 unoperated cysts 3 were cytologically associated with an adenolymphoma. The remaining 10 cysts were not interpreted as partial manifestation of a tumor (table X).

All inflammatory, traumatic or etiologically unclear retention cysts are characterized microscopically by diffusely distributed homogenous or granular basophilic or eosinophilic precipitates. One cystic preparation contained violet mucus. Lymphocytes (myoepithelial sialadenitis) or neutrophilic and eosinophilic granulocytes (chronic-recurrent parotitis and cysts of uncertain etiology) can be demonstrated in a few cases. Cell detritus and foam cells occur in one third of the aspirates. 7 out of 9 punctates contain epithelial cells. Squamous epithelia are found in 4 cases, and cylindrical epithelia with and without mucus formation as well as oncocytes (fig. 15a) in 1 case each (table XI).

The preparations of the two branchial cysts contain eosinophilic precipitates and foam cells. Cholesterol crystals, lymphocytes and squamous epithelia can be demonstrated in only one aspiration biopsy sample.

Diffuse eosinophilic or basophilic precipitates are also present in the microscopic picture of the 3 epidermal inclusion cysts. Squamous epithelia can be identified in only 2 punctates; in 1 of them numerous neutrophilic granulocytes can be observed in addition.

Table VIII. Preoperative cytological diagnosis of 14 histologically verified retention cysts, branchial cysts and epidermal inclusion cysts

Cytological diagnosis	Histological diagnosis					
	retention cysts				branchial cysts	epidermal inclusion cysts
	myoepithelial sialadenitis (n=2)	chronic-recurrent sialadenitis (n=2)	trauma (n=1)	unclear etiology (n=4)	(n=2)	(n=3)
Cyst				2		1
Cyst with squamous epithelial lining	1		1		1	1
Infected cyst with squamous epithelial lining	1					1
Cyst with squamous epithelial lining and granulomatous reaction					1	
Cyst with cylindrical epithelial lining				1		
Adenolymphoma		1				
Suspicion of mucoepidermoid tumor		1		1		

Table IX. Preoperative cytological diagnosis of 13 histologically verified tumor cysts of the parotid gland or the parotid region

Cytological diagnosis	Histological diagnosis							
	adeno-lymphoma (n=5)	papillary cystic adenoma (n=1)	basal cell adenoma (n=1)	pleo-morphic adenoma (n=2)	metastasis of squamous epithelial carcinoma (n=1)	neuro-fibroma (n=1)	hem-angioma (n=1)	lymph-angioma (n=1)
Cyst						1	1	1
Cyst (squamous epithelium)	1		1	1				
Cyst (squamous epithelium) in chronic-recurrent parotitis					1			
Cyst (cylindrical epithelium)		1		1				
Suspicion of adenolymphoma	3							
Adenolymphoma	1							

Table X. Cytological diagnosis of 13 cystic punctates of the parotid gland without subsequent operation

Cytological diagnosis	n
Cyst	6
Cyst with squamous epithelial lining and granulomatous reaction	1
Cyst with cylindrical epithelial lining	3
Adenolymphoma	3

The 13 tumor cyst biopsies, too, contain precipitates of different staining and structure. The aspirates of the 3 mesenchymatous tumors do not show any additional cellular or noncellular elements. In contrast to that one finds in the cyst biopsies of the 10 epithelial tumors a broad spectrum of cellular and noncellular elements. The latter include cholesterol crystals or rod-shaped crystals (fig. 16a) and metachromatic stroma particles in 3 cases (2 pleomorphic adenomas, 1 basal cell adenoma). Lymphocytes, centroblasts and neutrophilic granulocytes are only visible in punctates from adenolymphomas. Half of the cystic punctates show mono- or multi-nuclear foam cells. Oncocytes and squamous epithelia (fig. 16a) can be seen in 4 cases each, and cylindrical epithelia in 1 case. Basaloid epithelia in aggregates occur in 2 punctates (pleomorphic adenoma and basal cell adenoma). Retrospective anlysis permits tumor diagnosis in 6 cases (4 adenolymphomas, 1 pleomorphic adenoma, and 1 basal cell adenoma).

Discussion

According to our own experience, aspirates from cysts can be expected in 7–8% of biopsies taken from parotid swellings. Among the operated parotid swellings the cystic punctates constitute a portion of 8.3%. Excluding tumor cysts the incidence of parotid and extraglandular cysts of the parotid region is 4.3% in histologically examined material. This percentage agree well with the data of other authors who reported a range between 2 and 6% [30, 60, 72, 79]. The cytological literature does not yield comparable values.

Richardson et al. [60] recommended operative treatment of all parotid swellings that are clinically presenting as cysts. This concept seems justified since as much as one third of our cystic punctates came from tumors. It would be worthwhile to investigate if the general recommendation for operation could be replaced by special indications after application of punctate cytology.

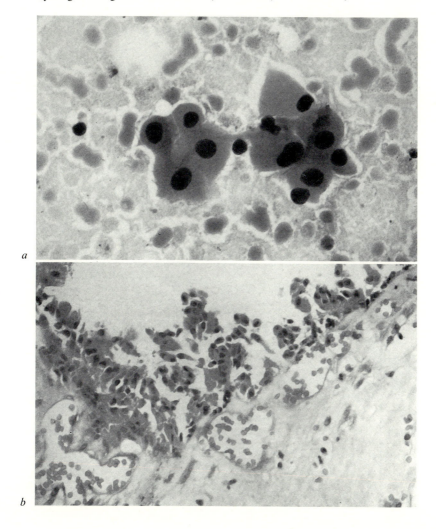

Fig. 15. Parotid retention cyst. *a* Eosinophilic protein precipitate and polygonal oxyphilic epithelia. Differential diagnosis: adenolymphoma. MGG. × 470. *b* Cyst with oxyphilic epithelial lining. HE × 290.

Table XI. Noncellular elements and cells in 27 cystic punctates of the parotid gland or the parotid region

Noncellular elements and cells	Frequency of occurrence				
	retention cysts	branchial cysts	epidermal inclusion cysts	tumor cysts	
				epithelial tumors	mesenchymal tumors
	(n=9)	(n=2)	(n=3)	(n=10)	(n=3)
Eosinophilic and basophilic precipitates	9	2	3	10	3
Mucus	1	1		2	
Cholesterol crystals	1			1	
Rod-shaped crystals				3	
Metachromatic stroma particles				2	
Cell detritus	2			4	
Lymphocytes	1	1		3	
Centroblasts				2	
Neutrophilic granulocytes	4		1		
Eosinophilic granulocytes	1	2		5	
Foam cells	3	1	2	4	
Squamous epithelia	4			1	
Cylindrical epithelia	1				
Mucus-forming cylindrical epithelia	1				
Oncocytes	1			4	
Basaloid epithelia in aggregates				2	

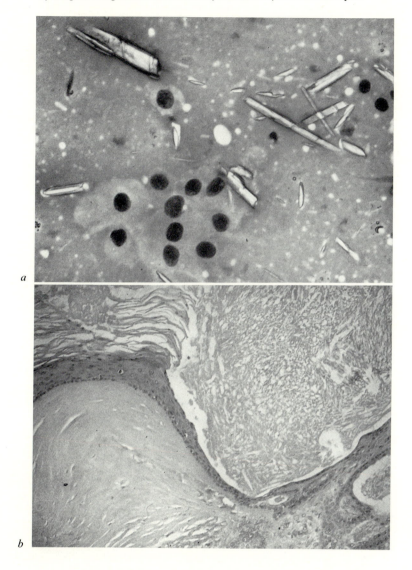

Fig. 16. Cystic pleomorphic adenoma. *a* Thick eosinophilic protein precipitate. Rod-shaped crystals and squamous epithelia. MGG. × 470. *b* Big cyst within a pleomorphic adenoma, lined with multiple-layered squamous epithelium. Inside the cyst eosinophilic secretion and rod-shaped crystals are present. HE × 120.

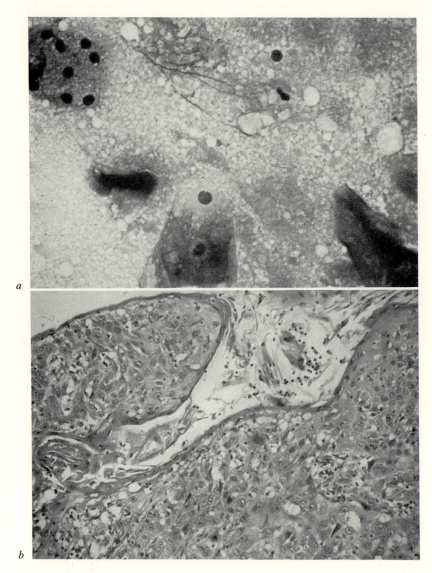

Fig. 17. Metastasis of a cystic squamous epithelial carcinoma within a paraglandular lymph node. *a* Basophilic protein precipitate, well-differentiated squamous epithelia without nuclear atypia and one basophilic keratinous plaque. Top left: one normal serous acinus. Differential diagnosis: branchial cyst. MGG. × 290. *b* Solid tumor cell formations are enclosing a cystic cavity with desquamated well-differentiated squamous epithelia and keratinous plaques. HE. × 120.

The common characteristic in the microscopic picture of all cystic punctates is the occurrence of diffuse precipitates of secretion or protein; further typical components of cysts are foam cells, cholesterol crystals or crystals appearing with different frequency, but they are all without importance for the morphological classification of the cyst. This also applies to inflammatory reactions. Eight punctates from cysts, nearly one third, merely contain diffuse protein precipitates. These specimens include retention cysts, branchial cysts, epidermal inclusion cysts as well as tumor cysts. In this connection the observation that benign mesenchymatous tumors may manifest themselves as cell-free cystic punctates deserves attention. In children this finding should always suggest the possibility of a hemangioma or lymphangioma.

The diagnosis 'cyst with squamous epithelial lining' was made in 9 instances, the biggest number of cases. They represent not only branchial cysts or epidermal inclusion cysts but also retention cysts in myoepithelial sialadenitis and after trauma, as well as tumor cysts. Particular attention must be focused on one punctate obtained from a metastasis of a cystic squamous epithelial carcinoma in an extraglandular lymph node (fig. 17). Carcinoma could not be diagnosed since the microscopic picture only revealed a nuclear squamous epithelial plaque and well-differentiated squamous epithelia without nuclear atypia. This case confirms the conclusions drawn by *Engzell* and *Zajicek* [37] form the results of a comparative study of branchial cysts and metastases of squamous epithelial carcinoma, that branchial cysts and metastases of highly differentiated squamous epithelial carcinomas cannot be safely distinguished by cytological investigation. The cytological diagnosis of a squamous epithelial cyst should always arise doubt in the clinician if the patient is over 30 years old because the majority of branchial cysts becomes manifest at a younger age. Besides, branchial cysts of the parotid gland are very rare. *Miglets* [51] found only 25 cases reported in the literature.

Nine cystic punctates with cylindrical epithelia or oncocytes came from nonneoplastic retention cysts or tumor cysts. If biopsy also involves solid tissue portions, the possibility exists that these cysts will be interpreted as partial symptom of a tumor or an inflammation. Retention cysts lined with oncocytes or mucus-forming cylindrical epithelia may be falsely diagnosed as adenolymphoma or mucoepidermoid tumor (cf. the section 'Sialadenitis') as shown by 3 of our own cases and the reports of other authors [56].

The ambiguousness of cytological findings in aspiration biopsies from cysts is reflected by the diagnostic results. Only 12 out of 17 cystic punctates were correctly classified with respect to choice between tumor or nonneoplastic change, and only 4 from 13 tumor cysts were identified as such.

Conclusions

This analysis permits the following conclusions: The value of punctate cytology consists in the possibility to verify the clinical diagnosis of a cyst by aspiration of fluid, and to make a preoperative assessment of the necessity of an operation and its type and extent, if proof of a benign or malignant tumor was obtained by microscopic examination. The diagnostic value of punctate cytology can be increased if after aspiration of cyst fluid also solid tissue components from the region of the cyst are included. Patients whose biopsy aspirates did not give evidence for the presence of a tumor should be reexamined 2–4 weeks later. Operative treatment will not be necessary if the follow-up examination reveals that the parotid swelling has subsided. Without this control investigation, recommended by *Zajicek* [80], morphological aspects always indicate an operation if tumor-negative biopsies cannot be etiologically classified even though clinical data were included in the diagnostic procedure.

References

1   Appaix, A.; Bonneau, H.; Sommer, D.: La cytologie des tumeurs des glandes salivaires. Presse méd. *67:* 600–602 (1959).

2   Arglebe, C.; Chilla, R.: Über ein biochemisches Modell neurogener Sialosen. Lar. Rhinol. Otol. *54:* 542–550 (1975).

3   Azzopardi, J.G.; Evans, D.J.: Malignant lymphoma of parotid associated with Mikulicz disease (benign lymphoepithelial lesion). J. clin. Path. *24:* 744–752 (1971).

4   Bark, C.J.; Perzik, S.L.: Mikulicz's disease, sialoangiectasis, and autoimmunity based upon a study of parotid lesions. Am. J. clin. Path. *49:* 683–689 (1968).

5   Batsakis, J.G.; Bernacki, E.G.; Rice, D.H.; Stebler, M.E.: Malignancy and the benign lymphoepithelial lesion. Laryngoscope *85:* 389–399 (1975).

6   Beck, C.: Zur Frage der Probeexcision aus der Ohrspeicheldrüse. Arch. Ohr.-Nas.-KehlkHeilk. *197:* 327–330 (1971).

7   Berge, T.; Söderström, N.: Fine-needle cytologic biopsy in diseases of the salivary glands. Acta path. microbiol. scand. *58:* 1–9 (1963).

8   Bernier, J.L.; Bhaskar, S.N.: Lymphoepithelial lesions of salivary glands. Histogenesis and classification based on 186 cases. Cancer, Philad. *11:* 1156–1179 (1958).

9   Böhme, P.: Die Parotischirurgie und ihre morphologischen Grundlagen (Thieme, Stuttgart 1966).

10   Bolognini, G.; Riva, G.: Lymphoproliferative Erkrankungen und Paraproteinämien beim Sjögren-Syndrom. Schweiz. med. Wschr. *105:* 1493–1506 (1975).

11   Bonneau, H.; Sommer, D.: L'orientation du diagnostic des tumeurs salivaires par la ponction à l'aiguille fine. Path. Biol., Paris *7:* 785–791 (1959).

12   Brands, T.: Diagnose und Klinik der Erkrankungen der grossen Kopfspeicheldrüsen (Urban & Schwarzenberg, München 1972).

13   Brechet, M.; Viellard, J.; De Brux, J.; Leroux-Robert, J.: La cytologie de ponction en pathologie ORL et cervico-faciale. Annls Oto-lar. *84:* 381–394 (1967).

14   Brizard, C.P.: Cytologie salivaire. Lyon méd. *231:* 303–306 (1974).

15   Castellain, G.; Castellain, C.; Lecoursonnois, C.: Cystodiagnostic et cytopronostic des tumeurs des glandes salivaires. Presse méd. *60:* 2302–2305 (1959).

16   Conley, J.: Salivary glands and the facial nerve (Thieme, Stuttgart 1975).

17   Cornillot, M.; Verhaeghe, M.; Clay, A.; Cappelaere, P.: L'examen cytologique par ponction-aspiration à l'aiguille fine des tumeurs de la parotide. Lille méd. *13:* 843–847 (1968).

18   Cruickshank, A.H.: Benign lymphoepithelial salivary lesions to be distinguished from adenolymphoma. J. clin. Path. *18:* 391–400 (1965).

19   Donath, K.; Seifert, G.: Ultrastruktur und Pathogenese der myoepithelialen Sialadenitis. Virchows Arch. Abt. A Path. Anat. *356:* 315–329 (1972).

20   Donath, K.; Seifert, G.; Pirsig, W.: Parotis-Sialadenose nach Langzeittherapie mit Antihypertensiva (Guanacline). Ultrastrukturelle Befunde. Virchows Arch. Abt. A Path. Anat. *360:* 33–44 (1973).

21   Donath, K.; Spillner, M.: Morphometrische und ultrastrukturelle Untersuchungen zur neurohormonalen Sialadenose. Verh. dt. Ges. Path. *58:* 494 (1974).

22   Donath, K.; Spillner, M.; Seifert, G.: The influence of the autonomic nervous system on the ultrastructure of the parotid acinar cells. Experimental contribution to neurohormonal sialadenosis. Virchows Arch. Abt. A Path. Anat. *364:* 15–33 (1974).

23   Donath, K.; Seifert, G.: Ultrastructural studies of the parotid glands in sialadenosis. Virchows Arch. Abt. A Path. Anat. *365:* 119–135 (1975).

24   Donath, K.: Die Sialadenose der Parotis. Ultrastrukturelle, klinische und experimentelle Befunde der Sekretionspathologie (Fischer, Stuttgart 1976).

25   Donath, K.: Wangenschwellung bei Sialadenose. HNO *27:* 113–118 (1979).

26   Droese, M.; Kempken, K.; Schneider, M.L.; Hör, G.: [131]J-induzierte Zellveränderungen im Follikelepithel der Schilddrüse. Verh. dt. Ges. Path. *57:* 336–338 (1973).

27   Droese, M.; Tute, M.; Haubrich, J.: Punktionszytologie von Speicheldrüsentumoren. Lar. Rhinol. Otol. *56:* 703–710 (1977).

28   Droese, M.; Haubrich, J.; Tute, M.: Stellenwert der Punktionszytologie in der Diagnostik der Speicheldrüsentumoren. Schweiz. med. Wschr. *108:* 933–935 (1978).

29   Droese, M.; Bähre, M.; Emrich, D.; Stubbe, P.; Jentsch, E.; Breuel, H.P.; Hofmann, S.: Zytologische Diagnose der Schilddrüsenentzündungen. Dt. med. Wschr. *104:* 875–881 (1979).

30   Eneroth, C.-M.: Histological and clinical aspects of parotid tumours. Acta oto-lar., suppl. 101, pp. 1–99 (1964).

31   Eneroth, C.-M.; Zajicek, J.: Aspiration biopsy of salivary gland tumors. II. Morphologic studies on smears and histologic sections from oncocytic tumors (45 cases of papillary cystadenoma lymphomatosum and 4 cases of oncocytoma). Acta cytol. *9:* 355–361 (1965).

32   Eneroth, C.-M.; Zajicek, J.: Aspiration biopsy of salivary gland tumors. II. Morphologic studies on smears and histologic sections from 368 mixed tumors. Acta cytol. *10:* 440–454 (1966).

33   Eneroth, C.-M.; Franzén, S.; Zajicek, J.: Cytologic diagnosis on aspirate from 1000 salivary gland tumours. Acta oto-lar., suppl. 224, pp. 168–171 (1967).

34   Eneroth, C.-M.; Zajicek, J.: Aspiration biopsy of salivary gland tumors. IV. Morphologic studies on smears and histologic sections from 45 cases of adenoid cystic carcinoma. Acta cytol. *13:* 59–63 (1969).

35   Eneroth, C.-M.; Jakobsson, P.A.; Zajicek, J.: Aspiration biopsy of salivary gland tumors. V. Morphologic investigations on smears and histologic sections of acinic cell carcinoma. Acta radiol., suppl. 310, pp. 85–93 (1971).

36   Eneroth, C.-M.: Die Klinik der Kopfspeicheldrüsentumoren. Archs Oto-Rhino-Lar. *213:* 61–110 (1976).

37   Engzell, U.; Zajicek, J.: Aspiration biopsy of tumors of the neck. I. Aspiration biopsy and cytologic findings in 100 cases of congenital cysts. Acta cytol. *14:* 51–57 (1970).

38   Evans, R.W.; Cruickshank, A.H.: Epithelial tumours of the salivary glands (Saunders, Philadelphia 1970).

39   Frable, W.J.; Frable, M.A.: Thin-needle aspiration biopsy in the diagnosis of head and neck tumors. Laryngoscope *84:* 1069–1077 (1974).

40   Franzén, S.; Giertz, G.; Zajicek, J.: Cytological diagnosis of prostatic tumours by transrectal aspiration biopsy. A preliminary report. Br. J. Urol. *32:* 193–196 (1960).

41   Godwin, J.L.: Benign lymphoepithelial lesion of the parotid gland (adenolymphoma, chronic inflammation, lymphoepithelioma, lymphocytic tumor, Mikulicz's disease). Report of 11 cases. Cancer, Philad. *5:* 1089–1103 (1952).

42   Haubrich, J.: Klinik der nichttumorbedingten Erkrankungen der Speicheldrüsen. Archs Oto-Rhino-Lar. *213:* 1–59 (1976).

43   Heckmayr, M.; Seifert, G.; Donath, K.: Maligne Lymphome und Immunsialadenitis. Lar. Rhinol. Otol. *55:* 593–607 (1976).

44   Jasper, A.: Parotidektomie und die Frage der Probeexcision. Arch. Ohr.-Nas.-Kehlk-Heilk. *194:* 313–316 (1969).

45   Kleinsasser, O.: Nervus fascialis und Glandula parotis. HNO *24:* 116–118 (1976).

46   Koivuniemi, A.; Saksela, E.; Holopainen, E.: Cytological aspiration biopsy in otorhinolaryngological practice. Acta oto-lar., suppl. *263,* pp. 189–192 (1970).

47   Kondratéva, T.T.; Petrova, A.S.: Cytologic diagnosis of salivary glands tumors. Vop. Onkol. *13:* 25–32 (1977).

48   Küttner, H.: Über entzündliche Tumoren der Submaxillarspeicheldrüsen. Bruns' Beitr. klin. Chir. *15:* 815–828 (1896).

49   Lindenberg, L.G.; Akerman, M.: Aspiration cytology of salivary gland tumors: diagnostic experience from six years of routine laboratory work. Laryngoscope *86:* 584–594 (1976).

50   Mavec, P.; Eneroth, C.-M.; Franzén, S.; Moberger, G.; Zajicek, J.: Aspiration biopsy of salivary gland tumors. I. Correlation of cytologic reports from 652 aspiration biopsies with clinical and histological findings. Acta oto-lar. *58:* 471–484 (1964).

51   Miglets, A.W.: Parotid branchial cleft cyst with facial paralysis: report of a case. Archs Otolar. *101:* 637–638 (1975).

52   Morgan, W.S.; Castleman, B.: A clinicopathologic study of 'Mikulicz's disease'. Am. J. Path. *29:* 471–503 (1953).

53   Münzel, M.: Ätiologische Aspekte der Sialadenosen. Lar. Rhinol. Otol. *50:* 389–393 (1971).

54   Nikitina, N.I.: The cytological diagnosis of the so-called mixed tumours of the salivary glands. Vop. Onkol. *7:* 43–48 (1961).

55   Paches, A.I.: Importance of the cytological method in diagnosis of tumors of the parotid gland. Lab. Delo *1:* 47–50 (1966).

56   Persson, P.S.; Zettergren, L.: Cytologic diagnosis of salivary gland tumors by aspiration biopsy. Acta cytol. *17:* 351–354 (1973).

57   Pfeiffer, K.: Die Röntgendiagnostik der Speicheldrüsen und ihrer Ausführungsgänge; in Diethelm, Olsson, Strand, Vieten, Zuppinger, Handbuch der medizinischen Radiologie, vol. VIII, p. 308 (Springer, Berlin 1968).

58   Räsänen, O.; Jokinen, K.; Dammert, K.: Sclerosing inflammation of the submandibular salivary gland (Küttner tumor). A progressive plasmacellular ductitis. Acta oto-lar. *74:* 297–301 (1972).

59   Rauch, S.: Die Speicheldrüsen des Menschen (Thieme, Stuttgart 1959).

60   Richardson, G.S.; Clairmont, A.A.; Erickson, E.R.: Cystic lesions of the parotid gland. Plastic reconstr. Surg. *61:* 364–370 (1978).

61   Seifert, G.; Geiler, G.: Zur Pathologie der kindlichen Kopfspeicheldrüsen. Beitr. path. Anat. allg. Pathol. *116:* 1–38 (1956).

62   Seifert, G.; Geiler, G.: Vergleichende Untersuchungen der Kopfspeichel- und Tränendrüsen zur Pathogenese des Sjögren-Syndroms und der Mikulicz-Krankheit. Virchows Arch. Abt. A Path. Anat. *330:* 402–424 (1957).

63   Seifert, G.: Die Sekretionsstörungen (Dyschylien) der Speicheldrüsen. Ergebn. Path. *44:* 103–188 (1964).

64   Seifert, G.: Mundhöhle, Mundspeicheldrüsen, Tonsillen und Rachen; in Doerr, Uehlinger, Spezielle pathologische Anatomie, vol. 1, pp. 1–415 (Springer, Berlin 1966).

65   Seifert, G.: Klinische Pathologie der Sialadenitis und Sialadenose. HNO *19:* 1–19 (1971).

66   Seifert, G.; Geier, W.: Zur Pathologie der Strahlen-Sialadenitis. Par. Rhinol. Otol. *50:* 376–388 (1971).

67   Seifert, G.; Donath, K.: Die Sialadenose der Parotis. Dt. med. Wschr. *100:* 1545–1548 (1975).

68   Seifert, G.; Donath, K.: Classification of the pathohistology of diseases of the salivary glands. Review of 2600 cases in the Salivary Gland Register. Beitr. Pathol. *159:* 1–32 (1976).

69   Seifert, G.; Donath, K.: Die Morphologie der Speicheldrüsenerkrankungen. Archs Oto-Rhino-Lar. *213:* 111–208, 371–380 (1976).

70   Seifert, G.; Donath, K.: Zur Pathogenese des Küttner-Tumors der Submandibularis. HNO *25:* 81–92 (1977).

71   Seifert, G.: Wangenschwellungen bei Speicheldrüsenentzündungen. HNO *27:* 119–128 (1979).

72   Shaheen, M.A.; Harboyan, G.T.; Nassif, R.I.: Cysts of the parotid gland. Review and report of two unusal cases. J. Lar. Otol. *89:* 435–444 (1975).

73   Sholley, M.M.; Sodicoff, M.; Pratt, N.E.: Early radiation injury in the rat parotid

gland. Reaction of acinar cells and vascular endothelium. Lab. Invest. *31:* 340–354 (1974).

74   Tarpley, T.M.; Anderson, L.; Lightbody, P.; Sheagren, J.N.: Minor salivary gland involvement in sarcoidosis. Report of 3 cases with positive lip biopsies. Oral Surg. *33:* 755–762 (1962).

75   Thackray, A.C.; Lucas, R.B.: Tumors of the major salivary glands. Atlas of tumor pathology, 2nd series, vol. 10 (Armed Forces Institute of Pathology, Washington 1974).

76   Thackray, A.C.; Sobin, L.H.: Histological typing of salivary gland tumours (World Health Organization, Geneva 1972).

77   Webb, A.J.: Cytologic diagnosis of salivary gland lesions in adult and pediatric surgical patients. Acta cytol. *17:* 51–58 (1973).

78   Westernhagen, B.: Aspirationsbiopsie oder Probeexzision zur Diagnostik von Parotistumoren. HNO *14:* 142–143 (1966).

79   Work, W.P.: Cysts and congenital lesions of the parotid gland. Otolaryngol. Clin. North Am. *10:* 339–343 (1977).

80   Zajicek, J.: Aspiration biopsy cytology. I. Cytology of supradiaphragmatic organs. Monogr. clin. Cytol., vol. 4 (Karger, Basel 1974).

81   Zajicek, J.; Eneroth, C.-M.; Jakobsson, P.A.: Aspiration biopsy of salivary gland tumors. VI. Morphologic studies on smears and histologic sections from muco-epidermoid carcinoma. Acta cytol. *20:* 35–41 (1976).

Priv.-Doz. Manfred Droese, MD, Pathologisches Institut, Medizinische Einrichtungen der Universität Göttingen, Robert-Koch-Strasse 40, D–3400 Göttingen (FRG)

Adv. Oto-Rhino-Laryng., vol. 26, pp. 97–234 (Karger, Basel 1981)

Biochemistry of Human Saliva

Christian Arglebe

ENT Department, University of Göttingen, Göttingen, FRG

Introduction

Salivary glands are widely distributed throughout the animal kingdom. They are found in many, but not all, groups of invertebrates as well as vertebrates. All mammals, which are the most highly developed group of vertebrates, are equipped with various cephalic glands which release their secretions into the oral cavity. Although differing considerably in their composition, the different fluids produced and secreted by these glands are commonly referred to as 'saliva'. This general, rather indistinctive term requires some further differentiation with respect to the several types of salivary glands involved. In man and the higher mammals, three pairs of salivary glands are arranged in a bilateral fashion. These are the sublingual, submandibular (or submaxillary) and parotid glands, the latter two being the major cephalic salivary glands as far as volume output is concerned. Among the vertebrates, the relative sizes of the two major glands are closely related to the type of food [for review see 5]. Herbivores, with bulky, carbohydrate-rich diet, have larger parotid glands, carnivores have smaller ones. Omnivores such as the rat and man possess parotid and submandibular glands of nearly equal size.

Besides the three types of salivary glands mentioned so far, there are inserted in the oral and labial mucosa a multitude of tiny salivary glands which are randomly distributed. The relative contributions of the different types of glands (under 'resting' conditions) to the total daily output of saliva in man are given in table I.

The weight of the cephalic salivary glands in the adult human being of average body weight amounts to altogether approximately 65 g, and a total volume of about 1–1.5 liters saliva is secreted per day [286]. *Mason and*

Table I. Contributions of the different cephalic salivary glands to total daily secretion of saliva [from 248]

Salivary gland	% of total saliva
Parotid	25
Submandibular	71
Sublingual	3–4
Minor (mucosal, labial)................................	traces

Chisholm [225] have cautioned against these high 'textbook values' that lack proper experimental evidence, and assume volumes between 500 and 600 ml/day as more realistic estimates [for references see 225]. Salivary gland secretion, however, is influenced by a wide variety of endogenous and exogenous (environmental) factors which will be dealt with briefly in the following section.

Apart from the quest for basic knowledge, the investigation of human saliva and its components has become of ever increasing importance as the chemical composition of saliva not only allows to draw conclusions about pathological changes of the salivary glands themselves but also about diseases of other organs, e.g. the pancreas. The most important functions of saliva comprise the following faculties.

(1) *Lubrication* of the mucous linings of the oral cavity and the upper digestive tract and their protection by mechanical cleansing and immunological defense. (2) *Digestion* of food by emulgation of the foodstuffs and cleavage of certain nutritive components by enzymes (mainly predigestion of starch by α-amylase). (3) *Excretion* of endogenous and extraneous (foreign) materials, e.g., iodine, antibodies, blood group reactive substances, coagulation factors, hormones, drugs, and viral pathogens, to name only a few. (4) *Protection* of teeth by mechanical cleansing, involvement in acquired pellicle formation, and by antibacterial action against cariogenic microorganisms. (5) *Other functions* of saliva include a mediator role in taste sensation, the support of swallowing, and a decisive role in the development of voice and speech.

The physiological role of saliva will be better understood only after a detailed description and discussion of the various components involved. As regards these, in this chapter we are concerned mainly with the sufficiently well characterized constituents of the secretions from the human major cephalic salivary glands, the parotid and the submandibular glands.

Collection of Saliva

General Remarks

Secretion of saliva results from stimulation of the respective salivary glands via their autonomic innervation or by the action of substances that mimic the effect of autonomic innervation. Under conditions of absolute rest (during sleep) saliva flow can altogether stop [221]. This had already previously been reported by *Schneyer* [305] and *Schneyer* et al. [307] who concluded from their studies that there is no truly spontaneous secretion from either of the salivary glands and thus, no true 'resting saliva'. The authors hold that saliva collected under the usual 'resting conditions' is entirely a product of glands stimulated by impulses arising in interoceptors. Fluctuations in the frequency and duration of these impulses would explain, in their opinion, the gross variation in flow rate of 'resting saliva'. It has nevertheless become an accepted custom to distinguish between 'resting saliva' sampled without any intentional stimulation ('unstimulated saliva'), and 'stimulated saliva' collected under the influence of an external stimulus of known intensity and duration.

Any collection of saliva has to be performed under strictly standardized conditions, with as many of the external and internal factors as possible under control. This is especially important since the concentration of most salivary components changes with flow rate [225, 312, 317] which in turn is influenced by a large number of different factors. These include circadian rhythms leading to diurnal variations [83, 115, 116, 133, 199, 248, 366], diet [97, 403], body weight [97] and size of the individual salivary gland [112], climate [311], physical activity [133, 307], gustatory, visual [160, 314, 315] and tactile stimuli [160], duration of stimulation [82, 299, 342], hormonal status [49, 217, 285], hyperhydration [313], and drugs [47, 55, 119, 178, 232, 255]. Age [6, 7, 75, 78, 366] and sex [203, 366, 367] of the donors have also been claimed to be responsible for variations in salivary volume and concentration of its constituents although, as far as sex differences are concerned, this has not remained undisputed [7, 8, 75, 233].

Separate Salivary Secretions

With all these experimental pitfalls in mind and the precautions they necessitate, the various methods employed in the separate collection of salivary gland secretions can now be dealt with. Although requiring experience and considerable skill of the operator, cannulation by the introduction of probes (plastic catheters) into the excretory ducts is the simplest procedure in technical terms. In this manner it is possible to obtain parotid saliva from inside Stensen's duct [8, 38, 39, 75, 76, 191], and submandibular saliva from inside Wharton's duct [7, 77] rather free from contaminating epithelia. The disadvantage of this technique is that, due to anatomical reasons, it is applicable only to those glands. The use of small glass capillaries (1–10 μl volume) permitted the collection of labial minor gland saliva [193, 341].

The technically more sophisticated methods involve the application of specifically constructed collection devices which also permit to obtain sublingual saliva not contaminated with submandibular saliva [304, 343]. As early as in 1910, *Carlson and Crittenden* [68] introduced the first appliance for the exclusive collection of *parotid saliva*. Although generally, but erroneously, credited with priority, *Lashley* [202] followed suit only in 1916. His device was a modification of *Carlson and Crittenden's* [68] original design as is the so-called *Curby* [81] cup. Figure 1 (of a collection device built in our clinic) reflects the common ancestry of the many versions of 'parotid cups' developed by numerous investigators and being used in many laboratories. Their common feature is the principle of a double well, the inner well being placed over the orifice of the parotid duct, and the outer well forming an airtight circular seal on the surrounding mucosa, thereby maintaining negative pressure and thus keeping the whole device in place.

An appliance for the collection of genuine *submandibular saliva* was described as a 'universal design' by *Truelove* et al. [362] and subsequently modified by *Stephen and Speirs* [341]. Its main features are a V-shaped undersurface, a wedge-shaped body, a central collection chamber and two outer suction chambers with the appropriate outlets.

As it is rather difficult to separately obtain submandibular and *sublingual secretions*, a device especially designed for this purpose would be of particular value. The specific requirements are met by the 'segregator' introduced by *Schneyer* [304] and later modified by *Block and Brotman* [52]. The construction of the 'Schneyer segregator' takes into account the specific anatomical situation to be reckoned with at the floor of the mouth. It permits the simultaneous but separate collection of secretions from the right and left sublingual glands, besides the combined secretions of both submandibular glands. This basic type of segregator has recently been modified to increase its stability [341, 343]. No suction is necessary to hold the appliances of this type in place as they are individually fitted for each subject.

All these collection devices offer an important advantage as they can be sterilized, e.g., by ethylene oxide at 30°C, [382] and thus permit to reduce the bacterial contamination of the samples, lowering the risk of microbially-

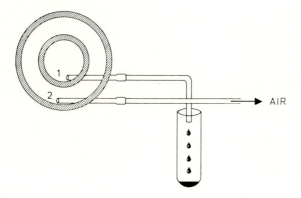

Fig. 1. Basic design of a device for collection of parotid saliva ('parotid cup'). Under-surface view. 1 = Inner (collection) chamber; 2 = outer (suction) chamber.

induced biochemical changes. But it must always be borne in mind that the, albeit slight, pressure inflicted by any such appliance might exert a certain degree of unintentional stimulation, although this will probably not exceed the stimulatory effect of cannulation.

If saliva is to be collected separately from individual glands by stimulation, the most frequently used stimuli are sapid ones, e.g., citric acid [7, 58, 75, 188, 221, 231, 306, 342], sour lemon candy [4, 11, 16, 283, 285, 331], or ascorbic acid [105, 106]. Cholinergic drugs such as pilocarpine have also been used to induce salivary flow [62, 216].

Whole Saliva

In many sialochemical studies the investigations were confined to *whole (mixed) saliva*. This appears justified in cases where the main interest is focused on whether or not the occurrence of a certain compound can be demonstrated in saliva, e.g., after drug application. As will be discussed in a later section of this chapter, rapid progress is being made in this field, and for a routine procedure to be developed, the sampling of saliva should be as simple as possible. Furthermore, knowledge of the course taken by the compound during excretion is not necessary for this specific purpose. On the other hand, the investigation of mixed saliva in biochemical studies on the nature of intrinsic salivary components unnecessarily misses the chance of a more exact elucidation of metabolic processes, sites of synthesis, and their implications.

For the collection of whole saliva rather coarse methods are resorted to since simultaneous tapping of all salivary glands by means of the above-mentioned appliances would involve technical difficulties and burden the patient with undue stress. Thus it is very frequently reported that whole saliva was obtained by expectoration [144, 332, 337] or 'spitting' into receptacles [231, 372, 378, 387]. More sophisticated techniques employ aspiration of saliva from the floor of the mouth by means of syringes [354], capillaries [141], or hemolysis tubes [118].

Since the use of liquid sapid stimulants is precluded in order to avoid contamination of the mixed saliva sample, masticatory stimulation of salivary flow is performed by chewing on a variety of inert substances such as paraffin wax [63, 132, 392], parafilm [293], washed elastic bands [310, 336, 340], washed, sterile pebbles [152], or even a piece of sterile rubber tubing [390] or Teflon [139]. It should be mentioned here that the use of lipophilic substances (paraffin, parafilm) involves an experimental hazard if lipophilic drugs are to be studied in the stimulated saliva [152, 354]. Whole saliva obtained under the above-mentioned conditions requires subsequent centrifugation to minimize its contamination with epithelia and oral microorganisms.

Composition of Saliva

Unlike the well-studied serum, the composition of saliva has only in the last few decades become a matter of detailed investigation. Thus it has become increasingly clear that not only blood but saliva, too, is indeed 'a juice of quality most rare', and a host of different compounds have been detected and partly, characterized. It stands to reason that this process is still far from completion.

The state of knowledge prior to this period of rapid progress in the identification of single salivary compounds can be best described, as did *Ellison* [415], by quoting from a contemporary dictionary: 'Saliva: A viscous, colorless, somewhat opalescent secretion that is usually alkaline in reaction, contains water, mucin, protein, salts, and often a starch-splitting enzyme...' While listing in elaborate detail a wide variety of substances found in blood, serum and erythrocytes, compiled in many tables, only one such list can be found for human saliva in a laboratory handbook of biochemical data, published as late as 1964 [187]. The constituents of saliva are only very summarily listed by subdivision into a few standard analytical classes, and some general physicochemical properties are given (table II).

Table II. Properties and constituents of human saliva [from 187]

Property/constituent	Average	Range	Dimension
pH	6.7	5.6–7.6	
Specific gravity		1.01–1.02	
Depression of freezing point		0.34–0.7	°C
Resting secretion	0.6	0.1–0.8	ml/min
Dry substance	0.6	0.1–1.0	g/100 ml
Ash	0.2		g/100 ml
Mucin	270	100–600	
Total N	90	40–125	
Nonprotein N	35	10–60	
Glucose	20	12–28	
Citrate	1.0	0.2–3.0	
Cholesterol	8	3–15	
Sodium	40	15–55	mg/100 ml
Potassium	55	45–60	
Calcium	6	4–10	
Inorganic phosphate	15	7–20	
Total phosphate	19		
Chloride	60	40–70	

It is evident that such a set of data is not very illuminating; although the information was probably derived from whole saliva, it is not stated under what conditions the saliva was collected and whether it was obtained from a single donor or a collective group. Considering the wide variations in saliva volume and in the amounts of individual salivary components encountered in different individuals, any quantitative data given for such components should be accompanied by detailed information as to sampling conditions, flow rate, age, sex, and health status as well as nutritional state of the test persons. If the influence of certain factors on salivary properties is to be investigated, it is essential that a not too small number ($\geqslant 15$) of persons be studied in order to obtain reliable information suited for statistical treatment.

Unfortunately, many investigations fall short of these demands. 'Normal values' were reported either for too small [83, 168, 186] or strongly selected groups of people, e.g., 'young men' [317] or 'students' [38, 39], flow rates were disregarded [186, 223], and data of a normal (de Moivre) distribution such as means ± standard deviation were computed without analyzing whether or not the measured individual values were normally distributed [38, 39, 191, 317]. All this contributes to a considerable variation of data reported for concentrations of salivary constituents.

Organic Components

Total Protein

Most of the organic components of saliva are of proteinic nature (e.g., enzymes, other proteins without enzymatic properties, immunoglobulins, many glycoproteins with varying amounts of carbohydrate). Since the overall concentration of protein is a standard parameter in the initial stage of characterization of any biological material, and since it is also essential for the calculation of specific enzyme activities, we will first give a few examples of protein concentrations reported for human saliva (table III).

In many reports on salivary protein concentration (and that of other constituents) it is the rule rather than the exception to give the mean ± standard deviation. However, this is not correct if nothing is known about the type of distribution of the data from which those parameters were computed. Without statistical analysis of distribution it is only permissible to give the median value including the range [300]. Of the protein concentrations listed in table III, attention to this restriction was given only in three studies [7, 8, 75]. Since many biological data are known to be lognormally distributed, these authors also analyzed the mode of distribution of their data and were able to demonstrate a lognormal distribution of flow rates, protein and amylase concentrations in stimulated [75] and unstimulated [8] human parotid saliva.

A lognormal distribution requires the logarithmic transformation of all values (x) according to $z = \log 10x$ and subsequent computation of the logarithmic mean $(\bar{z}) \pm SD$ before mean values and SD as the parameters of a normal distribution can be given. We performed this operation on all 90 protein concentrations because application of the distribution-free Kruskal-Wallis (H) test had revealed, on the 5% level of significance, no statistical difference between the three age groups tested (<30, 31–60, >60 years; for each group $n = 30$). All protein concentrations could therefore be regarded as one sample of size 90. The antilog of $\bar{z} \pm SD$ computed as described above yielded the true value for $\bar{x} \pm SD$ in the original dimension of milligram protein per milliliter saliva [8, 75]. Table IV compares the values for 'average'

Table III. Protein content of unstimulated and stimulated human parotid, submandibular and whole saliva (mean values)

Saliva	n	Subjects	Age years	mg/ml	Assay	Reference
Unstimulated						
Parotid	75	men		2.28	amido black	366
	73	women		3.14	amido black	366
	30	students		2.56	Lowry	38
				2.53	biuret	317
	7			2.72±0.29	Lowry	83
	90	45 men, 45 women	12–79	3.00 (0.68 – 12.1)	Lowry	8[a]
Whole	21		18–41	1.55±0.12	Lowry	144
				3.44 (1.88 – 4.06)	Kjeldahl (total N)	187
Stimulated						
Parotid	30	students		2.36	Lowry	39
	21			2.29	biuret	116
	90	45 men, 45 women	12–79	1.94 (0.24 – 8.88)	Lowry	75[a]
	26	men		1.91±0.58	Lowry	16
	52	women		1.79±0.93	Lowry	16
	33	men, women	adults	1.67±0.06	Lowry	392
Submandibular	30	17 boys, 13 girls	4–16	1.14 (0.53 – 3.09)	Lowry	7[a]
	30	11 men, 19 women	60–79	0.73 (0.33 – 1.83)	Lowry	7[a]
Whole	21		18–41	1.34±0.12	Lowry	144

[a] Median (including range).

protein concentrations of our 90 samples, arrived at by different procedures, and reveals the effect of incorrect statistical treatment.

The protein content of parotid saliva has been determined in many investigations, and a considerable body of data, both in health and disease, can be found in the literature. Owing to the greater difficulties involved in sampling submandibular as opposed to parotid saliva, information on the composition of the former is rather scant [366]. We [7] compared the protein content of parotid with that of submandibular saliva (table III) and found

Table IV. Protein concentrations (mg/ml) of parotid saliva from 90 persons without diseases of the salivary glands (45 men, 45 women; age 12–79 years), depending on the choice of statistic

Parotid saliva	Median (range)	Mean ± SD		Reference
		from $\bar{z}$ after log transformation (lognormal distribution demonstrated)	without log transformation (normal distribution incorrectly assumed)	
Unstimulated	3.00 (0.68–12.1)	3.18 $\bar{x} - SD = 1.77$ $\bar{x} + SD = 5.80$	3.77 ± 2.34	8
Stimulated	1.94 (0.24–8.88)	1.94 $\bar{x} - SD = 1.04$ $\bar{x} + SD = 3.51$	2.48 ± 1.87	75

the concentration of protein in stimulated parotid saliva to be significantly higher than in stimulated submandibular secretions (fig. 2).

Aside from the statistical considerations discussed above, another source of variation among the reported values of salivary protein is the choice of determination assay. The classic Kjeldahl procedure, although admittedly still the most precise technique, is rather tedious and time-consuming. It is therefore only rarely performed. According to tradition, the formula (N content × 6.25 = protein content) is in general use due to the tacit assumption that naturally occurring proteins contain 16% N by weight, but investigations of various protein fractions from serum or plasma have revealed that the conversion factors actually extend over a range from 5.9 to 12.5 [9, 346]. Protein species possessing lipid or carbohydrate moieties contain less N per weight and therefore require higher multiplication factors to arrive at a correct value for the protein content [66]. This is especially important to remember when dealing with saliva which is known to contain, to a considerable extent, protein-carbohydrate conjugates.

The two most frequently used analytic procedures today are the biuret [323, 398] and the Lowry [210, 323, 392] assays. Their common feature is the formation of a blue complex between bivalent copper ions and the peptide bonds occurring in all proteins. This type of linkage is also present in the biuret compound, $H_2N-(CO-NH)-CO-NH_2$, which has given this reaction its name. The Lowry type of protein assay involves still another principle,

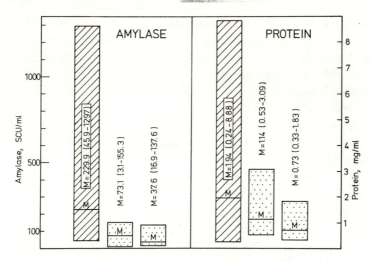

Fig. 2. Amylase and protein concentrations in stimulated submandibular and parotid secretions. According to our own investigations [75] the concentrations of amylase and protein are distinctly higher in parotid than in submandibular saliva. Submandibular saliva of old persons contains less amylase and protein than that of young persons. Left columns (dashed)=parotid saliva; middle columns=submandibular saliva (persons 4 to 16 years old); right columns=submandibular saliva (persons 60–79 years old); M=median; SCU=Street-Close units [from 7].

the reduction of phosphotungstic and phosphomolybdic acid (constituents of Folin-Ciocalteu's phenol reagent) to molybdenum blue and tungsten blue by both the preformed copper-protein (biuret) complex and by the two aromatic amino acids, tyrosine and tryptophan, present in protein. All these reactions operate in alkaline solution and, with the exception of Folin reagent reduction by the two aromatic amino acids just mentioned, are dependent on the presence of bivalent copper ions. The chelating properties of the K, Na-tartrate usually included in the reaction mixture support metal complex stabilization. A more detailed description and discussion of the problems involved in both procedures and their relative merits can be found elsewhere [66, 392].

Despite their considerable similarities, both assays may yield different values for protein concentration, depending on the species and source of protein. Since the Lowry procedure includes one additional feature which the biuret reaction lacks, one should expect the latter to give lower values, but the opposite seems to be true. *Mandel and Ellison* [220], for instance, state that the biuret reaction yields for parotid salivary protein a figure about

1.4 times the Lowry (Folin-Ciocalteu) value [222]. The existence and adherence to a goodly number of 'home-made' versions of these assays, separately developed in many laboratories to fit the specific requirements of particular problems, adds to the variability of results.

Another important factor is the choice of standard protein. Its composition with regard to relative amounts of the various amino acids and also nonprotein moieties should ideally correspond very closely to that of the protein actually investigated. Since in most cases these will present themselves as a mixture of a multitude of species, the above stated requirement will, at best, only be met approximately. An efficient although rather laborious procedure able to fulfil the demand of a standard protein similar to that whose concentration is to be determined consists in the taking and processing [e.g. lyophilization: 105, 468] of a representative sample and standardization of its protein content by Kjeldahl analysis [66].

The more or less universally accepted standard protein, however, appears to be bovine serum albumin (BSA) although the use of this substance will often be at best a compromise. For the determination of salivary protein, we now routinely use casein instead of BSA in our laboratory [7, 8, 75–77] as the amino acid composition of the former compound might approach that of the majority of salivary proteins more closely than BSA, the albumin content of saliva only amounting to 1–10% of total proteins present [144]. A comparison of both standard proteins reveals that with casein as the reference higher values are found than with BSA.

For the determination of salivary protein content, the Lowry assay seems to be the method of choice due to its high sensitivity which exceeds that of the biuret technique about 100-fold. This increased sensitivity is very advantageous in many instances when only small volumes of salivary specimens are available, sometimes with very low protein concentrations. This problem will frequently arise in clinical studies [77, 91].

One intrinsic source of error of the Lowry procedure ought not to be overlooked, i.e. its being prone to be influenced by nonprotein compounds containing organically bound nitrogen. These may be substances originally accompanying the proteins in the sample [468], or they may have been introduced during preparation (e.g., Tris buffer used for elution, addition of urea for the dissociation of protein complexes). Setting up blanks including comparable amounts of these interfering substances will often fail to be effective as the color development may become too strong and consequently small differences will be lost in the background. If possible, the addition of such organic N-containing compounds should therefore be avoided by diluting with water, saline or phosphate buffer, or the samples have to be dialyzed prior to protein determination, although this manipulation is not without risk [195]. A modified Lowry assay applicable to solutions containing detergents has been described [65]. When interfering nonprotein substances are occurring in a sample together with proteins, precipitation of the latter, mostly performed with trichloroacetic acid, but also with perchloric or sulfosalicylic acid [for references see 323] may serve as a remedy. If necessary, precipitation may be followed by one or more washings of the pellet with the precipitant. This technique of course requires the interfering substances to be soluble in the precipitating agent or else co-precipitation will occur [272], and, on the other hand, that precipitation of protein be complete.

Zipkin et al. [392] determined salivary protein by ultraviolet spectro-photometry. Appropriate sensitivity of their technique was attained by precipitation of the protein from saliva and subsequent dissolution in a sufficiently small amount of solvent.

All these sources of variability should be remembered when comparing reports on salivary protein concentrations laid down in the literature. In any case, the pertinent details always ought to be given, concerning choice of assay and reference (standard) protein, processing of sample and, if 'average values' for collectives were computed, mode of statistical treatment. We will not discuss here the many other methods for protein determination (e.g., gravimetry, dye binding, etc.) since these are of lesser importance, having only rarely been employed in the study of saliva.

Albumin

The main protein fraction of human plasma, albumin, is also found in saliva but in much smaller amounts [56, 82, 221, 229, 240]. Plasma albumin with a molecular weight of approximately 66 kdaltons and about 600 amino acid residues seems to be a uniform molecule although its solutions show a certain molecular heterogeneity, the physiological impact of which is still insufficiently known [441]. It is generally accepted today that albumin passively diffuses into glandular secretions from plasma [111] and that a significant extraglandular transfer may occur [266]. The biological role of salivary albumin has been a matter of speculation but it seems not impossible that it may be involved in some transport functions since plasma albumin acts as a carrier protein for a large number of endogenous and exogenous low molecular weight compounds.

There are some reports questioning the complete identity of plasma and salivary albumin. Thus McKean and Beeley [234] were unable to demonstrate

Table V. Albumin concentrations of unstimulated and stimulated whole human saliva from 21 volunteers of both sexes (18–41 years) [means taken from 144]

Assay technique	Whole saliva albumin, mg/l	
	unstimulated	stimulated
PAGE + amido black	294.5	210.0
Bromocresol green	264.7	219.1
Rocket immunoelectrophoresis	61.0	33.7

PAGE = Polyacrylamide gel electrophoresis.

antigenicity of salivary albumin in rabbits, and *Simons* et al. [322] failed to detect precipitin arcs corresponding to salivary albumin on immunoelectro-phoretograms, but these negative results could be explained [56] by the selection of an inadequate immunization technique to induce antibody synthesis. It has also been suggested that the salivary albumin molecule is not exactly identical to that of plasma, possibly owing to minor modifications occurring during passage through the salivary glands [114].

A recent study by *Hattingh* [144], undertaken to compare the results obtained for salivary albumin concentrations by the use of three different estimation procedures, tends to support the assumption of molecular differ-ences between the albumins from both sources. While plasma albumin gave nearly identical values (43.8–46.1 mg/ml) regardless of the type of assay, whole salivary albumin concentrations varied widely (table V), rocket immunoelectrophoresis yielding only about one fourth to one fifth of the amounts measured by the two staining techniques employed (densitometry of amido black stained electrophoretically separated albumin, and bromo-cresol green dye binding by albumin). The higher concentration found in unstimulated saliva as compared with stimulated secretion agrees well with the observation that increased salivary flow rates are associated with a decrease in albumin concentration [82, 221].

The conspicuous dependence of salivary albumin values on the choice of determination method had been obvious for some time even though, in most cases, various types of immunological techniques had been used. The very much higher values reported for paper electrophoresis can be easily explained by its comparatively low separating efficiency compared with modern electrophoretic systems. An extensive table listing details of the just mentioned differences can be found in the comprehensive paper of *Hattingh* [144].

It may be that salivary albumin is overestimated by dye-binding methods and underestimated by immunoelectrophoretic techniques [144]. On the other hand, only the second part of this statement may be true. The discrepancy between the results obtained with those two types of estimation can be interpreted as indication for an intrinsic disparity between human plasma and salivary albumins. Assuming a genuine molecular difference between the two proteins, salivary albumin could possibly bind certain dyes more strongly than plasma albumin, in stoichiometric proportion, but salivary albumin may not be able to react exhaustively to anti-serum albumin due to slight differences in certain antigenic determinants. The logical approach to a solution of this problem would seem to be the suggestion [144] to isolate and purify plasma and salivary albumins and then to study their chemical compositions and reactions to different dyes and antibodies.

Globulins

In contrast to albumin, this second major class of spherical proteins comprises a great variety of different species, for many of which molecular conformation and biological significance are well-studied. Besides their different solubility they are distinguished from albumin very characteristically by the covalent binding of various amounts of nonprotein moieties, mainly carbohydrates (glycoproteins). Since proteins of the globulin type play an important role also in human saliva, and since rapid progress is being made in this field of research, they will be dealt with later under their appropriate headings.

Enzymes

This huge class of biocatalysts is represented by many species in human saliva. The biological significance of their actions on the various substrates is, in many instances, not yet fully understood in terms of benefit for certain intraoral mechanisms, but there are on the other hand among the salivary enzymes quite a few for which such understanding has been gained owing to profound research that is still in full swing. α-Amylase, peroxidase, muramidase (lysozyme) and acid phosphatase may stand for those enzymes whose biological roles are reasonably well studied.

Some of the salivary enzymes that are known to occur in oral secretions but to which present knowledge does not attribute specific biological significance are possibly just passively permeating into saliva from plasma. Molecules with low molecular weights (up to the albumin range) would be likely candidates for this process. Although such behavior would not seem

to 'make sense' in biological terms, it is not inconceivable that nature, albeit
doing nothing without cause, may occasionally do something without
'purpose'. As an excretory route for no longer 'useful' components, saliva –
other than urine – would appear rather inefficient since most of it is swallow-
ed again [114], but it would in any case be futile to enter into teleological
interpretations. Further studies are likely to permit deeper insight into the
effects of many of those salivary enzymes that are as yet less well understood.

α-Amylase (EC 3.2.1.1)

Although not the first to be obtained in purified and crystallized form,
α-amylase (α-1,4-glucan 4-glucanohydrolase) which cleaves starch and
related substances, was the first enzyme to be recognized as a separate entity
of living matter. After *Kirchhoff*, in 1814, had described the involvement in
malt formation of an active principle which we may now refer to as malt
amylase [see 286], *Payen and Persoz* [449] discovered in 1833 that a substance
present in an alcohol precipitate of malt extract converted starch into sugar.
They called this thermolabile substance 'diastase' (from the Greek word for
separation) because of its ability to separate soluble dextrin from the otherwise insoluble envelopes of the starch grains. The first description of salivary
amylase action was given in 1826 by *Tiedemann and Gmelin* [462] who found
that crushed oats, mixed with sheep's saliva and left alone for a while, would
no longer be stained blue by added iodine. The presence in human saliva of
a similar principle ('ptyalin') was demonstrated in 1831 by *Leuchs* [439, 440]
in his studies on the formation of sugar from starch mediated by the action
of saliva. The use of the historic terms, diastase (for the amylolytic enzyme
present in plants and in blood) and the onomatopoeic ptyalin (for the
salivary enzyme), persisted far into the 20th century although in 1925, *Kuhn*
[438] had eventually proposed to call the enzyme, once and for all, α-amylase.

α-Amylase is the quantitatively most prominent enzyme in saliva. If the
textbooks are to be believed, the cephalic salivary glands secrete on the
average a total volume of up to 1.5 liters of saliva per day, with an amylase
content of 0.6 g [45] which equals about 10% of total salivary protein. 70%
of this amount is produced and secreted by the parotid gland where it
constitutes the main portion (30%) of the total protein [220], while submandibular saliva (fig. 2) is far less rich in this enzyme. The total daily
secretion of amylase in man is approximately 1.6 g [286] to which the
cephalic salivary glands contribute about 40%, the remainder being excreted
mainly by the pancreas.

Textbook data like these, however, can only convey a rough idea of the quantitative importance of α-amylase but fail to provide detailed information on its concentration in the various glandular secretions, indispensable for comparative clinical studies. Although amylase continues to be the pet enzyme of many researchers, surprisingly few quantitative data are available (in relation to the vast number of reports dealing with properties of amylase) on its content in parotid, and even less in submandibular saliva. Usefulness of quantitative data given in the literature (table VI) is somewhat restricted by the fact that the figures were derived from donor groups differing widely with respect to composition, manner of stimulation, and sampling times. What is more, with the exception of three reports [8, 75, 324], no analysis of the mode of distribution of amylase concentrations in saliva was performed. Since salivary amylase activity is log-normally distributed [8, 75, 76, 324, 326], only median and range may be given as acceptable statistical parameters without previous logarithmic transformation (cf. section on total protein).

The situation is further complicated by the circumstance that there is no universally adopted assay procedure for amylase. Table VI bears this out: 7 different assays were used by the 9 authors cited, and not in all instances were concentrations expressed in terms of activity units, otherwise the rule with enzymes. Amylase may well be the one enzyme for which the largest number of different estimation procedures were devised. This great diversity has historical reasons; α-amylase is a 'classical enzyme' both for its early identification and constant interest it has evoked. Accordingly, many differently termed arbitrary activity units have been introduced through the decades [209], and some of those are still frequently used despite all efforts made towards standardization. Commercially available test kits (e.g., Merckotest® α-Amylase) provide factors for conversion into the internationally established unit of enzyme activity, defined as $U = 1$ μmol of substrate transformed per minute under standardized conditions. But such factors can only serve as an approximation of the results obtained with assays directly measuring units. The choice of assay will always have to take into account the special demands made by certain fields of application, for instance on sensitivity, required time, number of steps involved and number of samples to be analyzed in one run. It is impossible to enumerate and discuss here all the different tests that were or still are in use for the determination of amylase activity, but we will try to give a classification of the different principles involved. Mainly four techniques can be distinguished that are employed in the measurement of enzymatic cleavage products.

Table VI. Amylase content of unstimulated and stimulated human parotid saliva (mean values)

Donors (n)	Stimulated (+)	Amylase concentration	Assay	Remarks	Reference
17	−	178.2 ± 84.5 U/ml	291	pancreas healthy subjects (18–76 years)	140
109	+	14.7–21.6–31.9[a] AU/min	iodine-starch method; 1 AU = E of 11.0 (after 'Deutsches Arzneibuch', 1970)	healthy subjects	324
29	− +	164.6 ± 13.9 163.7 ± 13.9	mg starch cleaved by 0.1 ml saliva in 5 min	students (19–23 years)	39
7	?	3,000 ± 166 Somogyi units/ml	333	women (20–26 years)	34
60	− +	m: 4,571.64 ± 1,835.21 f: 4,435.03 ± 2,368.20 m: 2,591.70 ± 1,432.77 f: 2,264.67 ± 1,130.18 (dimension SCU/ml)	345[c]	healthy subjects (20–40 years)	239
98	+	1,650 ± 661 U/kg body weight	67	pancreas healthy subjects (16 normal persons)	169
90	− +	402.9 SCU/ml[b] 240.9 SCU/ml[b]	345	each 45 men and women (no diseases of salivary glands)	8 75
16 11	− +	1.03 ± 0.11 mg 0.95 ± 0.15 mg (amylase/ml)	253	healthy men (20–30 years)	306

m = males, f = females.
[a] Range of $\bar{x}$ ± SD after log transformation.
[b] $\bar{x}$ after log transformation.
[c] Modified technique.

(1) *Iodometry* (amyloclastic procedures):

Photometric determination of the blue iodine-starch (amylose) inclusion complex whose formation depends on the availability of glucose [1, ↑ 4] chains of a certain minimum length [345]. Chain length is positively correlated to deepness of color within certain limits. Although subject to interference by various factors [135], amyloclastic methods represent today about 50% of routine amylase determinations in the United States and 60% in Germany [209] because they are simple, cheap, quick, and last but not least, very sensitive.

(2) *Reductometry* (saccharogenic procedures):

Estimation of the reducing ends liberated by the breakdown of starch or related substrates. The reducing terminals of dextrins and oligosaccharides (sugars) are mostly coupled with 3,5-sulfosalicylic acid yielding colored (yellow) products [46, 333, 334] but reduction of triphenyltetrazolium to red formazan has also been utilized [for references see 85]. Tests of this type are generally regarded as very accurate and sensitive [209] but, for instance in the United States, they account for less than 3% of all amylase assays as they are time-consuming and subject to interference by blood sugar [209].

(3) *Chromogenicity* (chromogenic or chromolytic procedures):

(a) One group of this class of assay utilizes various dyes [for a representative list see 85] covalently linked to starch or related insoluble polymers and measures the amount of solubilized, low molecular dye substrate. The Phadebas® method [123, 384, 407] where results are expressed as international (IUB) units, enjoys growing popularity and may be winning the day. Although only fairly recently developed, this group of techniques already comprises 30% of all routinely performed amylase determinations in Germany, and 40% in the United States [209].

(b) Another type of tests belonging in this class was introduced even more recently. It does not utilize the organic dyes mentioned above but involves the splitting off of 4-nitrophenolate *(p*-nitrophenolate) from enzymatically synthesized oligosaccharides. The appearance of the yellow-colored aromatic aglycon is monitored spectrophotometrically, thus permitting kinetic measurements. As a substrate for salivary α-amylase, *p*-nitrophenyl-α-maltoside [132] is to be preferred to α-(4-nitrophenyl)maltotetroside [373] since the salivary enzyme acts upon the latter substrate about 100 times slower than the pancreatic enzyme [373]. This group of chromolytic assays, too, expresses activity in IUB units.

(4) *Coupled assays* (continuous, kinetic procedures):

Common to the tests of this group is the coupling of cleavage products with NAD-dependent auxiliary enzymes (e.g., α-glucosidase and glucose-6-

phosphate dehydrogenase) and measurement of the resulting increase in extinction due to formation of reduced coenzyme NADH [85, 209]. Various well-defined oligomer substrates currently in use [383] are discussed in the Workshop Conference Report of *Lorentz* [209].

The remaining techniques, for instance measurement of the decrease in viscosity or turbidity of starch solutions, coulometry, radial diffusion, or the utilization of [^{14}C]-labeled starch as substrate are partly too insensitive and altogether of little practical importance [for review see 85].

As far as mode of action and substrate specificity of α-amylase are concerned, the reader is referred to the article of *Chilla* [this volume] and to various comprehensive reviews on this subject [274, 295]. The salivary enzyme has been obtained in purified and crystallized form utilizing a variety of different methods [for references see 238, 295] and is rather well characterized although knowledge of its complete amino acid sequence is still missing. Only one single polypeptide chain was found for human parotid amylase which contained one sulfhydryl group per molecule [181, 344]. Association of monomers as a source of isoenzyme heterogeneity could experimentally not be supported [238]. *Lehrner and Malacinski* [204] presented a model of the secondary structure of hog pancreatic amylase which is supposed to be very similar to the human enzyme. On this basis it was concluded that human amylases have five binding sites which would make maltopentaose the ideal substrate [381].

Human pancreatic and parotid amylases are very similar enzymes. They show antigenic identity [176, 264] and practically do not differ in their amino acid composition [179, 344]. The relative amounts of amino acids, calculated as number of individual amino acid residues per 1,000 residues, were shown to be virtually identical, with aspartic acid including asparagine (152/1,000) and glycine (98/1,000) being the most abundant amino acids. An apparent difference exists in carbohydrate content. While pancreatic amylase contains only very little covalently linked sugar [176], one portion of parotid amylase is glycosylated [179].

Already in 1954, *Muus* [251] had been the first to determine the amino acid composition of human salivary amylase. Her results differ somewhat from those of *Kauffman* et al. [179] probably because she investigated crystallized α-amylase from whole saliva which included also the enzyme secreted by the submandibular and other glands, but aspartic acid and glycine were again the most abundant amino acids (table VII).

Human α-amylase also contains at least 1 gram atom of calcium per mol which is of vital importance for its catalytic activity [121, 157]. The

Table VII. Amino acid composition of α-amylase prepared from human whole and parotid saliva

Amino acid	Number of residues per 1,000 residues		
	whole [251][a]	parotid [179][b]	
		family A	family B
Alanine	52	49	48
Arginine	55	58	59
Aspartic acid (+asparagine)	159	145	155
Cystine-SH	39	18	18
Glutamic acid (+glutamine)	71	69	68
Glycine	99	98	100
Histidine	23	22	23
Isoleucine	49	56	55
Leucine	48	49	49
Lysine	48	45	46
Methionine	18	18	21
Phenylalanine	48	53	53
Proline	34	51	53
Serine	81	67	64
Threonine	41	42	41
Tryptophan	39	36	32
Tyrosine	33	44	41
Valine	64	73	73

[a] Data computed from values (g residue/100 g protein) given by *Muus* [251].
[b] Family A parotid amylase contains carbohydrate while family B does not [179, 181].

enzyme is therefore to be classified as a metalloenzyme. Although the prevailing role of calcium as a stabilizing agent of α-amylases had been known for many decades [for references see 157] it was only in the sixties that the significance of calcium as a component part of amylase was demonstrated [157]. Removal of the metal by electrodialysis or progressive depletion by chelation with EDTA nearly killed the enzymatic activity (residual activity of the Ca-free enzyme = 10%) but by replenishment of calcium complete restoration of catalytic function could be achieved. It is assumed that the formation of a tight metal-chelate structure by calcium produces intramolecular cross-links similar in function to disulfide bridges which confer to α-amylase the structural rigidity required for effective catalytic activity [157], and that the metal protects the enzyme molecule from adverse physicochemical conditions and proteolytic attack by stabilizing its secondary and tertiary structure [121].

The presence of chloride ions and a pH of 6.9 are required for maximum activity. Other monovalent anions also activate α-amylase [250, 254] but with decreasing intensity in this order ($Cl^- = 100$): Br^- (80), I^- (50), NO_3^- and ClO_3^- (40). With the non-halides a shift of the pH optimum towards the alkaline side is observed and higher salt concentrations are needed (100 vs. 10–40 mM for the halides). When no anions are present, there is still found a residual activity of nearly 40% but the pH optimum has shifted to the acid side (pH = 6).

Several reports on the molecular constants of human salivary amylase have been published. *Muus* [251] and *Mutzbauer and Schulz* [249] both found the same sedimentation coefficient of $s_{20,w} = 4.60$ and, on the basis of amino acid composition [251], sedimentation and diffusion coefficients, and partial specific volume, a value of 55.2 kdaltons was calculated for the molecular weight of α-amylase from mixed saliva [249].

However, the enzyme is found both in parotid and submandibular secretions, and since the first multiple molecular enzyme system was identified [158] the existence of isoenzymes was also verified for human amylases. It seemed therefore not improbable that differences would be found in the composition of the isoamylases from both glands. Accordingly, a large number of reports have been devoted to this question. It is impossible to deal here with all of them but we will attempt to give an overview of the essential concepts. The rapid progress made over the last 25 years in the development of ever new separation techniques for complex biological material has led to the discovery of a host of multiple molecular forms making up enzymes and other macromolecules, and is also reflected by the increasing number of isoenzymes which could be demonstrated for human salivary amylase. *Mandel and Ellison* [219], using paper electrophoresis, found one band each in submandibular and parotid saliva, eluates from which exhibited amylase activity (the parotid zone sometimes separated into two bands). The utilization of polyacrylamide gel electrophoresis (PAGE) resulted in a much more efficient separation of proteins [269, 288]. Thus *Muus and Vnenchak* [252] demonstrated four amylase isoenzymes in whole saliva with the disc technique. Crystalline amylase from the same source had previously only given two peaks in free electrophoresis [250]. In the further course, up to eight isoamylases were detected in parotid [51, 53, 110, 179, 194, 196, 374, 386] but not more than six in submandibular saliva [110, 180, 194, 197, 230, 264]. The difference in numbers of individual isoamylases reported by the various authors may be due to the different electrophoresis media used, such as PAG [53, 179, 180, 194, 374, 386] or agar gel [264], and to different separation techniques, including gel filtration [12, 179, 180, 230], electrophoresis [53, 110, 179, 180, 194, 264, 374, 386] and isoelectric focusing [51, 230, 347, 369]. In our laboratory we have never found less than six different isoamylases both in submandibular [7] and parotid secretions [6, 75], employing an alkaline system of vertical slab PAGE [321, 339].

Kauffman et al. [179, 180], Keller et al. [181] and Stiefel and Keller [344] were the first to shed light on the nature of the molecular heterogeneity of human salivary amylase revealed by the existence of isoenzymes. By gel filtration on Bio-Gel P-100, followed by disc PAGE, they separated parotid amylase into two distinct groups which they called 'families' [179]. Family A comprising three isoenzymes (numbered 5, 3, and 1) contained sugar moieties firmly bound to the protein, while family B with two members (numbered 4 and 2) did not. This family, when applied to PAGE in high amounts, revealed the presence of two more, further anodally migrating, faint 'z bands' [179]. The isoenzymes were numbered according to the Standing Committee on Enzymes of the International Union of Biochemistry (IUB) which recommended that numbering start with the most anodal isoenzyme [161, 467]. Since the authors used a gel system where migration was towards the anode, the fastest isoenzyme carried the lowest number. The two families could also be demonstrated in submandibular saliva [180] but family A from both sources differed slightly in its carbohydrate content (table VIII). Whereas the glycoenzymes of parotid amylase had 7 mol of neutral sugar bound per mol of enzyme [181], only 6 mol were found in family A of submandibular amylase [180]. The content of 6 mol/mol amylase of glucosamine appeared to be the same for the family A isoenzymes derived from both sources. The similarity between parotid and submandibular isoamylases was also shown by the proportion of glycosylated vs. nonglycosylated isoenzymes (table VIII) which was the same (1 : 3) in both secretions [180, 230]. A comparison of the various amino acid analyses performed by the various research groups shows that the protein composition of the different isoamylases was essentially the same [179, 230], with the possible exception for four submandibular isoenzymes concerning aspartic acid, serine, glutamic acid, and proline [230]. Moreover, the specific enzyme activities and PAGE patterns of both families were virtually identical for submandibular and parotid amylases, and antigenic identity of the parotid isoamylases was severally reported [176, 177, 264].

There is, however, one striking difference concerning carbohydrate composition of the submandibular amylase isoenzymes. In contrast to the Kauffman/Keller group, Mayo and Carlson [230] found sialic acid (N-acetyl-

Table VIII. Molecular characteristics of parotid and submandibular α-amylase isoenzymes [data from 179–181, 230]

Family (A, B) or subgroup (1, 2)	Number/symbol of isoenzyme	% of total amylase protein	Mol. wt., kdaltons	Neutral sugars, mol/mol enzyme				Glucosamine mol/mol	Sialic acid mol/mol	pI
				mannose	galactose	fucose	total			
Parotid										
Glycosylated										
A	5	10								
	3	12.5								
	1	2.5								
		25	62	2	2	3	7	6	0	–
1	A	17								5.9
	B	12								6.4
		29	57	+	+	+		+	+	
Nonglycosylated										
B	4	60								
	2	15								
	z	+0								
		75	56					0	0	0	–
2	A	10								5.9
	B	61								6.4
		71	57					0	0	0	
Submandibular										
Glycosylated										
A	5, 3, 1	26	62	+	+	+	6	+	0	–
1	A	18		3	2	3	8	3	2	5.9
	B	10		3	2	3	8	3	0	6.4
		28	57							
Nonglycosylated										
B	4, 2	74	56					0	0	0	–
2	A	9								5.9
	B	63								6.4
		72	57					0	0	0	

+ = Present, but not separately determined.

neuraminic acid) covalently linked to one of the glycosylated submandibular enzymes, and only half of the glucosamine content (table VIII) reported by *Kauffman* et al. [180]. This could possibly be explained by the different purification procedures followed, and some component contributing to the glucosamine content of the isoenzyme population may have been removed during the purification. Besides, *Mayo and Carlson* [230] detected altogether only four submandibular isoamylases, separated by Bio-Gel P-60 filtration followed by isoelectric focusing. Two glycosylated and two nonglycosylated isoenzymes were found, with the same isoelectric points (at pH 5.9 and 6.4) in both groups. The relative amounts of isoamylases and the ratio between glyco- and aglycoenzymes coincided (table VIII) with the data of *Kauffman* et al. [180], and also the molecular weights which, owing to the sugar content, are higher for the glycoenzymes, can be taken to be identical within the limits of experimental error (table VIII).

It becomes apparent that the conflicting notation of isoenzymes is irritating especially if the results of different research teams are to be compared with further work. *Karn* et al. [174–176] have therefore suggested a definitive nomenclature for human salivary and pancreatic isoamylases, based on their studies on the mechanisms involved in isoamylase formation. They presented experimental evidence for the combined effects of the processes of glycosylation and subsequent deglycosylation and deamidation, acting alternately as posttranslational modifications on the primary product of a single allele, eventually creating two series of isoamylases, one of which contains carbohydrate while the other does not. The members of the glycosylated class of isoenzymes are slightly retarded in their electrophoretic mobilities on account of their higher molecular weights. Numbering starts with the slowest-migrating (most cathodal) isoenzyme. This arrangement (fig. 3) solves the dilemma encountered by *Kauffman* et al. [179] who had to use letters (z) for newly evolving isoamylases in their B family, and at the same time avoids labeling different 'families' by capital letters which conflicts with the established procedure of assigning capitals to variant alleles, respectively phenotypes [176, 238].

The representatives of the two series (= 'families') as appearing on an alkaline gel with anodal migration are arranged in alternating order, starting with a glycoenzyme. This results in the assignment of odd numbers to the glycosylated (= 'odds family') and of even numbers to the nonglycosylated (= 'evens family') isoamylases. Figure 3 presents a schematic outline of the mechanisms postulated for the stepwise formation of the individual amylase isoenzymes.

In a first step, a fraction of the primary amylase protein as coded for by one specific locus (Amy_1 for salivary amylase as opposed to Amy_2 for pancreatic amylase) is glycosylated by a mechanism or mechanisms (presumably enzymatic) as yet unknown. The suggestion that there might be a polypeptide alteration in one amylase family allowing its glycosylation [181] would imply the existence of at least two genes (alleles) coding for salivary amylase, one for the odds and one for the evens isoenzymes [176]. This assumption has to be rejected as shown by the genetical studies of *Karn* et al. [174–177] and *Merritt and Karn* [238]. The pattern of stable isoamylases constituting the phenotype is only formed after the primary, now partially glycosylated, gene product has passed through several transitory changes involving quasi-stable precursors or transitional isoenzymes [176, 238] moving slower than the final pattern and not normally seen on standard gels. They were identified using an asparagine-buffered special electrophoretic system [297].

In the evolvement of the final, relatively stable isoamylase pattern, the processes of deglycosylation and deamidation are responsible for the creation of more rapidly migrating species, in a variety of ways. One fraction of isoenzyme 1 ($=A 1$ in fig. 3) is preserved in its native state, a second portion is deglycosylated forming isoenzyme 2, and still another fraction is only deamidated producing isoenzyme 3. This in its turn follows the same deglycosylation/deamidation pattern as isoamylase 1, resulting in the formation of isoenzymes 4 and 5, and so forth. Thus all odds isoamylases are created only by deamidation of their own kin, whereas the evens isoamylases are derived both from the neighboring, slightly slower migrating odds species by deglycosylation (2 from 1, 4 from 3, etc.), and by deamidation from the evens enzyme preceding them (4 from 2, 6 from 4, etc.).

The creation of faster migrating isoamylases at the expense of slower ones was already observed by *Kauffman* et al. [179] when a sample of family A originally comprising bands 4 and 2 developed more rapidly migrating 'z bands' after prolonged storage in the cold. This effect, which appeared to involve deamidation, was nonenzymatic and could be enhanced in both families by incubation at elevated temperature (37 °C) in an alkaline (pH 9) medium [181]. Conclusive evidence for the spontaneous deamidation of salivary amylase was obtained by quantitative determination of the ammonia released from the purified enzyme incubated under similar conditions as above [176, 297], and faster moving species were created from slower ones when an isoamylase pattern, previously separated by electrophoresis in one dimension, was rerun in a second dimension in a warm (30 °C) gel. In a

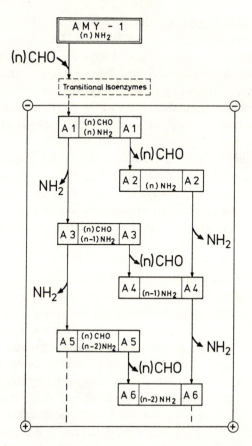

Fig. 3. Schematic outline of parotid isoamylase formation by sequential posttranslational deglycosylation and/or deamidation [modified after 176, 238]. After initial glycosylation of the primary gene product, alternating steps of deglycosylation (–CHO) and deamidation (–NH$_2$) progressively alter molecular weight and charge distribution, thus creating a set of differently migrating amylase isoenzymes.

cold (4°C) second-dimension gel the first-dimension isoenzymes retained their electrophoretic mobilities and new isoamylases did not appear [174, 297]. The high content (22%) in human amylase of aspartic and glutamic acids [179, 251] which very likely comprises a fair share of the respective amides [208] would seem to enable the amylase molecule to undergo a number of consecutive deamidation steps resulting in faster electrophoretic migration due to the increased negative net charge arising from the unmasking of dicarboxylic amino acids.

In contrast to deamidation, deglycosylation as proposed in the model from the laboratory of *Karn* and *Merritt* is not spontaneous. The conversion of odds to evens isoamylases, by an enzyme isolated from the oral bacterial flora, was demonstrated both by the altered electrophoretic behavior and by carbohydrate analysis [175]. The converted isoenzymes remained amylolytically active and it was concluded that the action of the salivary amylase modifier was restricted to the removal of carbohydrate moieties [175, 176].

The succession of modifying steps as stated in the model shown in figure 3 agrees well with the results of the *Kauffman/Keller* group who also found that glycosylated (odds: 5, 3, 1) always alternated with nonglycosylated (evens: 4, 2, z) isoenzymes [179]. Final proof by molecular characterization of all individual isoamylases would require their isolation in quantities not presently available.

Peroxidase (EC 1.11.1.7) and Catalase (EC 1.11.1.6)

Peroxidase (donor $:H_2O_2$ oxidoreductase) oxidizes substrates using hydrogen peroxide as the oxidizing agent, while catalase ($H_2O_2 : H_2O_2$ oxidoreductase) oxidizes hydrogen peroxide yielding oxygen and water. Both enzymes possess Fe^{3+}-protoporphyrin (hematin) prosthetic groups and can therefore also be classified as metalloenzymes. Since animal peroxidase contains a green hematin of unknown structure it has also been termed verdoperoxidase. A wide variety of substrates are oxidized, including phenols, cytochrome c, nitrite, etc., while catalase has a much narrower specificity by acting only on peroxides, particularly hydrogen peroxide, and can therefore be regarded as a peroxidase with a different specificity [90]. Since both enzymes are competing for H_2O_2 and since the general features of their mechanism of action are probably the same [90], they will be discussed here together.

Peroxidases are rather ubiquitously distributed among living matter. They were described for human saliva nearly 100 years ago [1896: *Carnot;* 1898: *Dupouy;* 1909: *Mac Donald and Smith;* references in 261]. Enzymology at that time was still in its infancy, and the reports conflicted regarding the source and the peroxidatic or oxidatic nature of the enzyme [261]. Although the physiological (in vivo) oxygen acceptor (hydrogen donor) is still unknown [280], ample experimental evidence has been presented for the in vitro oxidation of a large number of phenolic and heterocyclic aromates, in a reaction that requires the presence of hydrogen peroxide. The substrates used in the various peroxidase assays include pyrogallol [138, 261, 308], guaiacol

[69, 192, 246], orthodianisidine [162, 163, 182–185, 268], diaminobenzidine [141] and p-phenylenediamine [16, 280]. Oxidation of reduced nicotinamide adenine dinucleotide (NADH + H$^+$) in the presence of excess potassium thiocyanate (KSCN) has also been employed in the quantitative determination of salivary peroxidatic activity [155, 163, 164, 268]. Activity units are mostly expressed either as increase of extinction at 460 or 485 nm/mg of protein, caused by the formation of quinones from the corresponding phenolic precursors, or as decrease of extinction at 340 nm due to the disappearance of NADH. Oxidation of pyrogallol to purpurogallin is measured by the PZ value (Purpurogallin-Zahl = purpurogallin number) defined as the number of milligrams purpurogallin formed per milligram of enzyme (protein) in 5 min at 20°C.

The values reported for peroxidatic activity in saliva vary according to substrate and dimension of unit and are therefore difficult to compare. However, all studies agree on appreciable or even high peroxidase activity in human saliva, detected in whole [163, 164, 185, 192, 246, 261, 280, 414], parotid [92, 192, 261, 329, 414] and submandibular secretions [192, 261]. Only one investigation was performed on sublingual saliva whose peroxidase activity amounted to 50% of that measured in parotid, and to 20% of that of submandibular saliva [192]. Nickerson et al. [261] found activities to be slightly higher in parotid, and slightly lower in submandibular, than in whole saliva. After centrifugation whole saliva displays peroxidase activity not only in the supernatant but also in the sediment where it was reported to be strong [246, 414]. Histochemical examination of whole saliva sediment revealed a large number of peroxidase-positive cells that were subsequently identified as polymorphonuclear leukocytes mainly of the neutrophilic series, but these contributed only a small amount to the total salivary activity [261]. The different findings may be explained by different amounts of leukocytes present in the sediment owing to variations in sampling techniques and test persons. Although mixed saliva contains large numbers of streptococci said to possess bacterial peroxidase, its presence could be safely excluded [261]. While bacterial peroxidase is heat stable [406], the activity of the enzyme in whole saliva and separate glandular secretions was rapidly lost above 80°C with total inhibition at 90°C [261]. It could also be completely blocked by a number of inhibitors such as NaF, NaN$_3$, and KCN [261].

Salivary peroxidase is synthesized in the salivary glands themselves and is actively secreted by them. The histochemical demonstration of peroxidase in the human submandibular and parotid glands [292] indicated that their serous acinar cells are a rich source of tissue-specific animal peroxidase while plasma levels of peroxidase can be considered to be nonexistent [261]. Since salivary peroxidase is an enzyme with chemical and immunological properties very similar to those of purified peroxidase from bovine milk [244], salivary peroxidase was designated as *lactoperoxidase* [185, 245] in order to distinguish it from myeloperoxidase found in myelocytes. A molecular weight of 82 kdaltons [461] was determined for the crystallized enzyme from cow's milk [355].

Like the majority of enzymes, lactoperoxidase of human saliva is made up of several isoenzymes [16, 163, 164, 280]. Purification of parotid saliva by gel filtration on Sephadex G-200 followed by passage through Amberlite CG-50 resulted in a substantial increase of peroxidase activity due to the removal of inhibitory low molecular weight substances and yielded two peaks with peroxidatic activity [329]. One of these contained most of the enzymatic activity while the other had very little which may have caused the authors not explicitly to speak of isoperoxidases. At least two major active isoenzymes of peroxidase were detected in whole saliva of Japanese children [163] and three such multiple molecular forms of lactoperoxidase were demonstrated in parotid saliva of Japanese adults [164] by application of the two secretions to DEAE-cellulose columns and stepwise elution with NaCl of increasing concentration. Their peroxidatic nature was shown by substrate specificity and participation in an antibacterial mechanism. Heterogeneity was confirmed both by isoelectric focusing [164] and electrophoresis in agar gel [163, 164]. The lactoperoxidase isoenzymes were numbered, in anodal direction, from 3 to 1. Isoenzyme number 3 did not migrate at all [164]. Isoelectric focusing of whole saliva from European adults, using a microanalytical column, revealed the presence of three main isoenzyme components and of three minor fractions of peroxidase, with isoelectric points ranging from pH 3.8 to 9.5 [280]. The pI of three of them coincided, within the limits of experimental error, with those reported by *Iwamoto* et al. [164].

The presence of three peroxidase isoenzymes in human parotid saliva agrees well with the results of *Azen* [15, 16] who described three salivary peroxidase (SAPX) variants that are supposed to be formed by the action of certain acidic proteins (Pa proteins) occurring in parotid saliva and subject to genetic variation [15, 125]. Modification of SAPX by Pa takes place through direct protein-protein interaction, probably within the salivary gland [16]. Since it was demonstrated that the predominant acidic protein in parotid saliva is a dimer held together by a disulfide bond (Pa-S-S-Pa) and since treatment of the higher SAPX types 2 and 3 with 2-mercaptoethanol resulted in the formation of SAPX 1, the following mechanism has been postulated for the development of the three SAPX isoenzymes, respectively, variants [15, 16]. In the absence of the acidic protein (Pa 0) the only variant observed is SAPX 1. Pa 1 and Pa 2 monomers-SH complex with SAPX 1 through disulfide bridges to give SAPX 2 and SAPX 3 types. This mechanism would seem to correspond with an observation made by *Revis* [290] during immunoelectrophoretic identification of peroxidase in human parotid saliva. He attributed the less cathodal migration of parotid saliva peroxidase than bovine lactoperoxidase to complexing of the positively charged parotid saliva enzyme with one of the negatively charged proteins found in parotid saliva. This behavior resembled that of another basic protein, salivary muramidase [289].

The perfect correspondence between absence of Pa and SAPX 1, between presence of the common Pa 1 protein and SAPX 2, and between the uncommon variants Pa 2 and SAPX 3, as well as the finding that the frequencies of genes determining the SAPX types are the same as those for the corresponding Pa types [15, 126, 128] are strong arguments for the validity of this hypothesis. Although according to this mechanism the presence of only up to two isoperoxidases in one single sample of parotid saliva could be expected (assuming co-dominance of the alleles determining Pa), the three salivary peroxidases found in the preparation of *Iwamoto* et al. [164] can be explained by the circumstance that the authors worked with a combined sample derived from a group of donors while *Azen* [15, 16] investigated specimens from single persons.

The participation of salivary peroxidase in two of the several antibacterial mechanisms exerted by saliva [92, 182–185, 268] will be discussed later, together with other defensive principles.

In contrast to the well-studied peroxidase, the presence of *catalase* in human saliva has only sparsely been investigated and, despite some positive reports [for references see 261] in which catalase activity was attributed to whole and parotid [414] saliva, it seems now to be unequivocally established that all such activity when encountered in saliva must be assumed to be of bacterial origin [261].

Acid Phosphatase (EC 3.1.3.2)

Acid phosphatase (orthophosphoric monoester phosphohydrolase) hydrolyzes orthophosphoric monoesters yielding an alcohol and H_3PO_4. The enzyme has a very wide substrate specificity. Its pH optimum lies in the acid range. The activity of acid phosphatase is much higher in whole [74, 98, 301] than in parotid and submandibular saliva [for references see 225] due to its release from bacteria, leukocytes and epithelial cells present in whole secretions [38, 74, 301]. The enzyme was studied mostly in parotid saliva although it also occurs in submandibular saliva [72, 229], and marked activity on similar levels was observed in the secretions of both glands [72, 111]. The finding of *Benedek-Spät* [38] who reported low activity for an unstimulated parotid saliva sample comprising 16 specimens is difficult to interpret in relation to other studies where appreciable enzyme activities were demonstrated [72, 301], since different units were used for activity documentation. As could be expected, higher amounts of acid phosphatase were present in unstimulated than in stimulated parotid saliva [312].

Several investigations were carried out in order to determine the nature of the acid phosphatase found in parotid saliva [207, 258], with partly different results, especially regarding pH optimum for catalytic function. When a variety of substrates was used with unpurified stimulated secretions from 'normal males' the optimum lay between pH 4.5 and 4.7 [207], but a preparation of acid phosphatase which had been purified 700-fold from 8 liters of stimulated parotid saliva, by two ammonium sulfate fractionations with intermediate separation on DEAE-cellulose, exhibited an optimum as low as pH 3.3 [258]. Still another value was reported by *Saito and Kizu* [301] who determined it at pH 5.4.

Despite the many similarities existing among the phosphatases of various sources, it is reasonably well established that prostatic and blood enzymes are definitely different. As judged from the pH optima, reactivity to the substrate *p*-nitrophenylphosphate and inhibitory phenomena, it is evident that the parotid enzyme more closely resembles the prostatic variety [207, 258]. A possible bacterial origin could be excluded on the basis of substrate specificity and inhibitor studies [207, 258]. The parotid phosphatase was almost completely blocked by *L*-tartrate.

The heat stability of purified parotid acid phosphatase was very low at pH 7 and 50°C, decaying by more than 90% within 5 min, but the enzyme was reasonably stable at the same temperature in a buffer of reduced pH (3.3) where it only lost 50% of its activity during 1 h [258]. It appeared to be homogeneous as shown by sedimentation studies ($s_{20,w} = 1.6$) and disc gel electrophoresis where it consisted of only one band while ten such zones had been revealed after electrophoretic separation of crude parotid saliva. The pure enzyme was not inhibited by *p*-chloromercuribenzoate and therefore seemed not to possess any active sulfhydryl groups; from the sedimentation velocity it was speculated that the protein had a molecular weight of approximately 20–30 kdaltons [258].

Although multiple molecular forms of acid phosphatase are known to occur in other tissues [428], the enzyme preparation of *Nakamura* et al. [258] was characterized by the absence of isoenzymes. That they actually are present in human saliva was shown a few years later when experiments with whole saliva succeeded in establishing the presence of acid phosphatase isoenzymes [350] by a special zymogram technique involving horizontal slab PAGE in 10% polyacrylamide and subsequent staining for acid phosphatase activity. The observed strong sensitivity to inhibition by *L*-tartrate [434] safely excluded any contamination with bacterial phosphatase. Up to four isoenzymes, representing different phenotypes [350, 352], could be demonstrated in the zymograms from individual samples. Since three alleles each are to be assumed at the two separate loci (Sap-A and Sap-B) postulated [352], and since each one of those alleles at both loci are recessive null alleles not capable of expression, a total number of four different electrophoretic isophosphatase positions could be theoretically expected because the active alleles are co-dominant [350]. However, altogether five different positions were actually observed which was explained by the formation of a hybrid isoenzyme in *AA'* heterozygotes which was present in addition to the isoenzymes coded for by both the *A* and *A'* alleles [350]. The hybrid occupied an intermediate electrophoretic position between the two parent enzymes.

Alkaline Phosphatase (EC 3.1.3.1)

Alkaline phosphatase catalyzes the same type of reaction as acid phosphatase and is very similar to its twin enzyme as far as specificity for orthophosphoric monoesters is concerned but, as the name implies, its pH optimum lies in the alkaline range. A value of pH 9.1 was reported for the enzyme found in human saliva [74, 98]. It appears from the comparatively small body of literature that alkaline phosphatase is absent from submandibular saliva [225]. Many investigators altogether failed to detect alkaline phosphatase also in the secretion of the human parotid gland [38, 72, 74, 207, 350], attributing its presence in whole saliva to bacterial or cellular contamination [437]. *Saito and Kizu* [301] who used sodium β-glycerophosphate [320] as substrate at pH 8.6 found alkaline phosphatase to be present in parotid saliva, but its activity level was much lower than that of acid phosphatase determined in the same specimens. This confirmed another observation that acid phosphatase predominates in saliva [98] while in blood its activity is much lower than that of alkaline phosphatase [320].

Recently the enzyme was identified after gel filtration of parotid saliva on Sephadex G-150 where it was enriched 20-fold in the last of six eluted peaks [149], indicating a molecular weight of not more than 50 kdaltons which is about one half to one fourth of that assumed for alkaline phosphatase from animal tissues [29]. In *Escherichia coli* which also contains alkaline phosphatase of rather low molecular weight [29] the enzyme is dependent on the presence of certain bivalent cations (Mg^{2+}, Zn^{2+}, Co^{2+}) as cofactors. In this connection it is interesting to note that considerable amounts of zinc are present in human parotid saliva [149, 200].

Muramidase/Lysozyme (EC 3.2.1.17)

Muramidase (N-acetylmuramide glycanohydrolase) is still mostly referred to as lysozyme, its original name, since it is an enzyme dissolving (lysing) the cell wall substance of certain gram-positive bacteria of which *Micrococcus lysodeikticus* is the most sensitive. Although its traditional name characterizes the type of its action very fittingly, it seems indicated, for the sake of conformity, to generally adopt the term muramidase denoting its enzymatic nature and its substrate. Muramidase probably hydrolyzes β-1,4 links between N-acetylmuramic acid and 2-acetylamino-2-deoxy-*D*-glucose residues in a mucopolysaccharide or mucopolypeptide. Although detected in human saliva rather early (in 1922) by *Fleming* [122] of penicillin fame, salivary muramidase had to wait for about 40 years before it was isolated and chemically characterized [278]. Its nature was elucidated by chromatography on ion-exchange resin and CM-cellulose [278] and by isoelectric focusing [299]. The first isolation and purification from parotid saliva was reported by *Balekjian* et al. [25] who also analyzed the quantitative amino acid composition. Salivary muramidase is a basic protein (pI > 10) stable at acid and unstable at alkaline pH, consisting of a single polypeptide chain with the low molecular weight of approximately 15 kdaltons [25, 278]. The enzyme therefore is usually lost during dialysis and thus not to be found on electrophoretograms of dialyzed saliva [167, 195, 220].

The occurrence in saliva of a complex between muramidase and an electrophoretically more anodal 'carrier' has been suggested [289] by which the salivary enzyme differed from that of lacrymal origin, although otherwise both muramidases cross-reacted antigenically.

Owing to the difficulties regarding the availability of a well-defined, easy to handle and, if possible, soluble substrate for the measurement of muramidase activity, quantitative data are usually not given in terms of activity but as concentrations (mg/l). In principle, still another way could be followed leading to quantitative determination of enzymatic action by standardized estimation of bacteriolysis by muramidase-containing samples.

This, however, would be difficult to attain due to equipment requirements and problems arising in the standardization of *M. lysodeikticus* strains.

Even so, considerable variations must be noted when comparing the amounts of muramidase measured in salivary gland secretions by several authors. An overall concentration of 150–250 mg/l was reported for mixed parotid and submandibular saliva [278], the content in submandibular exceeding that of parotid secretion. Lower values and, if any, a predominance of parotid (4.5–80 mg/l) over submandibular (5–42 mg/l) muramidase concentration were found by other laboratories [153, 430]. In parotid saliva, enzyme content decreased distinctly upon stimulation, as shown both by determination of the muramidase levels of a group of donors (n = 117) and an individual sample [326]. Unstimulated parotid secretion collected from 'normal persons' had a concentration ranging from 26–80 mg/l that dropped after stimulation to values between 8 and 22 mg/l. A study of the changes in one single person revealed that after an initial muramidase concentration of 70 mg/l in unstimulated parotid saliva had been found, the enzyme level fell to 10 mg/l as a direct response to the onset of sapid stimulation although at the same time the concentration of total protein increased [326].

Besides the antibacterial action of salivary peroxidase already mentioned, the breakdown of bacterial cell walls by muramidase constitutes a second enzymatic principle of defense against oral microorganisms and disease.

Kallikrein (EC 3.4.4.21/EC 3.4.21.8)

Kallikrein is a peptidylpeptide hydrolase existing in several organ-specific forms. It is a member of a large group of enzymes acting on (poly)peptides that includes important digestive enzymes such as trypsin, pepsin, rennin and cathepsin, and whose systematic classification is still being discussed. This may be the reason why two different EC numbers for kallikrein are found in the literature. The kallikreins present in various tissues and body fluids (e.g., salivary glands, saliva, pancreas, kidney, urine) are differing from one another with respect to several characteristics [243] but, as opposed to most enzymes of this class, have a high substrate specificity [361]. Their common physiological role consists in the release from serum proteins of hormone-like substances that excite smooth musculature, reduce blood pressure and thus effect vasodilation. The kallikrein from human saliva acts on a kininogen to release blood pressure regulating kinins [for references see 458]. Stimulation of the chorda tympani nerve is supposed to induce kallikrein action resulting in the dilation of the glandular blood vessels, thus supplying the actively secreting salivary gland with the intensified blood flow required for this process [for references see 111]. Although the presence of kallikreins is established beyond any doubt, their essentiality for eliciting active secretion of salivary glands has not remained uncontested [for references see 111].

Human salivary kallikrein was detected rather early [379] and has since then stimulated continued interest [111, 149, 242, 243]. It was partially purified from human mixed saliva [243] by chromatography on DEAE-cellulose and subsequent fractionated precipitation with acetone. The enriched enzyme was completely resistant to heat treatment for 5 min at 55°C and pH 6. Salivary kallikrein is not related to trypsin (except that both are peptidases) since its activity is not blocked by the soybean trypsin inhibitor, but it is strongly suppressed by the Kunitz inhibitor from bovine glands [326, 416].

Vasoactive kinins were characterized after isolation from bovine plasma incubated in the presence of kallikrein from salivary glands [380], and from human plasma upon incubation with human kallikrein [279]. The kininogen on which the salivary enzyme acts during this process is a glycoprotein from the serum α_2-globulin fraction, kallidinogen, from which the active principle, kallidin, is cleaved off [279, 380]. Two polypeptides were isolated in this way, the nonapeptide bradykinin (kallidin I) and kallidin (kallidin II), a dekapeptide (mol. wt. = 1188.4) of the following amino acid sequence [279, 380]:

$$H_2N-Lys-Arg-Pro-Pro-Gly-Phe-Ser-Pro-Phe-Arg-COOH.$$

Subsequent synthesis of the dekapeptide and demonstration of its physiological activity [281] corroborated the previous findings.

Serum kallikrein cleaves the kallidinogen polypeptide chain between Lys and Arg residues (besides between Arg and Ser), producing bradykinin, while the kallikreins from salivary glands and pancreas preferentially attack the bonds between Met and Lys, and Arg and Ser residues, respectively, to yield kallidin. Although differences exist between the kallikreins from salivary glands, pancreas and urine, it has been suggested to classify them as isoenzymes [361] since their common reaction product is one and the same substance, kallidin.

For the in vitro determination of kallikrein activity, the synthetic compound N-α-benzoyl-L-arginine ethylester (BAEE) is used as a model substrate [106, 326, 361]. The enzyme is therefore also referred to as BAEE esterase but since other proteolytic enzymes, too, are able to hydrolyze this ester [106], the terms 'kininogenase' [361] or 'kallidinogenase' might be suggested as trivial names for kallikrein, signifying its physiological substrate and enzymatic nature.

High kallikrein activities were measured both in human parotid [312] and submandibular saliva [for references see 225] where the 'resting' concentration exceeded that of stimulated secretions. This observation was confirmed for parotid saliva, collected from 117 healthy donors by *Skurk* et al. [326] who also found kallikrein levels to be strongly dependent on flow rate, dropping to one sixth of the original value of 36.6 mU/ml upon stimulation. The total amount of the enzyme, secreted from the stimulated parotid gland per minute, was nevertheless 3-fold higher (7.1 mU/min) than under 'resting' conditions (2.1 mU/min) due to the increased salivary flow. The secretory behavior of kallikrein in the parotid saliva of 40 healthy persons had previously been studied by *Eichner* et al. [106] with essentially the same results as far as the changes of kallikrein activity secreted per minute, before and after stimulation of salivary flow, were concerned. The nature of the stimulus (oral administration of ascorbic acid or subcutaneous injection of pilocarpine) had no influence on the secretory behavior of the enzyme. Continued stimulation, however, led to exhaustion of secretory capacity of the parotid gland within 40 min. The high rate of synthesis of this organ, well documented for amylase, also became apparent for kallikrein formation when basal secretion rates were fully restored 15 min after cessation of stimulation.

Glucose-6-Phosphate Dehydrogenase (EC 1.1.1.49)

Glucose-6-phosphate dehydrogenase (G-6-PDH), one of the essential enzymes of carbohydrate metabolism, was identified in whole saliva by *Tan and Ashton* [351]. This enzyme (systematic name: *D*-glucose-6-phosphate: NADP oxidoreductase) oxidizes glucose-6-phosphate (G-6-P) to *D*-glucono-δ-lactone-6-phosphate, transferring hydrogen to NADP. The primary reaction product is transformed either spontaneously or by a specific lactonase to yield 6-phosphogluconic acid. In the human organism two different forms of G-6-PDH are found, the red blood cell type (G-form) which is sex-linked, has a strict specificity for G-6-P and is the only form present in red blood cells. The H-form which can act also on other hexose-6-phosphates, especially galactose-6-phosphate [48, 265], occurs together with the G-form in liver, kidney, and a number of other tissues [318, 319].

It could be demonstrated by substrate specificity studies that the G-6-PDH of human saliva was actually very similar to the galactose-6-phosphate utilizing H-form of liver [351] although for obvious reasons no biopsies could be taken from the saliva donors. Inhibition studies with the steroid hormones pregnenolone and dehydroisoandrosterone [224] confirmed that the salivary enzyme was of human and not of bacterial origin.

After genetic variants had already been demonstrated for the G-6-PDH from other sources [for references see 351], their existence in the H-6-PDH of human saliva was shown by horizontal flat slab electrophoresis in 10% acrylamide and by subsequent identification of isoenzymes by means of a special zymogram technique [351]. According to electrophoretic mobility, two isoenzymes could be identified pointing to three possible phenotypes depending on whether the donors were homozygous for one of the two alleles or heterozygous, containing both presumed alleles in their genome. It was concluded from family and population studies that salivary H-6-PDH is the product of an autosomal locus with two co-dominant alleles, *Sgd-1* and *Sgd-2* [351].

Arginase (EC 3.5.3.1)

Arginase (*L*-arginine amidinohydrolase) hydrolyzes the amino acid *L*-arginine yielding ornithine, an amino acid not found in proteins, and urea. It is specific not only for arginine but also for a limited number of other substrates with certain well-defined structural characteristics [29]. The enzyme was only recently discovered in human whole saliva by *Gopalakrishna and Nagarajan* [137] although its presence in various mammalian tissues, e.g. rat salivary gland, had previously been established [420, 424]. Total arginase activity in human saliva was unequivocally demonstrated by the absence from the enzyme preparation of arginine deimidase as well as ornithine carbamoyltransferase activities, and by the production of equimolar amounts of ornithine and urea [137]. Bacterial contamination as a source of whole saliva arginase seems unlikely since the saliva was centrifuged immediately after sampling and since its presence in bacteria seems to lack substantiation in the literature.

Salivary arginase was absolutely dependent on Mn^{2+} (optimum concentration 1.4 mM $MnCl_2$), had a pH optimum between 9.7 and 10.0 and a molecular weight of 120 kdaltons (determined by calibrated gel filtration on Sephadex G-100) which is similar to that of other mammalian arginases [29]. The enzyme was further characterized by a remarkable property. It was unstable in the cold but very stable at elevated temperatures [137]. Repeated freezing and thawing resulted in a 90% loss of activity that could not be compensated by either addition of Mn^{2+} or warming up, and storage at 4°C for 1 week led to an appreciable reduction of activity despite the presence of manganese ions. Heat treatment (10 min at 55°C) with added $MnCl_2$, on the other hand, resulted in a 10% increase over the activity of the native enzyme prepared from freshly collected specimens. The enzyme was stable for at least 1 h when incubated at 60°C in the presence of $MnCl_2$ but showed rapid loss of activity (80% after 15 min) when subjected to the same treatment without addition of Mn^{2+}. Thus, the conformation of the arginase molecule necessary for optimum catalytic function was strongly dependent on sufficient activation energy and presence of a kationic cofactor probably stabilizing arginase tertiary structure. Arginase dialyzed against a manganese-deficient medium lost 95% of its activity as compared to a loss of only 20% with Mn^{2+} present. Reactivation of 20% of original activity could be achieved by restoration of Mn^{2+} alone, and even of 80% when this process was supplemented by heat treatment [137].

Salivary arginase activities were in the range between 180 and 500 U/l which is about 400 times the value found in serum. This suggests a physiological role for this extrahepatic enzyme [137]. It may be involved in proline and glutamate, possibly also polyamine, biosynthesis [129, 388]. Since multiple molecular forms of arginase were reported for mammalian tissues including submandibular salivary gland [282], the presence of arginase isoenzymes in human saliva may be expected but is still a matter of speculation. It would not be surprising if this enzyme, too, showed the genetic polymorphism demonstrated and already discussed here for a number of other salivary enzymes.

Other Enzymes

A large number of different enzymes have been reported to occur in the oral cavity of human beings [for comprehensive lists see 70, 74, 220, 225, 353] but many of these are, in all probability, released from the bacterial colonization of mixed saliva. Thus only 2 of altogether 9 exoglycosidases found in human whole saliva were also present in sterile parotid and submandibular-sublingual secretions [237]. We will confine ourselves here to those salivary enzymes whose essentially glandular origin seems to have been established rather clearly [159] and enumerate the remaining enzymic constituents primarily of the parotid and submandibular (sublingual) secretions.

Lactate dehydrogenase (LDH), EC 1.1.1.27 (L-lactate:NAD oxidoreductase), is another metalloenzyme, containing Zn as an active group. It could be detected in parotid saliva by means of electrophoretic and spectrophotometric analysis but was absent from submandibular saliva [378]. The activity of LDH was much higher in whole than in parotid saliva where it was found to be inversely related to salivary flow rate. This would suggest an extra-acinar source for most of the LDH since the intrinsic parotid proteins tend to be independent of or vary directly with the flow [222]. Since there was no submandibular LDH activity it could be safely assumed that the source of the enzyme in whole saliva largely rested in bacteria and cells (leukocytes).

In both parotid and whole saliva, four isoenzymes were found occupying positions comparable to serum LDH isoenzymes 1–4, the most prominent zones in parotid saliva usually being comparable to serum LDH 3 and LDH 2.

Parotid LDH is susceptible to freezing and cannot be detected spectrophotometrically in saliva that had been stored frozen [own observation].

Ribonuclease (RNase), EC 2.7.7.16 (polyribonucleotide-2-oligonucleotidotransferase, cyclizing), was described for parotid as well as submandibular saliva [99]. Two varieties of salivary RNase could be distinguished according to the pH ranges determined for optimal catalytic activity of the enzymes. Acid RNase had the same pH optimum of 6.3–6.6 in both secretions while the alkaline RNase was characterized by the wide range of pH 7.8–8.3 in parotid, and by a narrower range of pH 7.8–8.1 in submandibular saliva. In the secretions of either gland both enzymes showed similar, high levels of activity when compared with each other, but total RNase activity of parotid saliva was about twice that of submandibular saliva.

These findings were largely substantiated upon investigation of centrifuged crude whole saliva [28] where pH optima of 5 and 8 were determined for acid and alkaline RNases, respectively. Enzyme levels were independent of flow rate. After purification of RNase by treatment with sulfosalicylic acid and subsequent KCl gradient elution (in pH 5.2 acetate buffer) of the dialyzed supernatant from an SE-Sephadex C-25 column, only alkaline RNase was found. Acid treatment had either destroyed or converted acid to alkaline RNase [28]. The 200-fold purified enzyme exhibited appreciable activity against double-stranded RNA amounting to about 5% of the rate for single-stranded RNA. It was acid- and moderately thermostable, losing only 60% of its original activity after boiling for 3 min at pH 5. The enzyme was activated by 50 mM NaCl and inhibited by Ca^{2+} (40%) and less by Zn^{2+} (10%), while Mg^{2+}, Cu^{2+} and EDTA had no effect.

Nonspecific Esterases belong to the *EC subgroup 3.1* (hydrolases acting on ester bonds) and comprise esterolytic enzymes without any marked (or known) substrate specificity. They are best identified by hydrolysis of naphthol compounds linked to a suitable group by an ester bond, and subsequent coupling of the released naphthol to a diazonium salt leading to the formation of a strongly colored azo dye [44, 353]. For the location of nonspecific esterases on polyacrylamide disc gel electrophoretograms a staining technique was developed by *Weinstein and Mandel* [377]. Such enzymes were moderately active in human parotid and submandibular saliva [70–72, 74]. The existence in saliva of membrane-bound (particulate) and soluble forms (possibly subunits) of nonspecific esterases has been discussed [149, 214].

Aliesterase is a synonym for an enzyme that catalyzes the hydrolysis of a wide variety of aliphatic esters, especially of short-chain fatty acids [70], but can also act as a transferase [29]. Its proper trivial name is *carboxylesterase*, EC 3.1.1.1 (carboxylic-ester hydrolase). The enzyme was described for human salivary gland [70].

Cholinesterase, EC 3.1.1.8 (acylcholine acyl-hydrolase), was found in parotid and submandibular saliva [70, 114] where its activity was even lower than the only moderate activity determined in parotid secretion (0.6–1.0 U/l after stimulation). The enzyme is occasionally termed 'pseudocholine esterase' to distinguish it from the 'true cholinesterase' *(acetylcholine esterase, EC 3.1.1.7)* acting on the neurotransmitter acetylcholine and mainly present in synaptic areas, but also reported for human saliva [70].

Acid and alkaline pyrophosphatases [70] were investigated in saliva and dental plaque with respect to a possible correlation between the activity of these enzymes and calculus formation [43]. Although the normal acid and alkaline monophosphatases are also able to catalyze the hydrolysis of pyrophosphate [29, 90] it seems likely that *inorganic pyrophosphatase*, EC 3.6.1.1 (pyrophosphate phosphohydrolase), was present in these experiments. The assumption was based on the requirement of Co^{2+} [368] by the acid form of the enzyme (pH optimum 5.5), and of Mg^{2+} by the alkaline (pH optimum 8.5) pyrophosphatase [43]. The pH curve pattern was modified by the different divalent cations added [368]. While a positive correlation between calculus formation and acid pyrophosphatase activity of saliva was observed [43, 93], the origin of the pyrophosphatases could not be clearly established. It was concluded that the weak activity in saliva compared to plaque might suggest a release of the enzymes from bacteria.

Two different species of *adenosine triphosphatase* (ATP phosphohydrolase) are known from several sources such as muscle and other animal tissues [29, 90]. The muscle enzyme (ATPase, myosin; EC 3.6.1.3) requires Ca^{2+} as a cofactor, while the other ATPase (EC 3.6.1.4) is dependent on the presence of Mg^{2+} for activity. Fractionation of human parotid saliva on

Sephadex G-150 revealed for the first time the presence of ATPase in this secretion [149]. Besides Mg^{2+}-dependent ATPase a Na^+- and K^+-dependent enzyme was identified, respectively. All these enzymes are particulate, membrane-bound proteins of very high molecular weight. Thus their occurrence in parotid saliva is somewhat surprising but their distribution in the elution profile agreed well with the postulated properties since about two thirds of the $Na^+(K^+)$- and Mg^{2+}-dependent ATPase activities appeared in the exclusion peak. The remainder was found in the very last peak comprising compounds of molecular weights up to 50 kdaltons, thus indicating either soluble forms of the enzymes or dissociation into subunits [149]. The latter could well have been the fact because the magnesium-dependent ATPase from beef heart mitochondria was shown to break up into subunits of 30 kdaltons [29] at an ambient temperature of 0°C, and gel filtration of parotid saliva had been carried out at low temperature. Although under these conditions the enzyme at once loses activity, the process is reversible [29], thus allowing determination of ATPase activity at the elevated temperatures employed in enzyme estimation procedures.

Another enzyme with a requirement for Mg^{2+} as cofactor, *5'-nucleotidase*, EC 3.1.3.5 (5'-ribonucleotide phosphohydrolase), characterized by a wide specificity for 5'-nucleotides, was also demonstrated for human parotid saliva after gel filtration [149]. The enzyme behaved very similar to ATPase being present in the first as well as the last peak of the elution profile.

The presence in human saliva of many other enzymes besides those discussed so far has become apparent during the last few decades. Since it would lead too far here to present detailed descriptions of all of them, and since in many instances knowledge is only fragmentary, these additional enzymes were compiled in table IX. All enzymes unequivocally originating only from bacterial colonization of the oral cavity were excluded from this tabulation.

Glycoproteins

The glycoproteins constitute the majority of three classes of macromolecules, the so-called glycoconjugates [450], the other two classes comprising the glycolipids and the proteoglycans. While the glycolipids, subdivided into the two major categories of glycosphingolipids and glycoglycerolipids, are composed of sphingosine (or glycerol), fatty acid or fatty ether, and carbohydrate, but do not contain any protein, the proteoglycans are characterized by having mucopolysaccharides attached to a protein core via a 'bridge' of two *D*-galactose units linked to *D*-xylose which connects the

Table IX. Further enzymic components of human saliva

Enzyme trivial name	systematic name	EC number	Source (gland)[a]	Reference
Succinate dehydrogenase	succinate:(acceptor) oxidoreductase	1.3.99.1	mixed[d]	70
	UDP-galactose:N-acetyl-glucosamine galactosyl-transferase	2.4.1.22[b]	P, SM/SL	259
	CMP-sialic acid: glyco-protein sialyltransferase	2.4.1.x[b]	P, SM/SL	256
	GDP-fucose: glycoprotein fucosyltransferase	2.4.1.y[b]	P, SM/SL	257
Lipase	glycerol-ester hydrolase	3.1.1.3	P	70–72, 74
Deoxyribonuclease	deoxyribonucleate oligonucleotidohydrolase	3.1.4.5	P SM	394 393
Neuraminidase	N-acetyl-neuraminate glycohydrolase	3.2.1.18	mixed[d]	275
α-*D*-Mannosidase	α-*D*-mannoside mannohydrolase	3.2.1.24	minor glands	225, 237
β-N-Acetyl-*D*-glucosaminidase	β-2-acetamido-2-deoxy-*D*-glucoside acetamido-deoxyglucohydrolase	3.2.1.30	P[c] P, SM/SL	375 237
β-Glucuronidase	β-*D*-glucuronide glucuronohydrolase	3.2.1.31	P SM	71, 72, 74 70
α-*L*-Fucosidase	α-*L*-6-deoxygalactoside deoxygalactohydrolase	3.2.1.51	P, SM/SL	237
Leucine aminopeptidase	*L*-leucyl-peptide hydrolase	3.4.1.1 3.4.11.1	P, SM/SL	270
Glycylprolyl β-naphthylamidase	–	3.4.11.x[b]	SM[c]	271
Aldolase	ketose-1-phosphate aldehyde-lyase	4.1.2.7	mixed[d]	70
Carbonic anhydrase	carbonate hydro-lyase	4.2.1.1	P, SM	70

[a] P = Parotid; SM = submandibular; SL = sublingual.
[b] Tentatively assigned (no EC number given in original reference).
[c] The enzyme was purified and biochemically characterized.
[d] At least in part of glandular origin.

Table X. Relative viscosities of the saliva of three different glands after stimulation with citric acid [from 304]

Salivary gland	Relative viscosity centipoise
Parotid	1.5
Submandibular	3.4
Sublingual	13.4

whole polysaccharide component to the protein by forming an O-glycosidic bond with a seryl residue [for references see 450].

In the true glycoproteins, two common types of covalent linkage of the carbohydrate moieties to the protein core are generally present, an O-glycosidic bond between N-acetylgalactosamine and the hydroxyl groups of either seryl or threonyl residues (predominating in glycoproteins of epithelial secretions), and an N-glycosidic bond between N-acetylglucosamine and the amide group of asparaginyl residues. Other bonding types may occasionally occur. To the N-acetylated amino sugars a varying number of different monosaccharide units are attached, forming carbohydrate side chains (that may be branched), ranging in length from 1 to 50 and more units (mucus glycoproteins). The use of the term 'prosthetic groups' for the carbohydrate moieties of glycoproteins as proposed by *Gottschalk* [418] has been discouraged [450] as having only a historical meaning. Instead, one should prefer to speak of 'oligosaccharide chains' or 'carbohydrate chains' [450]. It is impossible here and also beyond the scope of this article to deal extensively with the questions involved in biosynthesis, metabolism, purification procedures and criteria of purity, structural analysis, physiological role, and nomenclature of glycoproteins. For the pertaining details the study of the two monumental works of *Gottschalk* [418] and *Horowitz and Pigman* [429], both of which contain contributions from the most prolific researchers in this field, must be recommended. Current concepts of the structure and nature of mammalian salivary mucous glycoproteins were summarized by *Herp* et al. [150].

Glycoproteins are widely distributed in all animal tissues and secretory fluids. They fulfil diverse functions such as forming the 'glue' on cell surface membranes, being involved in transport processes as carriers of smaller molecules, constituting defense mechanisms, acting as lubricants, and forming structural proteins [113]. Numerous proteins contain bound carbohydrate, and a content of up to 4% is usually regarded as normal. Most 'typical' glycoproteins have a carbohydrate content between 10 and 25%, but this can extend to about 40% as in the acid α_1-glycoprotein (orosomucoid), and more. It will indeed not be far from the truth to say that the majority of protein species, including salivary proteins, are glycoproteins. Some of those have already been discussed in the preceding sections, e.g., the odds (formerly A) family of α-amylase isoenzymes, kallikrein, and RNase. The various secretions of the human salivary glands contain glycoproteins in different proportions which are responsible for the relative viscosities (table X) ranging from serous (parotid saliva) to mucinous (sublingual saliva). Thus the viscosity is directly proportional to the percentage of mucus-secreting cells in the various glands [225].

Some salivary enzymes probably involved in the synthesis and break-down of glycoproteins [256, 257, 259] are listed in table IX. There is various evidence for an initial synthesis of the protein core to which in a second step the carbohydrate chains are attached [for references see 218]. In membranes of the secretory granules of rat parotid acinar cells the amino acid profile was found to be very similar to that of the protein core of a major glyco-protein fraction (cationic glycoprotein) synthesized and stored in the acinar cells [3] which apparently use the same template for a variety of products. *Mandel* [218] consequently suggested that 'the economy of production and utilization in salivary glands could serve as a model during this age of depletion of resources and waste'. *Levine* et al. [206] observed that at very high flow rates of parotid saliva the protein core of the major parotid glycoprotein could be isolated. Under the conditions of strong gustatory stimulation the gland apparently synthesized incomplete glycoprotein molecules that were secreted as such. On the other hand, no variations in the carbohydrate content of the glycosylated species of α-amylase isoenzymes [433] and of two cationic glycoproteins of human parotid saliva [222] could be detected in stimulated secretions, regardless of flow rate.

Although in the last two decades an increasing number of salivary glycoproteins has been characterized, down to structural details, much work remains to be done in this rapidly expanding field of research which includes so important compounds as the immunoglobulins and the blood group specific substances. Earlier work utilizing paper electrophoresis [109, 219, 220, 222] already gave indications of considerable complexity of the glyco-protein constituents of human saliva, the total portion of submandibular exceeding that of parotid secretion. With the advent of more sophisticated techniques for the separation and purification of individual components making up mixtures of biological material, this complexity could be more satisfactorily resolved. We will now discuss in detail the sufficiently well-characterized glycoproteins present in human salivary gland secretions.

Immunoglobulins

Immunoglobulins are present not only in serum but also in a variety of body fluids and secretions, e.g. saliva. They form a heterogeneous group of glycoproteins with differences in charge, size, antigenicity, and function. According to their electrophoretic mobility they were first known by the term γ-globulins [463]. Separation of immunoglobulins by size had been achieved previously [423] in studies with horse antipneumococcal antibody. The larger component was then named IgM (immunoglobulin macro) and the smaller one IgG, reflecting size and electrophoretic mobility.

One basic structural principle is common to all immunoglobulins (Igs) and was elucidated mainly by studying IgG. It consists in the bilaterally symmetrical arrangement of two heavy (H) and two light (L) polypeptide chains. The H chains can be envisaged as long rods that start at the carboxyl terminal, run at first parallel and then form an outward angle at about mid-point (hinge region) where they are held together by several interchain disulfide bridges (fig. 4). Carbohydrate side chains are attached below the hinge region. The L chains are connected, near their carboxyl terminal, to the H chains by a disulfide bond inserted above the hinge region. H and L chains then run parallel to each other, ending in their amino terminals. The general formula of an Ig monomer is thus H_2L_2.

Five different classes of Igs can be distinguished according to the primary sequence of the H chain. The 4-chain molecular species is abbreviated Ig followed by a capital letter designating the individual class: IgA, IgD, IgE, IgG, and IgM. Any single H chain (for instance after the breakdown of the intact molecule into the four subunits) is identified by the lowercase Greek letter corresponding to the class. Thus the H chains of IgA are α, of IgG are γ, of IgM are μ heavy chains, and so forth. Light chains are of two different types, kappa (ϰ) and lambda (λ). Their isolated occurrence in urine (Bence-Jones proteins) was demonstrated in patients with multiple myeloma and was exploited for the elucidation of the complete amino acid sequence of an L chain [425]. *Edelman* et al. [413] determined the full sequence of an IgG myeloma protein and found for the H chain four homology regions (domains) of about 110 amino acid residues each, with each one intrachain disulfide loop. The entire H chain polypeptide was 446 amino acids long,

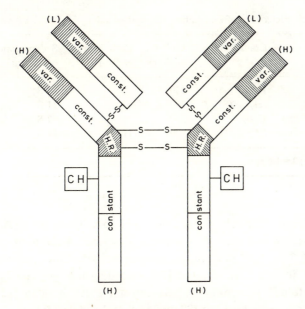

Fig. 4. Schematic drawing of the basic structure of an H_2L_2 immunoglobulin molecule of the IgG prototype [modified after 466]. H = Heavy chain; L = light chain; HR = hinge region; CH = carbohydrate; const. = constant region; var. = variable region.

comprising nearly exactly twice the number of residues making up an L chain (224 residues) which contained two homology regions.

The main carbohydrate moiety of IgG is covalently linked to the H chains at a segment located below the hinge region (fig. 4). Identification of glycopeptides obtained after extensive hydrolysis of various Igs revealed that carbohydrate may be attached also to other regions of the 4-chain prototype, varying with the Ig class studied [for references see 466]. The following monosaccharides are present in the five human Ig classes: fucose, mannose, galactose, N-acetylglucosamine (only in IgA and IgD), and sialic acid [466]. Sequence analysis of the O- and N-glycosidically linked oligosaccharide side chains was performed for one IgA subclass [21, 22]. Although it was suggested that the carbohydrate moieties might play an important role in the regulation of synthesis and secretion of Igs, the bulk of experimental evidence seems to attribute little or no functional involvement to the oligosaccharide units of Ig molecules.

Differences between the individual Ig classes involve configuration, molecular weight, and carbohydrate content (table XI). IgA can be divided

Table XI. Molecular characteristics of four human immunoglobulins

Class	Source	Configuration[a]	Mol. wt. kdaltons	Carbohydrate g/100 g	Sedimentation coefficient
IgA 1	serum	H_2L_2	150	8	7 S
IgA 2	saliva	$(H_2L_2)_2(SP)(J)$	390	12	11 S
IgG	serum, saliva	H_2L_2	150	3	7 S
IgM	serum, saliva	$(H_2L_2)_5(J)$	900	11	18 S

[a] SP = Secretory piece; J = J chain.

into two, and IgG into four subclasses. One of the IgA subclasses (IgA 1) occurs mainly in serum and corresponds to the described 4-chain model. Secretory IgA (IgA 2 or sIgA) predominates in external secretions and is the main Ig present in human parotid saliva [79], exceeding the IgG and IgM content about 100-fold [57]. In submandibular saliva it is less abundant [225]. The reported values range from 17 to 120 mg/l in stimulated parotid [57, 299] and from 5 to 27 mg/l in unstimulated submandibular saliva [470]. It has been estimated that a normal parotid gland is able to secrete about 25 μg sIgA/min in the initial stage of stimulation, while the corresponding value for IgG was only 1.3 μg/min/gland [299]. The mean IgG content, determined under the same conditions, amounted to approximately 0.4–4 mg/l [57, 299]. Of the two Igs, sIgA is produced by about 90% by the parotid gland itself while IgG originates from this organ by only up to 50%, the remainder being provided by transudation from serum [299]. The behavior of both Igs after prolonged stimulation is in good agreement with this assumption. Continuous monitoring of concentrations, performed over 30 min revealed a decrease of IgA and an increase of IgG [299]. This was explained by depletion of the glandular sources of IgA whereas the intensified blood flow due to the secretory stimulus could have promoted the transudation of IgG from serum where its concentration is very high compared to that of IgA 1. The same inverse relation between sIgA content and flow rate had already been observed earlier [221] and supported the assumption that IgA in saliva is produced by the plasma cells in the interstitial tissue of the parotid and submandibular glands [360].

While both plasma and salivary IgG are of the basic H_2L_2 configuration, IgA is characterized by some striking differences when molecules from the two sources are compared (table XI). Secretory IgA 2 has a much higher

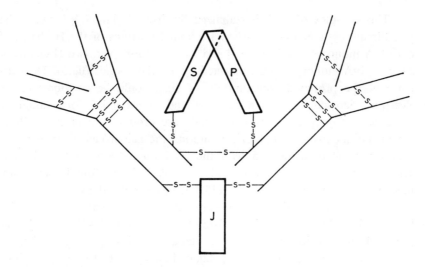

Fig.5. Schematic drawing of a secretory IgA molecule [modified after 466]. The complex consists of 2 IgA protomers and 2 smaller glycopeptides, secretory piece (SP) and J chain (J). The individual components are linked through disulfide bonds inserted near the COOH terminals of the protomer H chains.

molecular weight than plasma IgA 1 (about 390 vs. 150 kdaltons) which is also reflected by the different sedimentation constants (11 vs. 7 S) first determined by *Tomasi* et al. [360] whose continued studies of secretory Igs revived and greatly stimulated interest in this field of research. Only a small portion (roughly 10%) of the salivary IgA were 7 S molecules transudated from serum, while between 10 and 20% were found as higher polymers of IgA sedimenting as 18 S components [359, 360]. Isolation and purification of the main IgA species (11 S) from saliva was performed by applying stimulated parotid secretion [concentrated by ultrafiltration and then dialyzed against pH 7.5 phosphate buffer; 57] to DEAE-cellulose from which the IgA was eluted by stepwise exchange with buffer of increasing ionic strength but decreasing pH. The pH 6.4 fraction contained the bulk of sIgA and was further purified by gel filtration on Sephadex G-200 and/or sucrose gradient centrifugation [57, 360]. Investigations of the isolated product [57, 142, 358, 359] elucidated the following features of 11 S sIgA. Two 4-chain IgA monomers [with H chains of 55 kdaltons and L chains of 22.5 kdaltons each; 359] are joined to a dimer by a glycopeptide, the so-called secretory component (SC) or *secretory piece* (SP) and an additional polypeptide, the *J chain* (J for joining).

This complex of sIgA is stabilized by disulfide bonding between the penultimate cysteine of the carboxyl terminal portions of the H chains of both IgA monomers and SP [464] and J chain. Moreover, two H chains of adjacent IgA monomers are connected by disulfide bonds (fig. 5). The existence of the proposed configuration of sIgA could be corroborated by electron microscopy where a compact and an extended form could be visualized [359]. IgA dimers and J chain are produced in plasma cells in the interstitial tissue spaces. After entering the acinar cell cytoplasm, the complex becomes associated with the nonimmune subunit SP which is synthesized by serous epithelial cells [359, 360]. SP is also found in free form in saliva at a level of up to 20 mg/l [57]. It has a molecular weight of about 60 kdaltons and contains 6% carbohydrate when present in the complex [359, 464] while for the soluble form the content is 11–12% [357]. The principal amino acids are aspartic and glutamic acids, glycine, and leucine [218]. The smaller subunit, J chain [142], contains close to 10% carbohydrate and has a molecular weight of 20 kdaltons. Carbohydrate, comprising primarily hexoses and hexosamines but very little sialic acid [464], is found in all component parts of sIgA (overall content 10–12%) but is unevenly distributed among the complex [357]. The main portion was present in the H chains (63%), 28% in SP, and only 6.5% in J chain. L chains contained negligible amounts (2.5%).

IgA and IgG from human submandibular saliva were resolved into several fractions by Sephadex G-100 gel filtration and isoelectric focusing [229]. Heterogeneity of these moderately acidic proteins (pI values between 4.5 and 6.5) was suggested by the wide range in which they focused, from pH 5 to 6 for IgA and from pH 4.5 to 6.5 for IgG.

The J chain glycopolypeptide is also involved in the configuration of IgM, a pentamer of the basic H_2L_2 model, where it is supposed to induce a conformational change in the Ig protomers, leading to self-assembly of the full pentamer, with J chain in the center of the starfish-like structure [359]. This and the fact that IgM μ-chains are about 110 residues longer than γ-chains (possessing an additional domain) explains the very high molecular weight of IgM (table XI) which is the reason that its transudation from serum into saliva is largely blocked [359]. Consequently, its concentration in parotid saliva is very low, reaching only levels between 0.1 and 0.8 mg/l [57], and sometimes it cannot be detected at all.

The question whether or not IgD occurs in saliva has received controversial answers. *Dunnette* et al. [96], using a double-antibody radioimmunoassay, were unable to detect it in parotid saliva while *Sewell* et al. [309]

claimed to have found IgD in this fluid. Their technique, utilizing agglutination of antibody-coated cells, permitted them to determine IgD levels below 1 ng/ml, but it could not be entirely excluded that contamination of parotid with whole saliva (where IgD was identified in 3 out of 7 samples) had been responsible for the positive result.

Blood Group Reactive Substances

Substances with antigenic properties in the various blood group systems, such as the ABH(O) and Lewis systems, are present not only on the membranes of red blood cells but also occur as surface components of many tissue cells and in soluble form in a variety of secretions including saliva [376]. Since all of them, regardless of source, show serological cross-reactions with their corresponding antibodies from serum or plasma, and since such specificities may also be present in some other compounds such as disaccharidases or glycolipids [451], the simple term 'blood group substances' seems inaccurate and improper and should be replaced by the more characteristic names 'substances (or glycoproteins) with (A, B, etc.) blood group activity' [452] or shorter, 'blood group reactive (specific) substances'.

The ability to secrete blood group reactive substances (BGRS) is genetically controlled. For the BGRS of the ABH(O) system, where a pair of allelic genes *(Se* and *se)* independently of the ABO genes determines whether or not those substances are secreted [for references see 376], secretory ability is inherited as a Mendelian dominant trait. The dominant allele *Se* gives rise to secretion (in *SeSe* and *Sese* individuals) while homozygosity for the recessive allele *se* prevents it. Since *Se* is present in 3 out of 4 persons, 75% of the white population are secretors of BGRS of the ABH(O) system, involving the antigenic substances A and B and, in carriers of blood group O, the H substance without antigenic specificity. The synthesis of this compound is controlled by another set of alleles, *H* and *h*, and only homozygous carriers of the recessive allele *h* are unable to synthesize and hence, secrete H substance as well as A and B substances since these are formed by derivatization of the H component. The terms 'secretor' and 'nonsecretor' only apply to the BGRS of the classic ABH(O) system. Nonsecretors *(sese* homozygotes) nevertheless secrete a substance called Le[a] connected with the Lewis blood group system which is independent of *Se/se* alleles, if they possess in their genome the dominant allele *Le*. Individuals in whom both ABH(O) and Lewis blood group characters are present secrete still another substance, Le[b], which today is interpreted as an interaction product of the *H* and *Le* genes [for references see 376]. There are thus five blood group specificities,

A, B, H, Le[a] and Le[b], that are the products of three independent gene systems *(ABO, Hh* and *Lele)* and occur in a freely soluble form in tissue fluids and external secretions of individuals of the appropriate blood group and secretor type. We will in this section confine ourselves to a discussion of the BGRS of the ABH(O) system.

The antigenic determinants responsible for blood group specificity reside only in a very small part of the whole molecule, the terminal portions of the multiple-branched carbohydrate side chains. They are by now well defined. The A and B specific terminal configurations have their common precursor in the H substance from which they are derived by the action of genetically determined glycosyltransferases with the specificity and distribution required for their function. These enzymes were identified in a number of tissues [376] and modify H substance by covalent linking of a single monosaccharide to the terminal galactose unit. Thus A and B substances are formed by the addition of N-acetylgalactosamine (A) and galactose (B), respectively (fig.6). Members of blood group O are lacking those specific glycosyltransferases and therefore secrete the 'primitive' H substance.

Although the different specificities are primarily determined by the added monosaccharide unit, they are also dependent on the nature, sequence and linkage of the sugars already present in the chain [376]. There are, however, two forms in which A, B and H substances occur. Whereas in the red blood cell the BGRS are present as glycolipids consisting of carbohydrate, fatty acids and sphingosine (with the lipophilic moieties inserted in the erythrocyte membrane), they are found as true glycoproteins in saliva and secretions [for references see 376] where their carbohydrate content is extremely high (85%). The predominant portion of amino acids in the small polypeptide moiety is made up, in this order, by threonine, serine and proline [454]. Half-cystine is present only in traces, and methionine and tryptophan are altogether missing. In BGRS from human saliva, tyrosine and phenylalanine were to be added to the list of missing amino acids [432]. Five types of monosaccharides are observed, *L*-fucose (10–20%), *D*-galactose (45 to 60%), N-acetyl-*D*-glucosamine and N-acetyl-*D*-galactosamine (together 23–36%), and sialic acid which was found to be N-acetylneuraminic acid (1–5%). Although most of these data were derived from BGRS isolated from ovarian cyst fluid which is especially rich in these compounds, the close similarity in composition between BGRS from this source and from saliva seems to be unequivocally established [376]. The concentration of BGRS in saliva is rather low, amounting to only 10–130 mg/l [432], but differs within the secretions from the various glands proportional to the viscosity of the

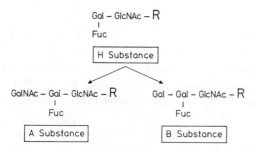

Fig.6. Array of units in the terminal portions of the carbohydrate side chains of blood group reactive substances determining antigenic specificity. Fuc = Fucose; Gal = galactose; GalNAc = N-acetylgalactosamine; GlcNAc = N-acetylglucosamine.

fluid. Thus the secretion from the minor labial salivary glands is particularly rich in these substances which has led to its utilization, under appropriate circumstances, in forensic medicine as a means of establishing an otherwise unavailable suspect's blood group, or for corroborative purposes. Parotid saliva only rarely contains very small amounts of BGRS [469].

The main glycoprotein portion of submandibular saliva ('high molecular weight glycoproteins') is apparently very similar in its composition to salivary BGRS [218, 397]. This and the observation that submandibular saliva of secretors had a higher concentration of protein-bound carbohydrate than that of nonsecretors [405] has prompted the assumption that both groups of substances may be the same [218]. However, differences found in the respective glycine contents [376] do not support this contention. Isolation of BGRS from saliva by means of gel filtration was severally attempted [120, 229]. After purification from human submandibular saliva by Sephadex G-100 chromatography and subsequent isoelectric focusing [229], these compounds were identified as strongly acidic glycoproteins (pI 1.8–2.8 with a peak at 2.3) with high molecular weights (elution in the exclusion peak). Analysis of their carbohydrate composition revealed that, in addition to the same sugars found in BGRS from ovarian cysts, mannose was also present. Sialic acid (N-acetylneuraminic acid) was detected at a level of 5%. Its isoelectric point and those of the two dicarboxylic amino acids lie within the observed pH range of 1.8–2.8 and 'undoubtedly accounted for the focusing of the macromolecules within this region' [229]. Heterogeneity of the BGRS or microheterogeneity of the carbohydrate side chains probably were responsible for the broad range of isoelectric focusing.

Other Glycoproteins

A variety of other glycoproteins are found in the secretions of the human cephalic salivary glands, but as many of them are not yet definitely characterized, their classification poses certain difficulties. *Mandel* [218] collected the information available on these compounds up to 1974 and summarized the pertinent details. We will mainly follow his classification and attempt to give a brief description of additional salivary glycoproteins as they occur (predominantly or exclusively) in the various secretions. For most references, the reader must be referred to the comprehensive article of *Mandel* [218].

Parotid Saliva. Cationic glycoprotein was first described by *Mandel and Ellison* [219] in 1961 and 1963 and partially characterized, on the basis of eluates from paper electrophoresis, a few years later [222]. Extended studies with more advanced techniques such as chromatography on DEAE-cellulose using stepwise elution with varying pH and ionic strengths, followed by gel filtration with Sephadex G-200, and final purification of the cationic glycoprotein by Sephadex G-25 filtration disclosed more exact details of the structure of this major component of parotid saliva, representing about 25% of its total protein and 75% of its total carbohydrate content. A protein core (mol. wt. 21 kdaltons) carries four polysaccharide units of about 3.4 kdaltons each. Similar to other saliva-specific nonglycoproteins that will be described later, the composition of the core polypeptide is characterized by the predominance of only a few amino acid residues (proline, glycine and glutamic acid/glutamine accounted for 80% of all amino acids) while eight others are altogether absent (Cys-SH, Leu, Ileu, Met, Phe, Thr, Trp, and Try). The carbohydrate moieties were made up by roughly equal portions of N-acetylglucosamine, fucose, galactose and mannose (18–22 residues each per 36.4 kdaltons mol. wt. of the glycoprotein) and only one tenth that amount (2 residues) of sialic acid. Apparently there were only N-glycosidic linkages (between GlcNAc and AsN) present. On a quantitative basis, the cationic glycoprotein consists of roughly 58% protein and 40% carbohydrate. The cationic character of the molecule and the observed, exclusively N-glycosidic, linkage between carbohydrate and protein suggest that the high content of dicarboxylic amino acids comprises a fair share of the respective amides.

Rapid stimulation of parotid saliva may lead to secretion of incompletely assembled cationic glycoproteins as observed by *Levine* et al. [206] who found 5–7% of total parotid protein to be present as an aglycoprotein. By virtue of its unusual amino acid composition (principal amino acids were

Pro, Gly and Glu and amounted to 75% of all residues) and on account of the absence of the same eight amino acids missing in the complete cationic glycoprotein, it was decided that this flow rate dependent constituent of parotid saliva was the protein core of the cationic glycoprotein. Immunological examination revealed identical reactions of the protein moieties of both substances. Core protein concentration in unstimulated saliva was always very low. On the basis of these findings it was proposed that the core is synthesized on the rough endoplasmatic reticulum and then transported to the Golgi apparatus where the carbohydrate side chains are sequentially attached by membrane-bound glycosyltransferases. Release into the acinar lumen may occur at different stages of assembly, depending on flow rate as well as type and duration of the stimulus applied.

From further experimental evidence it appears that besides this major cationic component there are a number of very similar glycoproteins present, in parotid saliva. All of them were identified as basic glycoproteins [10, 127 149] and would thus also be cationic at the physiological pH of saliva and under the conditions of the purification procedures applied to the 'cationic' parotid glycoprotein. What is more, the amino acid composition of the protein moieties again disclosed the strong preponderance of proline, glycine and glutamic acid (glutamine) residues, accounting for up to 80% of the entire polypeptide. Major differences were found in the portions of attached carbohydrate ranging from 2.5–53.5%, but only minor variations could be noted in the amino acid composition, sometimes within the confines of experimental error. The mechanism proposed for the synthesis of cationic glycoprotein would allow for such differences, and all experimental evidence seems to support the contention that the basic proline-rich glycoprotein fraction secreted by the human parotid gland constitutes a group of closely related but nevertheless heterogeneous glycoproteins [10, 127, 149, 206] of which the 'cationic glycoprotein' is the most abundant. Table XII summarizes data reported for eight such constituents of parotid saliva and compares them with those determined for cationic glycoprotein [206]. The purification steps applied to the various preparations include gel filtration on Sephadex G-150 [149], G-200 [127] or Bio-Gel P-100 [10], either followed by cationic ion-exchange chromatography with moderately acidic buffers [127, 149] or preceded by isoelectric focusing in a gradient ranging from pH 7 to 10 [10].

The most distant relatives among this group of basic parotid glycoproteins seem to be represented by the four glycoproteins isolated by *Henkin* et al. [149]. Two features in particular distinguish them from the other members of the family: the presence of an unknown, aminoacid-like uniden-

Table XII. Molecular characteristics of nine different preparations of cationic glycoproteins isolated from human parotid saliva [computed from 10, 149, 206]

	Reference								
	206	10				149			
	cationic glyco-protein	pI 9.5	pI >10			1	2	3	4
			I	II	III				
Amino acid residues per 1,000 residues[a]									
Proline	371	399	441	390	420	327	357	381	389
Glycine	231	176	171	199	189	224	225	229	206
Glutamic acid	190	186	183	201	192	180	187	179	194
Aspartic acid	48	46	44	38	36	50	54	47	44
Serine	42	45	41	44	41	48	37	35	29
Lysine	49	52	67	66	70	43	42	45	46
Arginine	44	58	31	32	32	37	36	37	44
Histidine	10	12	2	+0	+0	11	10	10	12
Alanine	8	5	18	30	22	16	0	4	6
Valine	7	7	+0	0	+0	0	0	0	0
Threonine	0	+0	+0	0	+0	12	5	6	6
Leucine	0	7	+0	+0	+0	8	0	3	4
Isoleucine	0	+0	+0	+0	+0	3	0	1	0
X[b]	–	–	–	–	–	40	49	41	20
Carbohydrate, g/100 g glycoprotein									
Neutral sugars	26.2	35	16	2.5	2.5	39	31	25	20
N-Acetylglucosamine	12.7	18.5	1	0	0	4–5 times the amount of mannose			
Sialic acid	1.7	0	0	0	0	2.8	1.3	0	0
Molecular weight, kdaltons	35.3	30–70	18	11.5	5–10	34	34	34	34

[a] Five amino acids (Cys-SH, Met, Phe, Trp, Tyr) were absent from all preparations.
[b] Unknown substance appearing after leucine.

tified substance 'X' which was found in appreciable amounts, and the unusual staining behavior. Amido black 10 B was not bound at all but the glycoproteins stained blue with Coomassie brilliant blue G-250, and pink-violet with Coomassie brilliant blue R-250.

The five glycoproteins only partially characterized by *Friedman* et al. [127] and therefore not listed in table XII were apparently much closer related to those of *Arneberg* [10] because of the absence of sialic acid and the wide variation observed in the quantitative relation of the different monosaccharides to each other. All five proteins were identified in the parotid secretions of single donors. Although the total amounts secreted at different sampling sessions varied, the general characteristics of the analyzed glycoproteins did not. Since the cationic glycoproteins seem to exhibit heterogeneity between individuals, genetic studies of a possibly heritable polymorphism were suggested [127].

Levine and Keller [205] recently isolated from parotid saliva a glycoprotein with a carbohydrate content of 6% whose amino acid composition closely resembled that of core protein [206]. It is not quite clear if this basic proline-rich glycoprotein is an individual species or merely represents an initial stage of glycosylation of the core protein.

Lactoferrin, an iron-binding glycoprotein, was demonstrated in many external secretions including parotid saliva, at levels between 2 and 10 mg/l. Its concentration was higher in unstimulated secretions. Lactoferrin apparently has properties similar to secretory piece (SP) because the two compounds were difficult to separate from each other [for details see 218]. The molecular weight (77 kdaltons) is similar to that of SP for which values between 60 and 75 kdaltons were reported. A carbohydrate content of close to 10% includes minor amounts of fucose and sialic acid [357].

The serum α_1-*acid glycoprotein* seems to transude into saliva in very low concentration as demonstrated by immunological examination. It has an isoelectric point of 2.7 and a molecular weight of 44 kdaltons.

Submandibular Saliva. High molecular weight glycoproteins (HMWG) of submandibular saliva and glands were so far largely studied in animals but not in man although the presence of substantial amounts of this type of glycoprotein had been recognized for some time. Only in the last few years some progress was made in the isolation of these substances from human submandibular saliva and partial characterization was achieved. After dissolution in 3 M NaCl of a mucin clot formed by the treatment of submandibular secretion with cetyltrimethylammonium bromide (CETAB) and removal of CETAB by passage of the dissolved clot through CM-Sephadex, further purification was attained with Sephadex G-200 from which the HMWG eluted in the exclusion peak [397]. The yield from 100 ml saliva was about 20 mg of HMWG, 50% of which was carbohydrate. The main hexose present was galactose, besides small amounts of mannose and glucose, with a galactose to fucose (deoxygalactose) molar ratio of 3:2, varying with flow rate and secretor status. Such variations were also noted for the hexosamines where the average molar ratio between N-acetylglucosamine and

N-acetylgalactosamine was roughly 2 : 1. Sialic acid was entirely N-acetyl-neuraminic acid, and small amounts of sulfate were also detected. Principal amino acids were threonine, serine, proline and alanine; the amino acid profile is thus similar to the HMWG isolated from other species. Sequencing was not yet performed on the core proteins of different species but in view of the just mentioned similarity, comparative phylogenetic studies would seem quite interesting.

In quantitative terms submandibular HMWG is the mucinous counterpart of parotid cationic glycoprotein, contributing 12% of total N, 23% of total carbohydrate, and even 70% of total sialic acid present in the secretion. Cationic glycoprotein itself occurs in submandibular saliva only in minor amounts.

The investigation of HMWG by gel electrophoresis is hampered by the high molecular weight (between 500 and 1,000 kdaltons) and probably also by its molecular shape since it does not migrate at all. Only a smaller component, possibly a disaggregation or dissociation product, showed some electrophoretic mobility.

Very similar, but not entirely identical, glycoproteins were isolated from homogenates of human submandibular glands. The substances could be heated to 100°C without being destroyed. A minimum molecular weight of 300 kdaltons was estimated. The marked similarity to other 'mucin' preparations from submandibular/sublingual saliva described in the literature [229] suggested that the mucins are secreted as HMWGs. All these substances are strongly acidic proteins and therefore carry, at physiological pH, an excess of negative charge which makes them also strongly anionic. The same characteristics apply to a preparation of blood group reactive substances which focused at pH 2.3 [229], and identity of submandibular HMWG and BGRS has indeed been postulated. Although undoubtedly strong similarities exist, the view also finds experimental support that these two groups of compounds are closely related but not virtually the same (cf. section on BGRS). The strongly anionic character obviously derives from the presence of the two dicarboxylic amino acids and from the high concentration of sialic acid, while the sulfate content of about 1.6% of total glycoprotein contributes little to the acidity of HMWG of human submandibular saliva.

A number of *other anionic glycoproteins* (at pH 8.3–8.9) were demonstrated in submandibular saliva by carbohydrate staining and analysis of eluates from paper and polyacrylamide gel electrophoretograms [219]. This diversity of glycoproteins includes, besides minor components with comparatively low molecular weights still awaiting further elucidation, also rather well-defined species already described in more detail elsewhere in this chapter, e.g., immunoglobulins, the glycosylated family of isoamylases, free secretory piece, and others.

A phosphorus-containing glycoprotein found in submandibular and parotid secretions of normal (healthy) persons and children with cystic fibrosis [404] exhibited great affinity for calcium and hydroxyapatite surfaces and was therefore named *calcium-precipitable protein* (CaPP). Purification was achieved by salting out with ammonium sulfate, gel filtration on Bio-Gel P-10, and subsequent preparative PAGE. This phosphoprotein was also acidic (pI 4.4) and thus, anionic under physiological conditions. Its molecular weight was determined at 12 kdaltons. The principal amino acids were serine, glycine and glutamic acid; hexose content amounted to slightly over 5% while only traces of hexosamines and sialic acid, and no sulfate, were present. The phosphorus content, responsible for the ability of CaPP to bind calcium and become attached to hydroxyapatite, was 0.85%. CaPP was also identified by isoelectric focusing of submandibular/sublingual saliva previously separated into several peaks by gel filtration [229]. The sample of submandibular saliva obtained from a single donor revealed the presence of altogether three *phospho(glyco)proteins* which were only partially characterized (pI 4.3–4.4). One of them was only detected in stimulated secretion, together with two basic (pI>10) and an unidentified protein (pI 7.1).

As yet *unidentified glycoproteins* of submandibular saliva were reported by several investigators [for references see 218]. They were characterized by positive PAS staining and an anionic mobility somewhat greater than that of the glycosylated isoamylases [219] and include two substances with a pI of about 5 and carbohydrate moieties comprising mannose, galactose, fucose as well as glucosamine and galactosamine in a molar ratio of 2:1 [229]. An even more anionic glycoprotein, isolated in 1975, was also a phosphoprotein with a P content of 0.8% and a molecular weight of 13–14 kdaltons. The main amino acids were glutamic and aspartic, followed by serine and glycine. Tyrosine and proline were present in low amounts. Since sialic acid was only found in traces (besides nearly 6% hexose) the anionic character of the molecule is determined by the predominance of the dicarboxylic amino acids and possibly also by the phospho-moieties. The isoelectric point was not determined. Although the amino acid profile was similar to CaPP, the two phosphoproteins were not identical. Both occur in submandibular saliva in much higher concentration than in parotid saliva from which the most anionic glycoproteins may be altogether absent.

Sublingual Saliva. The major human *sublingual glycoprotein* was isolated and partially characterized. Earlier studies had shown that this fraction of sublingual saliva inhibited the hemagglutination of influenza virus and this property (HI) was used as a standard of purity of the preparation. Purification included treatment in boiling water which did not precipitate the HI fraction, present at a level of 20% of the total protein. Filtration on Bio-Gel P-300 excluded the HI fraction in the void volume, together with the BGRS of the secretion. The sublingual glycoprotein has a molecular weight of 560 kdaltons and is a very acidic substance with a pI of about 2. Aspartic and glutamic acids were the main residues present, followed in amount by glycine, serine and threonine. Although molecular size (18.9 S), insensitivity to high temperature and high levels of dicarboxylic amino acids might suggest a close relation to the HMWG of submandibular saliva, the two are different compounds since the HMWG have a much lower content of aspartic acid and are not so strongly anionic. Carbohydrate made up 50% of sublingual glycoprotein, comprising neutral sugars, fucose, glucosamine, galactosamine, and sialic acid. Besides by blood group and HI activities, this component of sublingual saliva was also characterized by its strong affinity for hydroxyapatite and its high calcium binding capacity. Like CaPP and a number of other saliva-specific proteins to be discussed later, it may therefore play a role in acquired dental pellicle formation.

The affinity for calcium seems to be a common property of the strongly acidic (anionic) glycoproteins of the mucin type of human saliva. Acidity is mainly caused by the presence of moieties with very low pK_a values, sialic acid and sulfate, and consequently sialo- and sulfomucins are distinguished [298]. The prevalently negative charge carried by these components results in the strong attraction to the positively charged calcium of hydroxyapatite (dental enamel). The study of *sulfated glycoproteins* [389] has been newly stimulated by the identification of a variety of such components in saliva [for details see 298]. Presence of sulfated glycoproteins in human saliva had previously only sporadically been reported [389] without definitive characterization. Whereas their concentration in parotid saliva was very low, rather high amounts had been found in submandibular/sublingual saliva, and even higher ones in the secretion obtained from the minor salivary glands. Sulfate content may extend up to 6% by weight. Sulfated or sialylated glycoproteins may be the predominant acidic type within a secretory cell population but, as in human salivary glands, both types are found together in the same gland [229]. In that case sialic acid and sulfate may occur on the same oligosaccaride side chain. Most of the sulfated HMWG of human salivary gland secretion are just beginning to be studied in closer detail so that definitive molecular characteristics cannot yet be given. For additional information and the main references on this subject, the reader is referred to the review article of *Roukema and Nieuw Amerongen* [298].

Whole Saliva. Besides those originating from and described for the secretions of the individual cephalic salivary glands, several other glyco-proteins are found in mixed secretion [218]. They are derived from mucous cells of the glands but were identified and investigated so far only in whole saliva. There are a number of reports describing HMWG with variable carbohydrate, sialic acid and sulfate content and certain differences between amino acid profiles. Some of them closely resembled the HMWG of sub-mandibular/sublingual saliva but others apparently were distinct. While all these constituents of whole saliva may indeed represent different species originating from other than submandibular or sublingual sources, the mostly slight dissimilarities to the HMWG (mucins) from the secretions of those two glands might also suggest bacterial alteration operating in whole saliva. Like other acidic glycoproteins, the HMWG of whole saliva strongly adsorbed to hydroxyapatite surfaces.

Another acidic (pI 4.75), calcium precipitable glycoprotein was isolated from filtered whole saliva by adding calcium ions, collecting the precipitate and dissolving it. The purified substance was of moderate size (mol. wt. 61 kdaltons), rich in dicarboxylated amino acids, and contained 15% carbohydrate [399]. Quite remarkably, it shares a number of properties with the glycoprotein described in the following paragraph, although it would be too farfetched to state that the two substances are identical.

A substance with the ability to bind cobalamin (vitamin B_{12}) had long been known to occur in human saliva. Its identification was based on immu-nological studies. This *vitamin B_{12}-binding protein* which is similar to trans-cobalamin I of serum and gastric juice had a molecular weight of 50 to 65 kdaltons revealing considerable heterogeneity, and a pI around 5.0; its principal amino acids were aspartic and glutamic acids with lower contribu-tions of leucine and threonine. A variable content of sialic acid (about 0.5 mol/mol of complex) was accompanied by 15% total hexose. The vitamin B_{12}-binding capacity of this glycoprotein suggests the presence of 'intrinsic factor' (apoerythein) in human saliva. Resorption of 'extrinsic factor' (B_{12}) requires its association with apoerythein. Sialic acid functions in the binding of the vitamin by dimerization of two intrinsic factor monomers and attachment of 1 mol cobalamine per mol of monomer. The presence of intrinsic factor in whole saliva [225] would attribute to this fluid another important physiological role.

Carcinoembryonic antigen (CEA), isolated from normal adults' saliva by extraction with perchloric acid and gel filtration on Sepharose 6-B, was not in any way connected with blood group and secretor status. The antigen was found to be immunological identical to an antigen specific to mucus-producing cells which may explain that its concentration in saliva exceeds that in blood about 100-fold. Differences between the human salivary CEA-like glycoprotein and CEA isolated from normal tissues, not including salivary gland, mainly concerned carbohydrate content which was lower in salivary (25%) than in tissue CEA (42%).

Saliva-Specific Proteins

The secretions mainly from the human parotid but also from the sub-mandibular salivary glands are distinguished by the occurrence of certain saliva-specific proteins that are in most cases characterized by only a few amino acids making up the main portion of the polypeptide chain. Thus a variety of proline-rich, histidine-rich and tyrosine-rich proteins of rather low molecular weight were isolated, some of which are phosphorylated and exhibit strong affinity towards calcium, preventing its precipitation from human saliva which is supersaturated with respect to this ion. They are involved in acquired pellicle formation on the one hand and agglutination of bacteria on the other, and therefore play an important role in caries etiology [435]. More about this physiological aspect will be said in a later section. The saliva-specific proteins include acidic and basic species and are subject to genetic polymorphism, a property making them readily accessible sources of genetic markers. Since glycoproteins with similar distinctions were already described in the foregoing section, only saliva-specific proteins that are not glycoproteins will be discussed here.

Proline-Rich Proteins

The first report on proline-rich (non-glyco) proteins from human parotid saliva was given in 1971 by *Oppenheim* et al. [267]; they are sometimes referred to as the 'four classic proline-rich proteins' (PRP), since different proline-rich proteins species were detected later. PRP *(Pr proteins)* were isolated from stimulated parotid saliva, after lyophilization, by ammonium sulfate fractionation, gel filtration on Sephadex G-75 of the 35–50% fraction and ion-exchange chromatography on DEAE-Sephadex A-25 equilibrated with Tris buffer (pH 8.5). A shallow NaCl gradient separated four PRP whose

Table XIII. Molecular characteristics of the four proline-rich proteins [267] and of acidic protein [125]

	PRP (=Pr proteins)				Acidic (Pa) protein
	I	II	III	IV	
Amino acid residues per 1,000 residues					
Aspartic acid (asparagine)	76	77	107	103	21
Threonine	12	3	5	12	2
Serine	43	39	49	59	72
Glutamic acid (glutamine)	194	255	256	195	197
Proline	271	261	212	220	223
Glycine	220	213	197	211	185
Alanine	10	8	12	11	22
Valine	28	21	29	35	63
Cystine	0	0	0	0	0
Methionine	0	0	0	0	+0
Isoleucine	21	13	18	23	34
Leucine	27	22	34	38	55
Tyrosine	0	0	0	0	0
Phenylalanine	9	8	10	12	27
Lysine	17	16	11	12	18
Histidine	25	22	21	14	26
Arginine	47	42	39	45	53
Tryptophan[a]	0	0	0	0	0
Molecular weight, kdaltons	12.3		6.1		50–150
pI	4.71	4.59	4.14	4.09	3.9–4.5
Phosphorylated	+	+	+	+	+

[a] Not determined (destroyed by acid hydrolysis).

purity was checked by disc gel electrophoresis. The yields from 5 g of freeze-dried parotid protein were 21 mg (PRP I), 8 mg (PRP II), 22 mg (PRP III), and 10 mg (PRP IV). The purified proteins only stained properly with amido black while Coomassie blue was not bound. Isoelectric points between 4.1 and 4.7 were determined by column isoelectric focusing and molecular weights between 6 and 12 kdaltons by analytical (equilibrium) ultracentrifugation. Investigation of the amino acid composition revealed a close similarity among all four PRPs, with proline, glycine, glutamic and aspartic acids amounting to 75% of all residues (table XIII). The dicarboxylic acids were present almost entirely in their amide forms. Four amino acids (cystine, methionine, tryptophan and tyrosine) were absent from the purified material;

in a later report [448] threonine, too, was stated as nonexistent in the four PRPs (= Pr proteins).

The observed cross-reaction of antisera raised in response to PRP I and III with all four human PRPs as well as with the primate PRP from *Macaca fascicularis* suggested their origin from a common precursor molecule [189]. Preliminary studies on the N-terminal amino acid sequence also indicated a significant degree of sequence homology between the human and primate Pr proteins [448]. A striking difference nevertheless exists in that the primate PRP is a glycoprotein, containing 10% neutral sugars, 10% hexosamines and 15% sialic acid [189, 448]. A possible evolutionary advantage of this loss of carbohydrate by the human Pr proteins is not obvious.

Similar if not identical proline-rich proteins designated A–D were described by *Bennick and Connell* [42] and their primary structure partially elucidated [400]. Two of them (A and C) were also found in submandibular saliva [41], and in addition six minor variants of this class (PRP A–F) could subsequently be identified [147]. Like the other acidic polypeptides belonging to the group of proline-rich proteins (acidic and double-band proteins), the Pr proteins (PRP) are phosphorylated [17, 41].

An acidic proline-rich protein *(Pa protein)* was isolated by *Friedman and Merritt* [125] from parotid saliva by ion-exchange chromatography of lyophilized protein on DEAE-cellulose with a steep (0–0.4 *M*) linear NaCl gradient in pH 7.5 Tris buffer, followed by ascending Sephadex G-200 gel filtration. Purity was checked by anionic disc gel electrophoresis and staining with amido black. Column isoelectric focusing in a sucrose gradient containing ampholine in the range from pH 3 to 10 disclosed a pI 3.9–4.5 for the purified Pa protein fractions. Besides Pa, another protein (Pa-II) was isolated whose amino acid composition distinctly differed from that of Pa and closely resembled PRP III and IV judged from its electrophoretic behavior. The amino acid compositions of the four Pr proteins and the Pa protein are juxtaposed in table XIII. While the proline content resembles that of Pr, aspartic acid (asparagine) is much less. Methionine was present in Pa only in traces (if at all), and cystine, tyrosine and tryptophan were not found. A molecular weight of 50–100 kdaltons was estimated on the basis of gel filtration data [125].

Although the Pa protein could be detected in whole, submandibular and parotid secretions from the same individual regardless of time and day of collection, it was only present in 1 out of 4 persons where it constituted approximately 9% of parotid salivary proteins [125]. This finding is due to a genetic polymorphism [18–20, 128] owing to the presence or absence of an autosomal, dominant allele Pa^1. The phenotypic expression is then Pa 0 (for absence) or Pa 1 (for presence). A second, very rare variant, Pa 2, was described by *Azen* [15] who concluded, from the identical gene frequencies for the three Pa and the three SAPX (salivary peroxidase) variants as well as from experimental evidence, that SAPX are produced by disulfide bonding with Pa (cf. section on peroxidase/catalase). Treatment with 2-mercapto-ethanol degraded Pa 1 to a single, faster-migrating product suggesting that the Pa 1 protein might be a dimer with a disulfide linkage [15]. Labeling available thiol groups with radioactive iodoacetamide supported these findings. Since the proposed mechanism would require the presence of cystine in Pa which was not found [125], the Pa-SAPX relationship merits further investigation to resolve this obvious paradox.

A third member of the group of proline-rich proteins is the double-band protein *(Db protein)*, so called because of its appearance on gel electrophoretograms as two widely separated bands, one of them (slow Db) located cathodal from Pa 1 and the other (fast Db) more anodal between Pr 2 and Pr 3 [17, 19, 448]. The two bands of Db protein always occur together (in 12% of Caucasians) or not at all (88%). Db is thus another genetically polymorphic protein, its presence being dependent on the allele *Db+* [19, 128]. Other than Pr, Db stains well with Coomassie blue [15]. To be judged from their electrophoretic migration, the two Db components must widely differ in their negative charge densities in an alkaline gel system and probably also in their molecular weights. Since exact data on amino acid composition and molecular size are lacking, these differences must at present remain unresolved. Their inclusion into the group of proline-rich proteins is based on evident biochemical and genetical relationships [17–20].

Finally another acidic, probably also proline-rich protein must be mentioned which migrates anodal of the slow Db band and very close to Pa 1/Pr 1 [15, 448] and was designated *X (non-Pa) protein* [15, 17, 19]. Based on multiple experimental evidence, a close biochemical and genetical relationship is assumed [17] for all proline-rich, phosphorylated nonglycoproteins of human saliva, comprising Pr 1–4, Pa 1 and 2, Db, and X (non-Pa). They are regarded as the products of separate but closely linked loci.

The occurrence of so many different but nevertheless related proteins is rather confusing and consequently standardization (typing) has been proposed utilizing an alkaline (pH 8.9) PAGE system. At an acrylamide concentration of 7–7.5% [128], the consecutive order in anodal direction is (Pa 2), Db slow, non-Pa/Pa 1, Pr 1, Pr 2, Db fast, Pr 3, Pr 4 [17, 124, 448].

Histidine-Rich Proteins

This group of mostly basic proteins also comprises a whole set of different polypeptides, characterized by high proportions of basic amino acid residues and low molecular weights. The strongly basic (cationic) members are closely related and within each group may evolve from each other [276, 415].

The isolation from human parotid saliva of a group of basic proteins whose principal amino acids were histidine, lysine and arginine was reported from two different laboratories [24, 276]. Subsequently available experimental evidence strongly suggested that both materials were the same. *Balekjian and Longton* [24] purified three 'histones' by elution of parotid saliva from Bio-Rex 70. After discarding an initial protein fraction, three histone peaks were eluted by an alkaline (pH 8) phosphate buffer of increased ionic strength. The isolated histones were subjected to cationic disc gel electrophoresis to establish their purity. *Peters and Azen* [276] applied lyophilized parotid saliva protein to gel filtration (Bio-Gel P-10) under strongly acidic conditions (pH 3), followed by ion-exchange chromatography on CM-cellulose at pH 8.5 with a steep gradient of ammonium formate (0.1–1.0 M). Two peaks of parotid basic proteins *(Pb proteins)* were obtained; electrophoresis in an acid urea-starch gel and subsequent staining with a high-sensitivity arginyl stain revealed the presence of several (up to 5) Pb bands [276, 277].

The Pb proteins are the fastest migrating parotid proteins and also show genetic polymorphism [13, 14]. Their heterogeneity (table XIV) was explained by a combination of allelic differences and post-translational modifications through deamidation and proteolysis [14, 18, 276] involving changes of tertiary structure [276]. Pb proteins a–b and d–e are derived from Pb 1e by a succession of steps, while Pb protein c evolves from the other primary gene product, Pb 2, which is similar to Pb 1e, in a single step [276].

The amino acid compositions of the Pb proteins (histones) isolated by the different authors are compared in table XIV together with that of another parotid basic polypeptide (post-Pb protein) to be described later. Six amino acids (cystine, methionine, proline, threonine, tryptophan and valine) are not found or present in very low amounts. By flatbed isoelectric focusing a pI higher than 9.5 was determined [266]. The molecular weights, estimated after electrophoresis in gels containing sodium dodecylsulfate, ranged from 5.8–7.2 kdaltons [266]. The Pb proteins are *not phosphorylated* [17, 276].

Another basic protein with a lower pI than 9.5 was termed *post-Pb protein (PPb protein)* because it characteristically eluted from Bio-Gel

Table XIV. Molecular characteristics of parotid fluid histones [24], parotid basic (Pb) proteins [276] and human post-Pb (PPb) proteins [277]

	Histone			Pb-1[a]		Pb-2[a]	PPb
	1	2	3	a–b	d–e	c	
Amino acid residues per 1,000 residues							
Lysine	84	133	169	155	120	164	76
Histidine	178	254	319	259	207	225	186
Arginine	106	132	130	131	124	103	104
Aspartic acid (asparagine)	123	111	61	49	115	73	131
Threonine	4	0	0	2	2	2	0
Serine	79	86	78	57	66	105	46
Glutamic acid (glutamine)	88	37	40	56	43	91	91
Proline	42	1	0	2	2	3	26
Glycine	88	63	72	89	76	94	93
Alanine	7	28	26	42	35	41	+0
Isoleucine	2	0	0	1	1	2	0
Leucine	29	26	4	6	31	4	30
Tyrosine	92	101	74	79	112	56	126
Phenylalanine	73	30	28	41	31	44	78
Tryptophan[b]	0	0	0	0	0	0	0
Valine	0	0	0	3	2	0	0
Cystine	0	0	0	3	4	0	0
Methionine	0	0	0	0	0	0	0
Molecular weight, kdaltons	ND	ND	ND	5.8	7.2	6.1	8.3
pI	ND	ND	ND	>9.5	>9.5	>9.5	9.5
Phosphorylated	ND	ND	ND	–	–	–	+

[a] Postsecretory conversions transform the primary gene products Pb-1 and Pb-2 into Pb proteins a, b, c, d, and e.

[b] Not determined (destroyed by acid hydrolysis). ND = Not determined.

columns immediately after the Pb proteins [277]. It was further purified by gel filtration on Sephadex G-75 equilibrated with pH 3 ammonium formate. Post-Pb protein is biochemically and immunologically related to the Pb proteins as shown by its amino acid composition (table XIV) and sequence, partially elucidated for both proteins [277]. The content of the three basic residues (His, Lys, Arg) is a little less than in Pb proteins or histones, while the Asp (AsN) content is higher. Because of the similarity in size and certain differences between the amino acid sequences of Pb and PPb, any product-precursor relationship between the two proteins was considered unlikely [277].

Table XV. Molecular characteristics of histidine-rich acidic protein [146] and of tyrosine-rich acidic protein = statherin [459]

	Histidine-rich acidic protein	Tyrosine-rich acidic protein
Amino acid residues per 1,000 residues		
Aspartic acid (asparagine)	144	23
Threonine	0	23
Serine	73	47
Glutamic acid (glutamine)	89	233
Proline	26	163
Glycine	86	93
Alanine	0	0
Valine	0	23
Cystine	0	0
Methionine	0	0
Isoleucine	0	23
Leucine	31	47
Tyrosine	85	163
Phenylalanine	83	70
Lysine	81	23
Histidine	190	0
Arginine	111	70
Tryptophan[a]	0	0
Molecular weight, kdaltons	4.5	5.38
pI	7.04	4.22
Phosphorylated	+	+

[a] Not determined (destroyed by acid hydrolysis).

Other than Pb, post-Pb protein is phosphorylated [17]. A molecular weight of 8.3 kdaltons was estimated [277]. Upon cationic electrophoresis in urea-starch gel it trails behind the bands of Pb proteins which agrees well with its lower isoelectric point.

PPb protein is probably identical [415] to HRP 1, one of the four histidine-rich proteins *(HRP 1–4)* described by *Baum* et al. [33]. The principal amino acid residues of both PPb and HRP proteins are His, Asp/AsN, Tyr and Arg, and the molecular weights are also very similar (HRP: 5.8 kdaltons; PPb: 6–13 kdaltons). The single primary gene product HRP 1 is apparently modified by postsecretory conversions yielding HRP 2–4 [33, 415].

An even smaller histidine-rich phosphoprotein (mol. wt. 4.5 kdaltons) was isolated by *Hay* [146] from 13 liters of stimulated parotid saliva by anionic exchange chromatography. Histidine, asparagine and arginine were the principal amino acids of this *histidine-rich acidic peptide* (table XV). This phosphopeptide was shown to have a pI of 7.04 which would let it appear rather 'neutral' but compared with the very strong basicity of the other histidine-rich proteins it is certainly an acidic molecule. The acidic phospho-peptide has an especially high affinity for hydroxyapatite [146].

Another histidine-rich protein, identified in human parotid saliva by *Holbrook and Molan* [156] and shown by them to be particularly active in enhancing the glycolytic activity of salivary microorganisms, differs from the other histidine-rich proteins by its comparatively low content of aspartic acid (asparagine).

Tyrosine-Rich Protein (Statherin)

This acidic phosphopeptide was also identified and isolated by *Hay* [421] who termed it '*statherin*' (from the Greek verb stathero = I stabilize) because of its high capacity to prevent precipitation of calcium phosphate salts from supersaturated solutions. Although glutamic acid (glutamine) is the most frequent amino acid residue and although the content of proline equals that of tyrosine (table XV), the compound was appropriately labeled 'tyrosine-rich protein' since this aromatic amino acid otherwise occurs only in small quantities in the saliva-specific proteins. Tyrosine-rich protein is present in parotid saliva at a concentration of 2–6 μmol/l [421]. Its amino acid sequence was completely elucidated [459]. Statherin is composed of 43 residues and has a molecular weight of 5,380 daltons. One quarter of the residues is made up by the aromatic and another by the dicarboxylic amino acids among which the amide/acid ratio is 8:4. The relatively low pI of 4.22 is caused by the charged amino acid residues together with two phosphoserines.

Free Amino Acids

While in early reports exclusively dealing with whole saliva the test subjects had been asked to spit into receptacles [for references see 296], the first experiments separately investigating unstimulated parotid and sub-mandibular saliva by cannulation of the excretory ducts were performed in 1958 by *Rose and Kerr* [296]. The amino acids were separated by two-dimensional paper chromatography of ultrafiltrated samples (2 ml) and identified by the usual ninhydrin color reaction. Altogether 10 different amino acids were detected in this way. The sulfur-containing compounds (cystine and methionine) were absent throughout despite previous oxidation with hydrogen peroxide and ammonium molybdate of the samples to be analyzed. Four amino acids (glutamic acid, glutamine, glycine and serine) were shared by both secretions while the parotid constituents leucine, lysine, phenylalanine and tyrosine were absent from submandibular saliva; alanine and aspartic acid, present in submandibular secretion, were not found in parotid saliva. Both secretions revealed the presence of two other ninhydrin-positive substances, taurine (an amino acid with a sulfo- instead of a carboxyl acid group) and phosphoethanolamine.

The observed absence of ten naturally occurring amino acids cannot be taken as conclusive proof since the study was hampered by the circumstance that the two secretions were derived only from each one individual donor [296]. Additional amino acids were indeed found in another investigation of stimulated parotid and submandibular saliva from 3 male donors who were between 30 and 40 years old [31]. The amino acids in the salivas of these persons were studied by two-dimensional chromatography in three experiments conducted separately on 3 alternate days. The ninhydrin-positive spots were eluted and spectrophotometrically determined. Again, cystine and methionine were not found except in whole saliva where their concentration was very low. Parotid saliva showed very small amounts (0.1–0.2 mg/l) of only seven amino acids (aspartic, glutamic, alanine, glycine, phenylalanine, leucine and isoleucine) invariably detected in much higher amounts (up to 4 mg/l) in submandibular saliva. Here the most prominent substances were glycine, aspartic and glutamic acids, serine and alanine, while threonine, arginine, lysine, valine, phenylalanine, tyrosine, leucine and isoleucine were present mostly at somewhat lower levels. Only traces of proline were found in 1 individual. The number of amino acids detected totaled 14 different compounds, 12 of which were invariably found.

Still another amino acid, tryptophan, not previously reported for either human glandular saliva [31, 296], could be determined in normal parotid saliva collected from 33 persons by ultraviolet absorption techniques [392]. Tryptophan was accompanied by tyrosine, and while both were present in appreciable amounts (31 and 73 mg/l, respectively) in normal persons, their concentration was reduced in albinos. Since these two aromatic amino acids are involved in melanin formation by enzymatic oxidation to colored quinone-like condensation products, the result of *Zipkin* et al. [392] could be interpreted in terms of a lack of precursors but not necessarily of the oxidative enzymes (phenol oxidases such as tyrosinase). Other amino acids were not looked for [392].

Summarizing, it can be said that a mere three studies based on relatively few donors revealed the presence in human parotid and submandibular saliva of altogether 16 amino acids. Further extended investigations might disclose that all 20 naturally occurring amino acids can indeed be found although rarely in one single person. The occurrence of these compounds in saliva appears to follow a rather erratic pattern; it is unlikely that the major source of salivary amino acids derives from the breakdown of salivary proteins since proline, abundantly present in many salivary proteins, was also quantitatively one of the rarest freely soluble amino acids in saliva.

Free Carbohydrates

Carbohydrate in saliva is nearly exclusively protein-bound and non-dialyzable. Only small amounts of freely soluble, dialyzable carbohydrates can be measured which are thought to be enzymatic breakdown products from glycoproteins [109, 444]. Submandibular saliva with a higher proportion of glycoproteins indeed is richer in free sugars (30 mg/l) than parotid saliva (5 mg/l) [109, 111, 114]. Calculated per 100 mg protein, parotid saliva only contained 23 mg nondialyzable carbohydrate whereas the value for submandibular saliva was 43 mg [109]. Storage of submandibular saliva prior to dialysis enhanced the portion of dialyzable carbohydrate while the addition of enzyme inhibitors and storage in the cold lowered it [109].

While most of the free carbohydrate of parotid saliva was glucose whose concentration was related to serum glucose concentration [111, 114], galactose, mannose, fucose, hexosamines and sialic acid were additionally found in submandibular saliva [109]. Free sialic acid was also detected in stimulated parotid saliva [312] and small amounts of hexoses other than glucose, fucose or hexosamines could be demonstrated in submandibular saliva [405].

Hormones

It appears from the literature that mostly steroid hormones were studied in saliva. The favorite fluid was whole saliva while parotid saliva was only rarely analyzed [316, 372], predominantly by *Shannon* and his colleagues [for references see 316]. The majority of reports deal with the sex hormones, in attempts to assess hormonal status and gonadal function by a routine procedure using material that can be repeatedly obtained by stress-free, non-invasive techniques.

Estrogens [108, 148], androgens (testosterone) and two precursors, progesterone and 17α-hydroxyprogesterone, were studied in human saliva [108, 199, 332, 363, 371, 372], revealing close correlations between free hormone concentrations in matched samples of saliva and plasma [332, 363, 371, 372]. Small volumes of saliva (200 μl) are needed to determine hormone levels by radioimmunoassays [199, 332, 371, 372] or enzyme immunoassays [363], and the sensitivity of the tests may be as low as 0.5 pg [371]. It was concluded that determination of steroids in saliva could well replace determination in plasma. Testosterone concentrations showed marked diurnal variation, being highest in the morning and lowest at night [199, 371, 372]. The circadian rhythm of testosterone was even better defined in saliva than in plasma [371]. The level of free progesterone in saliva from normal women was at its peak in the late luteal phase and reached the lowest values in the follicular phase [371].

The investigation of free 17-hydroxycorticosteroids in parotid fluid and serum also disclosed an excellent correlation between the two sources [316]. Discharge of this adrenocortical hormone into parotid saliva was promoted by graded doses of ACTH gel, administered intramuscularly, and the results substantiated the premise that parotid fluid steroid levels may be employed to assess adrenocortical status.

Lipids

Compared to many other salivary constituents, reports on concentration and individual components of lipids (other than steroid hormones) in human saliva are rather scant. *Dirksen* [411] has summarized the available data and given a detailed account of the history of lipid research in saliva. Both total lipids and individual lipid classes (fatty acids, cholesterol, triglycerides, phospholipids) are represented in roughly equal amounts (20–30 mg/l) in submandibular as well as parotid saliva [443]. Higher values for total lipids in parotid saliva were reported in a different study [455] where no influence of flow rate could be demonstrated; the average concentrations ranged from 60 to 70 mg/l regardless of stimulation.

The major portion of salivary lipids (about one half) is made up by *fatty acids* which comprise saturated as well as mono- and polyunsaturated, exclusively even carbon chain fatty acids ranging in length from 10 to 22 carbon atoms. The proportion of *free* fatty acids, however, is much lower [455] and the distribution of the individual fatty acids varies between the two major salivary secretions. It may also be dependent on sampling conditions and donors. The acid spectrum analyzed for parotid and submandibular saliva by *Mandel and Eisenstein* [443] differs very much from that determined for parotid saliva alone by *Rabinowitz and Shannon* [455] who used a strongly selected group of donors (58 fasted men between 17 and 22 years of age).

While in the latter sample there was a strong preponderance of palmitic and stearic, as well as oleic acids (each amounting to roughly 30% of all fatty acids), the total fatty acids in a pool of parotid and submandibular secretions [443] had as their main component (40%) an acid with 20 carbon atoms and 5 double bonds (eicosapentaenoic acid, $C_{20:5}$). Another polyunsaturated fatty acid, docosahexaenoic acid ($C_{22:6}$), was second in amount (10%) and the concentration of docosatetraenoic acid ($C_{22:4}$) was still higher (8%) than those of the three saturated fatty acids, arachic ($C_{20:0}$), stearic ($C_{18:0}$) and palmitic ($C_{16:0}$) acids. In constrast, the proportion of unsaturated fatty acids in pure parotid saliva from young males [455] was very low (with the exception of oleic acid, $C_{18:1}$ cis) compared to that of the saturated acids whose chain lengths varied between 10 and 22 carbon atoms. Based on iron and DNA content, less than 2% of total lipids was attributed to blood and cellular contamination.

A number of additional organic acids were found in unstimulated whole saliva [465] but the sample was derived from only 4 male subjects between the ages of 20 and 25 years, and it is not improbable that bacterial contamination contributed to the reported spectrum. (Although no true lipids, the different organic acids are included here because of their relationship to the lower members of the series of fatty acids.) Besides four fatty acids (myristic, palmitic, stearic, and oleic) six other organic acids (lactic, hydroxyisocaproic, succinic, phenylacetic, hydroxyphenylacetic, hydroxyphenylpropionic) and a phenolic compound (2,6-di-t-butylcresol) were found but no relative amounts were stated. The presence of the phenolic derivative may be attributed to its use as an antioxidant in foodstuffs [411]. Pyruvic and citric acids were noted by others [225].

Cholesterol was present in parotid saliva in free and derivatized form and in a number of esters [455], representing 11 and 17%, respectively, of total lipids. In a different report 20 years earlier it had been suggested that whole human salivary mucin was in fact a glycolipoprotein containing 1–1.5% cholesterol on a weight basis. This, however, could not be confirmed in a later study, possibly due to differences in the organic solvent extraction procedures employed [for references see 411].

Lecithin occurred in parotid saliva at about the same, and *triglycerides* at twice the level of free fatty acids and cholesterol esters [455]. Only minor amounts were found of fatty acid methyl esters, mono- and diglycerides, as well as of phospholipids other than lecithin (phosphatidylcholine), namely, the phosphatidyl compounds of serine, inositol and ethanolamine, lysolecithin, phosphatidic acid, and sphingomyelin [455].

Cyclic Nucleotides

The presence of cyclic nucleotides (cyclic nucleoside 3′,5′-monophosphates) in human saliva was first demonstrated in 1971 by *Stefanovich and Wells* [338] who detected cyclic AMP (cAMP) in whole secretions. Cyclic nucleotides, first discovered in 1959, play an important role as 'second messengers' in protein biosynthesis and are also essentially involved in the secretion of α-amylase from the cephalic salivary glands (see article of *Chilla* in this volume). Whole and parotid saliva levels of cAMP and cGMP were found to equal those of serum [172, 173, 302] and to be dependent on stimulation. Gustatory stimulation during a meal [11, 213] or application of acid stimulants [302] significantly increased the amount of cAMP secreted per unit of time in whole [213] and parotid saliva [302]. Of the two cyclic nucleotides present in human parotid saliva, cAMP is the far more abundant, exceeding concentration and secretory rate of cGMP about 100-fold [11]. *Asakura and Kataura* [11] investigated cAMP and cGMP in the parotid saliva from 31 normal persons between 19 and 50 years, before and after stimulation with sour lemon drops. While in unstimulated secretions (flow rate 0.03 ml/min) the concentrations of cAMP (24 pmol/ml) and cGMP (0.3 pmol/ml) were both about 3-fold higher than in stimulated saliva (flow rate 0.52 ml/min), an inverse relation was found when the amounts secreted per minute were measured. Under the conditions of stimulation, both cAMP (3.8 vs. 0.64 pmol/min) and cGMP (0.04 vs. 0.008 pmol/min) were secreted at a 5-fold higher rate than in unstimulated saliva.

Cyclic nucleotides are also of pathognomonic value [11, 303].

Other Organic Components

A considerable variety of other organic components were described for human saliva but as most of them were only sporadically reported we will just enumerate them here for parotid, submandibular and whole secretions.

Parotid and Submandibular Saliva

Gustin, a zinc-containing, apparently slightly basic (cationic) protein with a molecular weight between 50 and 100 kdaltons was obtained from parotid saliva by gel filtration on Sephadex G-150 and further purification on DEAE-Sephadex A-50 and CM-cellulose [149]. The protein obviously did not contain any bound carbohydrate; with Coomassie blue it stained different (blue) from the glycoproteins (pink-violet) present in the same fraction. Gustin showed electrophoretic mobility in a pH 8.9 polyacrylamide gel.

The concentration of *urea* varies within the secretions from different glands [114] and is highest (280 mg/l) in saliva from minor (accessory) labial glands, and lowest (100 mg/l) in submandibular saliva [73]. Parotid saliva contained an intermediate amount (250 mg/l). The concentration of urea varies inversely with the rate of flow [312].

Of the small heterocyclic compounds several reports have been given on the purine derivative *uric acid* [195, 312, 392], mostly for parotid saliva. Measurements undertaken in 314 parotid saliva samples obtained from normal males (17–25 years) revealed that uric acid concentration (30–40 mg/l at the onset of stimulation) was only moderately decreased by extended stimulation, but the amounts secreted per minute were positively correlated with increasing flow rate [312]. Similar levels (25 mg/l) were reported by *Zipkin* et al. [392]. The salivary levels of urea and uric acid seem to be related to serum levels [392]. *Creatinine* is present in parotid saliva in minimal amounts [312]. For the determination of whole saliva creatinine a modified high-performance liquid chromatographic assay was developed, permitting to detect levels below 0.3 mg/l [284].

The sulfo β-amino acid *taurine* occurs in parotid and submandibular saliva [296].

Whole Saliva

The lipoprotein *thromboplastin* (tissue factor, factor III) was identified as the coagulant of normal human saliva [390]. The salivary tissue factor (STF) was related to cells and cell fragments present in mixed saliva. Centrifugation at 1,000 g reduced the cell count to zero, leaving roughly 20% of the initial STF coagulant activity in the supernatant, and virtually all STF activity was lost upon filtration of saliva supernatant fluid through filters of 0.2 μm pore size [390]. Other blood-clotting factors with analogues in saliva are pro-activator (factor VII), antihemophiliac globulin (factor VIII), Christmas factor (factor IX), and a platelet factor [for references see 114].

Variable but mostly low amounts (between 1 and 600 μg/l) were found of *choline, histamine,* and of several *vitamins* [for references see 225]. The latter comprise the group of B vitamins, B_1 (thiamine or aneurin), the B_2 complex (riboflavin, nicotinic, folic and pantothenic acids), B_6 (pyridoxine), B_{12} (cobalamin), and vitamins C (ascorbic acid), H (biotin) and K (menaquinone).

Inorganic Components

The quantitative and qualitative composition of salivary electrolytes determines pH and buffering capacity of saliva. Salivary pH, an important factor of intraoral environment, is dependent on the ratio between acids and their corresponding conjugated bases, e.g., between di- and monohydrogen phosphate. Ammonia [31, 220, 312] and carbon dioxide [82, 115, 191] are both present in saliva and their ratio also contributes to salivary pH. Although reports on measurements of salivary pH vary slightly [82, 115, 116, 191, 312, 342], they more or less agree on values not far from either side of the neutral point differing between 'resting' and stimulated secretions. Unstimulated saliva from the parotid and submandibular glands has a moderately acidic pH [82, 115] which rises upon stimulation, a change positively correlated with flow rate [82, 312]. While unstimulated parotid saliva had a pH of about 5.8, this value was increased to 7.4 following stimulation, and the shift towards alkalinity coincided with an increase in hydrogen carbonate output and a decrease of dihydrogen phosphate [82, 365]. In a comparative study of three different secretions of the human cephalic salivary glands, the increase in pH was found to be most marked in stimulated parotid saliva (pH 7.85–8.30 at flow rates of 1–3 ml/min), followed by sublingual saliva (pH 7.5–8.0 at flow rates of 0.01–0.1 ml/min) and submandibular saliva (pH 6.85–7.60 at flow rates of 1–4 ml/min), measured in 'normal volunteers' [341, 342]. In a different investigation the electrolyte compositions of parotid, submandibular and sublingual secretions were compared [73].

The electrolytes of human saliva comprise differently charged proteins and inorganic cations and anions whose concentrations are characterized by marked circadian rhythms in parotid [83, 116] and submandibular saliva [115]. The time of day at which sampling is performed is therefore of profound influence, and comparative data on concentrations of salivary electrolytes ought to be interpreted with caution unless they were determined in individual samples where all components are present with their relative amounts corresponding to a certain phase of the diurnal cycle, or unless saliva was collected at identical times from a sufficiently high number of donors. In unstimulated submandibular saliva, studied in separate specimens from 15 persons, a combination of a fundamental sine wave of 24 h and its first harmonic was found to fit the data in 164 of the 180 data cycles studied [115]. It is a common feature of most circadian rhythms in man that variables show one maximum and one minimum separated by a 12-hour interval, and that a closely fitting sine wave of 24 h returns to approximately the same value every 24 h [115]. The extent of circadian variation from maximum to minimum was about 40–50% of the mean value for most constituents of submandibular saliva. The changes in concentration due to circadian variation were likely to be least in the early afternoon but considerable variation between subjects in timing of rhythms was observed. It is interesting to note that the rhythms of salivary pH, flow rate, and inorganic and organic phosphate content coincided with the rhythm observed for intraoral temperature, with a high in the early morning (06.00 h) and a low in the late afternoon (18.00 h). While sodium and chloride concentrations followed a perfectly opposite rhythm (high at 06.00 h, low at 18.00 h), potassium exhibited a somewhat intermediate behavior, with low levels at 07.00 and 17.00 h, a minor peak at noon and a major one around midnight [115].

Cations

Monovalent Cations (Sodium, Potassium)

While sodium ion concentration in plasma (expressed as mEq/l) by far exceeds that of potassium ion, the opposite is true for unstimulated parotid saliva (table XVI) which resembles intracellular fluid in this respect [38]. Na^+ and K^+ concentrations are strongly influenced by stimulation which causes a sharp rise of salivary Na^+ and a very marked decline in salivary K^+ [82, 312] resulting in similar levels of both monovalent cations (table XVII). The diurnal rhythms discussed above are to be considered in this connection; the times for Na^+ and K^+ maxima and minima are very similar in parotid and submandibular saliva [115, 116] but almost exactly 12 h out of phase [83, 115]. Sodium is high when potassium is low, and vice versa. This was attempted to be explained in terms of an aldosterone rhythm dependent on posture and hence sleep-wakefulness cycles [115, 116]. The lower amplitude of the K^+ rhythm compared to that of the Na^+ rhythm could be expected, assuming the plasma aldosterone rhythm as the main causative factor, since aldosterone has a more pronounced effect upon sodium reabsorption by the salivary duct than it does on potassium secretion [83]. In unstimulated submandibular saliva, Na^+ content varied between 6 and 13 mEq/l and K^+ concentration between 8 and 14 mEq/l [115].

Divalent Cations

Only a portion of divalent cations (Me^{2+}) is found as free inorganic components in saliva; another portion is firmly attached to proteins where

Table XVI. Electrolyte (sodium, potassium) composition of *unstimulated* human parotid saliva (mean values)

Donors (n)	Na+ concentration mEq/l	K+ concentration mEq/l	Flow rate ml/min	Remarks	Reference
513	2.65	25.5–46.3	0.027	summer	317
527			0.042	winter	317
18–32	3.14 (n = 18)	29.7 (n = 29)	0.048 (n = 32)	students (morning, fasting)	38
35	2–8	25	0.03–0.11	'patients' (18–35 years old)	102
7	1.3	28.4			83

The values are scattered over a wide range owing to differences in number and age of donors, and collection procedure employed.

Me^{2+} may be essential constituents of enzymes, e.g. in the calcium-metallo-enzyme α-amylase.

Calcium was studied in saliva rather early [370] but implications of the ratio between its ionized and protein-bound fractions were only recognized later. The concentration of total Ca was found to be higher in unstimulated submandibular (2–8 mEq/l) than in unstimulated parotid saliva where it was present at a level of approximately 0.2–2.5 mEq/l [82, 83, 115, 328]. Studying ionized and total Ca in parotid saliva from 10 healthy males, *Maier* et al. [215, 216] found that with increasing flow rate the concentration of Ca^{2+} rose exponentially from 1.13 to 1.76 mEq/l forming a plateau at very high flow rates (2.5 ml/min). The remaining (protein and phosphate bound) calcium fraction was enhanced under the same conditions from 2.2 to 3.6 mEq/l. Concentrations of total and free ionic calcium were closely correlated with a ratio of 0.54 for Ca^{2+}/Ca total remaining nearly constant at all flow rates.

The other divalent cations of human saliva were less extensively studied, and with the exception of zinc [27, 149, 200] hardly any attention was given to Me^{2+} protein binding. *Magnesium* is present in saliva at very much lower levels than calcium [83, 328] and its concentration is inversely related to salivary flow rate [327]. Other trace metals of submandibular and parotid saliva are *iron* (both Fe^{2+} and Fe^{3+}), *copper* and *zinc* [327, 328]. The presence of *manganese* in sialoliths and whole saliva [328] seems of particular interest

Table XVII. Electrolyte (sodium, potassium) composition of *stimulated* human parotid saliva (mean values)

Donors (n)	Na$^+$ concentration mEq/l	K$^+$ concentration mEq/l	Flow rate ml/min	Remarks	Reference
125	64.41	18.15	1.18		317
18–32	21.1 (n=18)	28.1 (n=29)	0.57 (n=32)	students	39
6	22	8.0–10.5	1.10	children	168
22	29.8	21.8		children	223
35	8–40	25	0.2–0.5	'patients' (18–35 years old)	102
21	42.6	26.5	1.22		116
11	41.4	13.3	1.0	students (20–27 years old)	191
3 (?)	50.4	45.3		students (20–26 years old)	186

The values are scattered over a wide range owing to differences in number and age of donors, and collection procedure and type of stimulant employed.

since the discovery of the strongly Mn^{2+}-dependent enzyme arginase in this secretion [137]. Cu^{2+} could be identified in only 80% of cases [327]. *Cadmium* was found to be associated with zinc [200].

Several authors have devoted research to the presence of *zinc* in whole [27] and parotid saliva [149, 200]. Sephadex G-150 gel filtration of an ultrafiltrate of centrifuged mixed normal human saliva yielded three separate zinc-containing peaks. The first Zn peak of the elution profile (8% of total Zn) corresponded to proteins with molecular weights of 120 kdaltons and more; the second and third fractions eluting as closely neighboring peaks (20% of total Zn) most probably comprised low molecular weight peptides [27]. 72% of total Zn remained in the pellet obtained after centrifugation of whole saliva. There are several zinc-containing enzymes with molecular weights in the range of the first Zn-protein peak (alcohol dehydrogenase, EC 1.1.1.1; lactate dehydrogenase, EC 1.1.1.27; triosephosphate dehydrogenase, EC 1.2.1.12; glutamate dehydrogenase, EC 1.4.1.3). Of those enzymes only lactate dehydrogenase is known to occur in pure human saliva, but as whole secretion was investigated [27] the zinc-containing proteins (enzymes) may have been derived from bacterial contamination.

Similar results were obtained by investigation of parotid saliva also employing fractionation on Sephadex G-150 columns [149, 200]. The second peak of the elution profile, corresponding to proteins with apparent molecular weights ranging from 50 to 150 kdaltons, contained the main portion (68%) of the total amount of Zn applied onto the column [149]. *Langmyhr and Eyde* [200] determined the distribution and total content of cadmium (3.5 ppb), copper (88 ppb) and zinc (49 ppb) in the protein fractions of stimulated parotid saliva. Again the highest concentration of Zn was found in high molecular weight proteins where it was associated with Cd, while Cu was present in a relatively narrow range of proteins of intermediate molecular weight.

Anions

Halides

Among the halides, *chloride* is found in saliva at the highest concentration. One of the main physiological roles of this anion is the activation of α-amylase. Mean Cl^- levels between 17 and 22 mEq/l were observed in unstimulated parotid [82, 83] and submandibular saliva [115]. In both secretions Cl^- follows the same rhythm as Na^+; its concentration is highest in the early morning and lowest in the late afternoon. On the other hand, Cl^- (like K^+) levels are markedly reduced by stimulation of salivary flow [82]. At low flow rates (0.25 ml/min) the Cl^- concentration fell at once and continued to decline although at a lower rate. Higher flow rates (0.5 ml/min) resulted in an initial slight increase preceding concentration decrease, and a flow rate of 1 ml/min elevated Cl^- within the first 2 or 3 min to a value about 60% higher than that of unstimulated samples. The 'resting level' was reached again after 15 min. At any time after onset of stimulation, Cl^- concentration was directly related to flow rate [82]. The changes of Cl^- levels and those of Na^+ and HCO_3^- are reciprocally connected; an exchange mechanism between chloride and hydrogen carbonate operating at higher flow rates during passage of saliva down the salivary duct is discussed as an explanation for Cl^- levels being initially increased at high flow rates [82].

Fluoride, with very low saliva levels of approximately 5 μEq/l [114, 317] but important in caries control, *bromide* and *iodide* are the other three halides found in human saliva. The level of iodide is dependent on the capacity of the human salivary glands (similar to the thyroid gland) to concentrate this ion from blood [2, 64, 143, 203, 226]. Iodine is not organically bound in the salivary glands and is excreted as inorganic I^- [203]. Concentration of halides by salivary glands is determined by ionic size; thus Br^- with a much smaller ionic size than I^- is concentrated to a much lesser extent [2]. The ratio between the saliva and plasma concentrations of iodide (S/P ratio) and its relation to flow rate has been the object of extensive studies [64, 226]. It decreases with increasing salivary flow [143] and a similar relationship was found for other, non-halide anions of similar size, e.g., clinically administered pertechnetate [2, 143]. Other than in animal (mouse) salivary glands, no sex differences exist with respect to the iodide concentrating ability of the human parotid gland and the S/P ratio [203]. The relationship between S/P ratio for bromide and flow rate differs from that for the bigger anions owing to transport of Br^- from the acinar as well as from the duct cells of parotid gland [203].

Chloride and iodide are involved in enzymatic defense mechanisms against oral microorganisms to be discussed later.

Other Monovalent Anions

Hydrogen carbonate ('bicarbonate') acts as the conjugated base of carbonic acid and as such constitutes an important factor in the buffering capacity of body fluids. The major portion of H_2CO_3 is present as the anhydride CO_2. While unstimulated parotid saliva was shown to have a pH of 5.8 and a very low HCO_3^- concentration accompanied by pCO_2 values around 45 mm Hg, stimulation increased the hydrogen carbonate level from 1.0 up to 28 mEq/l resulting in elevation of pH to a value of 7.4 [82]. The stimulation-elicited increased HCO_3^- concentration was directly related to flow rate. The levels of pCO_2 in unstimulated saliva corresponded to the normal arteriovenous range of plasma but could not be calculated very accurately owing to equipment insufficiencies. Apparently they did not change significantly throughout the period of stimulation [82]. The human parotid gland possibly behaves different from the parotid glands of other species such as the dog, where the salivary HCO_3^- concentration was dependent on the pCO_2 of the blood; increase in pCO_2 was always accompanied by an increase in HCO_3^- [for references see 82]. The main effect of human salivary hydrogen carbonate possibly lies not so much in the participation of this anion in an intrinsic H_2CO_3/HCO_3^- buffering system (since stimulation does increase pH) but rather in providing a protective mechanism guarding against abrupt pH changes towards acidity provoked by extrinsic (bacterial) factors.

The salivary glands also secrete *thiocyanate* (SCN⁻) which is an essential constituent in the peroxidase-mediated bacteriostatic action of saliva. (The term 'rhodanide' found in the German literature is synonymous with thiocyanate.) Investigating stimulated parotid saliva from donors of different ages and smoking habits, *Azen* [16] found a variety of significant correlations between the parameters studied. The concentration of SCN⁻ was reduced as a linear response to flow rate (about 1 ml/min) but older persons and smokers had higher amounts of SCN⁻ in their saliva. In smokers a 3-fold higher average level of this ion (1.8 mEq/l) was observed compared to nonsmokers (0.6 mEq/l). A sex difference as previously reported [460] and characterized by significantly higher salivary SCN⁻ concentrations in males was not observed.

Phosphates

Salivary phosphate (orthophosphate), like calcium, can be divided into two categories, free ionic (inorganic) and protein-bound phosphate. Saliva contains a variety of phosphoproteins which were already described in detail; a considerable portion of phosphate exists in organically bound form. Inorganic phosphate (mean concentration 5.63 mmol/l) constituted about 71% of total phosphate (mean concentration 7.92 mmol/l) in unstimulated submandibular saliva [115]. Both fractions were governed by a similar but not entirely identical daily rhythm resembling that of intraoral temperature. A significant phosphate rhythm was also demonstrated for parotid saliva [83].

Since salivary inorganic orthophosphate comprises two differently charged anions, monohydrogen phosphate (HPO_4^{2-}) and dihydrogen phosphate ($H_2PO_4^-$) which form another buffering system, their combined concentration cannot be expressed in terms of mEq/l (unless the exact proportions of both ions are known) but is given in the dimensions mg/100 ml or mmol/l. A mean inorganic phosphate concentration of approximately 11 mmol/l was measured in unstimulated parotid saliva [82]. It was significantly reduced by stimulation, reached a stable level after 3 min and was not further influenced by prolonged stimulation. An inverse relation to all flow rates elicited (0.25–1.0 ml/min) could be observed. The finding that the concentration of HPO_4^{2-} in parotid saliva is rather constant regardless of pH and flow rate while the level of $H_2PO_4^-$ decreases [365] agrees well with the results of *Dawes* [82] and the observed rise in salivary pH after stimulation of secretion.

Salivary Defense Mechanisms

In human saliva, like in other external secretions, several defense mechanisms are effective which are directed against a variety of different agents such as allergens, viruses and bacteria. These protective mechanisms can be divided into enzymatic and nonenzymatic systems. The latter comprise immunoglobulin action and the effects of many saliva-specific proteins that are involved in protection of dental surfaces against potentially cariogenic bacteria. Another nonenzymatic protective mechanism provided by whole saliva shall only be mentioned in passing, namely the empirically encountered phenomenon that 'licking' is effective to some extent in stopping the bleeding of smaller wounds. This may be explained by some cellular components of whole saliva and by the presence in this fluid of a number of blood-clotting factors [114, 390] already mentioned. Anticoagulant warfarin therapy reduces the coagulating activity of the salivary tissue factor, thromboplastin [390].

The enzymatic defense mechanisms depend on the action of various salivary enzymes, namely, peroxidase, muramidase and α-amylase, on their appropriate substrates. Peroxidase exerts its bacteriostatic effects by means of reaction products originating from enzyme-substrate interaction, muramidase and amylase directly attack substances incorporated into the cell walls of certain bacteria.

Immunoglobulins

For a better understanding of immunoglobulin (Ig) action it is worthwhile to recall the basic structural features common to all Ig classes (fig. 4). A portion of roughly 105–120 amino acid residues extending from the hinge region up to the amino terminals of both H and L chains is very variable in its sequence. These so-called hypervariable regions are responsible for the specificity of an Ig molecule, creating certain steric configurations near the NH_2 terminal where antigen binding takes place by noncovalent combination. The molecule segments between hinge region and amino terminals are also known by the term Fab, for fragment, antigen binding. The universality of the different Ig classes consists in their pronounced ability to adjust to the requirements of specific antigen binding by changing the steric configuration of the hypervariable regions, tailored to fit different antigens. Thus a certain class of immunoglobulins will always consist of a population of slightly different molecules, depending on the antigens in response to which their synthesis was elicited.

The two carboxyl terminal homology regions of the H chains below the hinge region are constant in their amino acid sequence and were identified as mediators of biological activity [for references see 466]. This portion of an Ig molecule is termed Fc, for fragment, crystallizable, because it could be isolated in crystallized form after cleavage of the intact Ig near the hinge region. Mediation of biological activity involves several functions such as complement fixation, opsonization (enhancement of phagocytosis), skin fixation, attachment to macrophages, and membrane transport. The molecular mechanisms operating these biological effector functions have not yet been clearly defined, but the biological activities presumably result from the interaction of a portion of the Ig molecule and a membrane or enzyme receptor site [466].

Brandtzaeg et al. [57] have pointed out that, although secretory IgA (sIgA) is a minor component of salivary protein, the ratio of IgA to IgG in parotid saliva which is 570 times that of serum, emphasizes a selectivity inherent in the secretion of sIgA. This and the unique structure of the molecule (fig. 5) suggests that its presence in external fluids is of particular biological significance [57]. An intrinsic advantage of sIgA, enabling it to function more effectively in external secretions than monomeric Igs, seems to rest in its complex polymer structure (especially in the presence of bound secretory piece) assumed to confer to sIgA resistance against proteolytic degradation [for references see 57].

The general biological role of secretory Igs (11 S IgA and 19 S IgM) is believed to consist in furnishing polyvalent antibodies especially effective as a first line of defense against bacterial or viral antigens [57, 359]. As far as local hypersensitivity reactions against allergens or in autoallergic diseases of the secretory systems are concerned, much is left to learn about the Ig-specific mechanisms involved, but sIgA probably delays entry of antigens or allergens into mucous membranes [57]. In the secretions of the respiratory tract of hayfever patients suffering from ragweed allergy, IgA-type anti-ragweed antibodies could be identified but their biological relevance was not established [359]. Secretory fluid antibodies with specificities for non-living antigens commonly ingested with food possibly limit access of these antigens to the general circulation [359].

The implications of human secretory Igs in resistance to viral diseases are better understood. After settling on the mucosa at their portal of entry viruses undergo an initial stage of replication but their further fate runs different courses with different virus species. Some go on to produce systemic infection or disease (polio, ECHO, measles), others remain confined to their original site of infection (adenoviruses, influenza viruses, rhinovirus), blocked by secretory antibodies specifically directed against them [359]; glandular Ig synthesis seems to be effectively stimulated by infectious agents proliferating on an adjacent mucous membrane [57], e.g., the oral cavity linings. Prophylactic local immunization may strengthen the membranous line of defense against certain viruses by eliciting early secretion of Igs, particularly sIgA. In these cases secretory antibodies establish immunity by preventing colonization of mucous membranes. Patients with sIgA-type antibody deficiency are not immune to viral agents producing superficial local diseases [359] although in their secretions sIgA may be replaced by IgM or IgG. It has been found that local immunization produces better immunity to certain respiratory viruses (e.g., influenza and rhinovirus) than systemic immunization [359]. The mechanisms involved in virus elimination very likely include cooperation between secretory antibodies and phagocytic systems as well as other cellular functions. Additional inflammation may participate in the process of recovery by facilitating transudation of serum antibodies [359].

True bacteriolysis by salivary Igs lacks strong experimental evidence; in order to produce bacteriolysis, antibodies must have the capacity to fix complement. This property was found to be absent from sIgA but even if the combination of this antibody with oral bacteria does not result in lysis of bacteria, it may lead to the *in vivo* formation of long chains of growing streptococci or enhancement of bacterial phagocytosis. Both phenomena possibly contribute to rendering the indigenous microorganisms harmless and may in this way be involved in host resistance [57]. The finding that colostral antibodies to *E. coli* in combination with complement and muramidase did in fact produce bacteriolysis [57] may be of some importance also in the human oral cavity, muramidase being a regular constituent of salivary secretions; a complement factor not detected in parotid saliva occurs in whole saliva, probably originating from gingival exudation [57].

Saliva-induced aggregation of streptococci, both *in vitro* and *in vivo*, has been the object of many investigations since strong experimental evidence points to an important role of these ubiquitous oral bacteria in caries etiology [for references see 58, 59, 241, 435]. Application of an enzyme-linked immunosorbent assay revealed that human parotid saliva invariably contained IgA antibodies reacting with different serotypes of *Streptococcus mutans* [59]. Another investigation of salivary agglutinin and secretory IgA reactions with four different strains of streptococci disclosed, independently of blood group and secretor status, the ability of parotid saliva to induce aggregation particularly of two strains of oral streptococci, with a high degree of interindividual similarity [58]. Secretory IgA antibodies reacting with all four strains *(Streptococcus mutans, salivarius, mitis,* and *sanguis)* were identified in the subjects studied, but in contrast to parotid saliva some interindividual variation was noted for a few strains with submandibular/ sublingual saliva.

According to present knowledge, two mechanisms seem to operate in bacterial and antigen disposal. They are represented by the glycoprotein factors sIgA-type antibody and salivary (secretory) agglutinin [for references see 58, 241]. These components probably impair attachment of bacteria to intraoral epithelial cells and to hydroxyapatite (HAP) surfaces, either in conjugation or independently of each other [58]. Variations between individuals in salivary agglutination capacity might therefore be due to different specificities or mutual absence of these factors. With regard to microbial colonization of the oral cavity this would give an ecological advantage to microorganisms with distinct surface receptors [58]. Foreign agglutinins such as wheat germ agglutinin (WGA) which very specifically binds to N-acetylglucosamine (GlcNAc) may interfere with salivary aggregation of certain bacteria. Pretreatment of whole saliva with WGA inhibited aggregation of three *S. mutans* strains due to reversible binding of the wheat lectin to a salivary agglutination factor containing GlcNAc [241]. The inhibitory effect could be eliminated by restoration of GlcNAc.

The ability of sIgA to promote phagocytosis (opsonization) is not yet definitely and unequivocally established but according to *Tomasi* [359] it is very likely that IgA-type antibodies actually do opsonize, particularly through monocytes. This mechanism would probably mainly concern particles that have penetrated into submucosal layers where the majority of phagocytic histiocytes are located [359]. In any case the polymeric structure of sIgA and IgM furnishes these salivary immunoglobulins with particular features favoring the formation of polyvalent antibodies. Since antibody specificity rests in the sterically adjustable amino terminal sequences of the L chains, the presence in the dimeric sIgA of 8, and in the pentameric IgM of even 20 light chains may be of particular value.

Finally it should be mentioned that drug treatment may affect the amounts of oral IgA. Controversial findings were obtained when the influence of the antiepileptic compound phenytoin (diphenylhydantoin) on salivary IgA was studied. A positive effect could be noted in one report where phenytoin treatment resulted in a significant increase of sIgA secretion rate by the parotid glands of epileptic patients although the proportion of the immunoglobulin relative to total parotid protein secretion remained unchanged [331]. On the other hand, phenytoin-induced depression of salivary IgA was also noted [1] but this investigation was based on examination of unstimulated whole saliva.

Saliva-Specific Proteins

Constant interplay takes place in the human oral cavity between tissues, salivary proteins and colonizing microorganisms, mostly bacteria. The various interrelationships and the factors by which they are influenced are at present only partially understood. For many of the salivary proteins which continue to be detected and differentiated, clear-cut physiological roles remain to be established. The difficulties encountered in attributing functional significance and mechanisms of action to all these salivary constituents are best defined by quoting *Ellison* [415] who had to state that 'we may have too few functions and too many components'. For a detailed discussion of the problems looming in this rapidly expanding field of research, especially concerning caries etiology, the reader must be referred to the various contributions gathered in the volume edited by *Kleinberg* et al. [435]. We will try to give in this section a brief review of basic principles involved in dental environment control. Since the more important aspects of interaction between bacteria, oral structures and immunoglobulins were already covered in the preceding section, the following paragraphs will deal with the role of the unique saliva-specific proteins and the factors by which they are influenced.

There is a plethora of experimental evidence for the involvement of saliva-specific proteins in protection of teeth by covering them with a proteinaceous layer, the 'acquired dental pellicle'. Especially acidic, phosphorylated and sulfated proteins and glycoproteins were demonstrated in vitro to have high affinities for HAP [145, 146, 260]. Blood group reactive substances of saliva were identified as part of the in vivo formed dental pellicle [for references see 456]. The common principle governing the attachment to dental enamel of all these acidic proteins is most likely the interaction through ionic forces between the dental surface material with its high content of complex calcium phosphates (HAP) and the acidic protein moieties. Due to their low isoelectric points they carry a negative net charge at the physiological pH of saliva and are thus attracted by the positively charged calcium incorporated into HAP. Cationic basic proteins for which in vitro binding to HAP was also demonstrated may displace the cations in the hydration shell of HAP and in this way become adsorbed to the enamel surface [456]. HAP thus has the properties of an ion-exchanger.

The so-called calcium-reactive proteins include the glycoproteins of mixed saliva, the calcium-precipitable protein (CaPP) of submandibular secretion, the major sublingual glycoprotein and statherin. They all are characterized by a high affinity for calcium and are capable of preventing or delaying precipitation of calcium phosphates from supersaturated solutions such as saliva [145, 146, 422]. These salts are thus kept available for incorporation into dental enamel. Saliva-specific proteins identified as HAP-binding components comprise statherin, the parotid phosphoproteins (Pr proteins), the histidine-rich (pI 7) acidic peptide, calcium-reactive acidic glycoproteins, and both mucous acidic submandibular and parotid basic glycoprotein [for summary and references see 415].

The protein layer covering the dental surfaces affords no permanent protection since it is subject to degradation by masticatory action and attack by oral bacteria. Acquired pellicle is the matrix to which oral bacteria become attached, thus initiating the formation of dental plaque. Several mechanisms have been proposed for this process. They were summarized as follows. After formation of the pellicle the more negatively charged bacterial surface interacts with the pellicle which allows diverse molecules on the bacterial surface to approach the salivary polymers. In a third phase molecules with specific affinities to each other form tighter bonds and initiate formation of the attached plaque [457]. The interbacterial spaces contain both bacterial and salivary polymers [408]; experimental evidence points to the possible role of salivary BGRS of various antigenic specificities in bacterial colonization of teeth, suggesting that they may serve as receptor molecules for bacterial attachment [131].

The conditions under which bacteria transcend from the initial rather innocuous aggregation stage to demineralization of the dental surfaces have been the object of many studies [for references see 435]. The intact acquired pellicle which has to be penetrated as a first step was shown in in vitro experiments to form a membrane permeable to ionic transport [114, 391]. Salivary pellicles artificially produced on pressed disks of HAP displayed ionic permselectivity, i.e. ionic transport is slower than that of neutral molecules [391]. This would still permit in vivo ionic exchange by HAP; the physical properties of the proteinaceous membrane may also act to inhibit caries development since enamel subsurface demineralization by *S. mutans* was significantly reduced by pretreatment of teeth with saliva for 7 days [391].

The main factor controlling integrity of the dental pellicle apparently is salivary pH. Low pH values caused by metabolic products of bacteria will result in a decrease of negative net charge of the anionic saliva-specific proteins and diminish therefore the ionic binding forces between the anionic protein moieties and their HAP counterparts. An acidic environment also favors the proteolytic activity of bacterial [80] and fungal enzymes [130]. The observation that a wide range of anionic parotid saliva proteins, particularly the proline-rich proteins, were prone to extensive proteolytic degradation by *S. sanguis* [80] is of special interest in this connection. Exposure of denuded enamel to bacterial action will then facilitate demineralization leading to the formation of cariogenic lesions. Salivary pH and buffering capacity of stimulated saliva are thus of paramount importance, constituting a further defense mechanism involved in host resistance. The devastating effects of xerostomia regarding dental decay are well known. The overall effect of saliva has been defined as the capacity to limit pH drop and accelerate the rise [431]. Several substances exerting divergent influences on salivary pH have been identified, for instance sialin, a tetrapeptide of the sequence Gly-Gly-Lys-Arg, which is a major 'pH rise factor' in saliva; its content of both lysine and arginine enables it to produce base over a broad pH range [436]. Ammonia, released by the enzymatic action on urea of certain caries-suppressive bacteria *(Enterobacter* sp., *Proteus mirabilis, E. coli)* acting as antagonists of streptococci and lactobacilli, also contributes to maintenance of sufficiently high salivary pH levels. It was found that dental caries-inactive persons usually showed high salivary urease activities while caries-active patients showed less [426].

On the other hand, acid production by glycolysis of other bacteria (streptococci, lactobacilli) runs counter to these pH elevating mechanisms. Interesting enough the main end product of human protein metabolism, urea, is again involved in these antagonistic effects. Urea is utilized as a major nitrogen source by the salivary microorganisms and was identified as one of the low molecular weight factors enhancing glycolysis [427]. Another factor promoting bacterial glycolysis was subsequently isolated and characterized as a small basic peptide (mol. wt. 3 kdaltons) with the principal amino acids lysine, histidine and arginine [156]. Due to the constant synthesis of such 'pH drop factors' by the human and microbial organisms countering the action of host resistance mechanisms, inhibition of acid-producing glycolysis is not easy to attain. The most important factors still are proper oral hygiene and sensible dietary habits. In this connection the observation should be mentioned that nuts and cheese, but not apples, greatly reduced salivary pH changes [431]. Sialin may be present in cheese, and dietary stimulants of saliva which are not themselves acid (celery, raw carrots) have given promising results [457]. Attempts to supplement glycolytic substrates such as sucrose with other carbohydrates possibly interfering with sucrose degradation in human saliva have failed. Addition of xylitol to mixtures of sucrose and saliva both under aerobic and anaerobic conditions did not succeed in inhibiting sucrose degradation by commensal bacteria [211].

There is thus in the oral cavity a delicate balance between several microbial and salivary gland-specific metabolic influences. Saliva-specific proteins, although playing an important role in host defense, are only part of the factors controlling dental integrity. The protective pellicle formed by them on the dental surfaces provides by no means a durable shield; it must permanently be newly acquired to combat the lifelong processes of abrasion and decay which are accelerated by poor or faulty oral hygiene.

Salivary Peroxidase

Salivary peroxidase is the enzymic component of two similar antibacterial (bacteriostatic rather than bacteriolytic) defense mechanisms utilizing different ionic factors besides hydrogen peroxide as a substrate. The ionic components are thiocyanate on the one hand and halides on the other. The two principles can be characterized as a lactoperoxidase-thiocyanate-H_2O_2 system and as a myeloperoxidase-halide-H_2O_2 system. Both apparently do not contribute directly to caries control but probably function by limiting the extent of bacterial action. Comparison of several species revealed that the requirements of effective antibacterial action of the thiocyanate-dependent system are only fulfilled in human and guinea pig saliva [141].

Thiocyanate-Dependent Lactoperoxidase System

The existence of an antibacterial principle in human saliva inhibiting the growth of microorganisms such as *Lactobacillus acidophilus* had been known for several decades. Its physicochemical characteristics remained in the dark until 1959 when experimental evidence was presented that this system which was then termed 'bactericidin' comprised two components, one of which was heat-labile and nondialyzable while the other was heat-stable and dialyzable [for references see 185, 329]. Subsequent studies disclosed that the latter component was thiocyanate (SCN⁻) ion [for references see 329] whereas the former was identified as a peroxidase [185]. Corroboration of this conclusion was obtained by the observed inhibition of the antibacterial salivary system by catalase, an enzyme competing with peroxidase for H_2O_2 substrate [185]. Since peroxidase purified from bovine milk (lactoperoxidase) could replace the heat-labile fraction and since it was further shown that salivary gland and milk peroxidase are very similar enzymes [329], this bacteriostatic, peroxidase-dependent principle retained the name lactoperoxidase-thiocyanate-H_2O_2 system. Halides can replace SCN^- only when added in amounts exceeding normal salivary concentration [185]. Horseradish peroxidase is unable to oxidize SCN^- [268].

Several reaction products derived from the oxidation of thiocyanate were suggested as active bacteriostatic principles. One of those was identified by *Oram and Reiter* [268] as $S(CN)_2$ (sulfur dicyanide), together with a number of other intermediary reaction products, OCN^- (cyanate), sulfite and 'compound 235'. Addition of pure sulfur dicyanide to bacterial cultures inhibited growth in the same way as the complete lactoperoxidase-thiocyanate-dependent system. The final products of lactoperoxidase-mediated oxidation of SCN^- by H_2O_2 were found to be sulfate, CO_2 and NH_3. The 'compound 235', so-called because of its high absorption at 235 nm, was not identidal with $S(CN)_2$ but both were reduced by resistant strains. They may be structurally related [268] and act as electron acceptors for an $NADH_2$-sulfur dicyanide oxidoreductase present in resistant strains [268]. In susceptible streptococci the intermediates of SCN^- oxidation interfered with glycolysis by completely inhibiting the activity of hexokinase and partially of glucose-6-phosphate dehydrogenase and aldolase.

Another dialyzable inhibitory compound, hypothiocyanate ($OSCN^-$) was identified in a different study [for references see 447]. The substance exerted its effect by blocking glucose transport through bacterial membranes. *Dogon and Amdur* [92] reported the presence of two different SCN^--dependent antibacterial systems in saliva, one of which was the previously described lactoperoxidase-mediated system. The other principle was nonperoxidative, functioned anaerobically as well as aerobically and was not inhibited by catalase. Both systems differed in the reaction products created, although cyanate [268] and hypothiocyanate were probable intermediates. Whereas the peroxidative system converted thiocyanate to a volatile product which had hypothiocyanate, hydrocyanic and cyanic acids as possible precursors, the nonperoxidative system involved formation of a nonvolatile product and was further distinguished by the absence of sulfite and sulfate as the final products of the reaction.

Halide-Dependent Myeloperoxidase System

An antibacterial effect of myeloperoxidase, a halide such as iodide, bromide or chloride ion, and H_2O_2 was described by *Klebanoff* [183, 184]. The system could be inactivated by heating or enzyme inhibitors such as HCN or NaN_3, acted against *E. coli* or *L. acidophilus* and was most active at acid pH values. Addition of hydrogen peroxide was not necessary with the lactobacillus since it was generated by the microorganism itself. The optimum of the reaction at pH 5.0 suggests for it a role as defense mechanism particularly under conditions where salivary acidity pervails. Leukocytes present in the oral cavity were the probable source of the myeloperoxidase operating in the system, and the most potent halide was I$^-$, followed in activity by Br$^-$ and Cl$^-$, in this order, while F$^-$ was ineffective [184]. Patients without any peroxidase activity in the leukocytes which normally contain myeloperoxidase and concentrate iodine, are sensitive to infections [for references see 192].

Although lactoperoxidase could substitute for myeloperoxidase, the presence of the latter component was required for full activity of the system [184]. On the other hand, I$^-$ potentiated the antibacterial effect of lactoperoxidase [183, 184] suggesting a synergistic relationship between the two enzymes [192]. The coincidence between iodine concentrating ability and peroxidase activity in salivary glands is rather interesting in this connection; peroxidase may function in the transport of iodide through the cell membrane [192].

Iodination of the bacteria by the myeloperoxidase-iodide-H$_2$O$_2$ system most likely involved labile intermediates of iodide oxidation rather than more stable end products of oxidation such as iodine [183]. More recent research suggested the generation of oxygen singlets as the active principle of the myeloperoxidase-halide-dependent system [for references see 447].

In conjugation with a halide (I$^-$, Br$^-$, Cl$^-$) both myelo- and lactoperoxidase also form a potent virucidal system which was shown by *Belding* et al. [35] to be effective against polio and vaccinia virus, especially at low pH values. This peroxidative system may be functioning in the host defense against certain viral infections of the oral cavity. The synergistic effect between myelo- and lactoperoxidase in the oxidation of halides which was discussed [183, 184, 192] could well be of special importance in this connection.

Muramidase, Amylase

Muramidase (lysozyme) activity in human saliva was reported in 1922 by *Fleming* [122] along with his discovery of this enzyme. Using sediment-free secretions of the individual salivary glands it was found that muramidase titers in the mixed secretions of the submandibular and sublingual glands were considerably higher than in parotid saliva [153]. The same authors reported competitive inhibition of parotid muramidase activity by a 'mucopolysaccharide component' (BGRS?) isolated from submandibular/sublingual saliva and suggested the possibility that diminished quality or quantity of salivary 'mucopolysaccharide' and/or an abnormally high parotid muramidase titer could play a role in the etiology of ulcerative gingival disease.

In contrast to the other salivary defense mechanisms discussed above, muramidase brings about genuine lysis of the microorganisms (at least in mammalian cell systems) since it directly attacks substances incorporated as highly cross-linked macromolecules into the cell walls of certain bacteria using them as substrates for enzymatic hydrolysis. The preferred substrate is the cell wall peptidoglycan polymer (for description of the enzymatic mechanism, cf. the section on muramidase in this chapter). The primary effect of the lytic enzyme on bacteria consists in an initial rapid interaction with the microbial membrane which involves leakage of electrolytes and smaller organic molecules; in contrast to mammalian cell systems gross lysis with release of macromolecules (DNA, proteins) does not necessarily follow [453]. The rapid kinetics of release of ions and low molecular weight substances is quantitatively correlated with loss of cell viability, usually referred to as cell 'killing' [for references see 453]. Whereas the peroxidase-dependent bacteriostatic mechanisms probably act by immitting into bacteria poisonous reaction products of halide or thiocyanate oxidation, the bacterio-semilytic mechanism of salivary muramidase seems to obey an opposite pattern by depletion of bacterial cells of vitally essential ions and smaller organic molecules. An extended discussion of the problems and possible pathways of bacteriolytic muramidase activity in the salivary medium was given by *Pollock* et al. [453].

Another, very specific, bacteriolytic mechanism could be attributed to a different salivary enzyme, α-*amylase*, when it was found that saliva was a powerful and specific inhibitor of *Neisseria gonorrhoeae* [236]. Other species of this genus which were also tested were insusceptible to treatment with saliva. Amylase, extracted from parotid saliva and hog pancreas, was strongly inhibitory to gonococci and was thus identified as the active antigonococcal principle of saliva. The enzyme was assumed to act on the outer cell wall rather than passing into the gonococcus, a possible target for hydrolytic action being the polysaccharide component of the lipopolysaccharide moieties [236]. The difference observed in the susceptibilities of various *Neisseria* strains suggested that the structure of the gonococcal lipopolysaccharide is different from that of other, commensal, *Neisseria* species and/or that the integrity of these moieties is particularly important to the gonococcus *N. gonorrhoeae* [236].

Saliva as a Diagnostic Tool

Salivary Changes in Disease

Cystic Fibrosis

Cystic fibrosis (mucoviscidosis), a not uncommon congenital disease in Caucasians, is inherited as an autosomal recessive trait. It is clinically characterized as generalized dysfunction of the exocrine glands leading to inspissation of secretory products and thus deficiencies in vital body functions. Salivary changes in cystic fibrosis homozygotes are well studied but recognition of the heterozygous carriers of the mucoviscidosis allele, e.g., by measuring salivary constituents, has so far been rather unsuccessful [for review see 28].

The salivary changes prominent in cystic fibrosis (CF) patients include calcium [395, 396, 401, 445], sodium [445], protein [395, 396, 417], amylase [409, 417, 446], acid and alkaline RNase [28, 409], hypersecretion in parotid [28, 395, 396, 401, 445] and submandibular saliva [402, 404, 409, 446]. *Mayo* et al. [446] observed in the submandibular saliva of children with CF also the increased secretion of an acid phosphatase-containing fraction and an unidentified protein with a pI of 7.1 which was already mentioned in the section on submandibular salivary glycoproteins. The increased calcium and protein levels of CF saliva were held responsible for the formation of insoluble precipitates of calcium-phosphoprotein complexes, leading to turbidity of parotid and submandibular secretions upon cold exposure [395, 396, 401, 402, 404]. The parotid saliva from healthy persons and from CF patients differed in this respect since the turbidity forming at an elevated temperature (37°C) was only observed in calcium-rich specimens and was stable (irreversible) in the CF saliva, although it could be prevented by addition of EDTA [395].

Electron microscopy of calcium phosphate precipitated from submandibular CF saliva revealed that the initially observed amorphous calcium phosphate globules transformed on standing in vitro to stellar clusters of HAP crystals [402]. The calcium-phosphoproteins obtained from centrifuged pellets of cold-induced turbid saliva were found to comprise proline-rich proteins and a calcium-precipitable protein [396]. *Boat* et al. [404] purified and characterized this phosphoprotein (CaPP) from CF submandibular saliva and found it not to be different from the normal salivary CaPP (cf. section on submandibular salivary glycoproteins). The phosphate could be removed by treatment with alkaline phosphatase. Formation of insoluble complexes between calcium and a variety of proteins with high affinities for this metal in CF results in obstruction of acinar lumina and small ducts of the salivary glands [401, 404].

Age- and sex-dependent differences between the secretion in CF of amylase and total protein were noted by *Gillard* et al. [417], emphasizing the importance of age- and sex-matched controls in all studies of salivary composition. All hypersecretors were CF patients and were in the 14- to 24-year age group. While CF males were hypersecretors only up to an age of about 10 years, female CF patients exhibited elevated amylase levels in their saliva at all ages up to 30 years.

Electrolyte abnormalities in the saliva of CF patients may result from the action of an ATPase inhibitory factor present in saliva and inhibiting various components of this enzyme in the ducts of the salivary glands [410]. Ultrafiltrated CF saliva decreased the portion of ouabain-sensitive ATPase by 16% compared with filtrated control saliva [410]. It was concluded from these experiments that a factor in CF children's saliva interferes with active cation transport as a result of inhibition of one or more components of the ATP hydrolyzing enzyme system. Similarity of this factor with the ciliotoxic factor identified by other investigators in serum and saliva of patients with CF was suggested [410]. Inhibition of the oyster ciliary beat had been ascribed earlier to an enzymatic factor identified as amylase [412]. Addition of heparin to serum or saliva from CF patients complexed and precipitated amylase from CF saliva and reversed the inhibitory effect on cilia. Restitution of CF saliva with the enzyme or addition of purified parotid amylase from CF children to serum of normal subjects again resulted in inhibition of ciliary beat [412]. The phenomenon may be due to the increased concentration of amylase in the saliva of hypersecretors or to an unknown modification of the enzyme molecule secreted by patients with CF.

Unfortunately there are no such obvious differences to be found between the salivary gland secretions of 'normal' persons and heterozygous carriers of the CF allele. If the latter could be identified with certainty, the risk of giving birth to a child with CF could be calculated and genetical counsel could be given to the parents who are phenotypically devoid of any symptoms. The finding that in parotid saliva of 11 children with CF 'fast isoamylases' could be identified by alkaline PAGE in 10 cases, while an appropriate control group showed these components in only 2 instances, prompted the attempt to develop a screening test for heterozygous carriers of the disease by utilizing 'fast isoamylases' as markers [91]. Fast isoamylases are amylase isoenzymes not always found in parotid and submandibular saliva and characterized by their greater anodal mobility compared to that of the constantly observed basic pattern consisting of 6 isoamylases [6, 7, 75]. After preliminary studies in 16 parents of CF children had yielded promising results [91] the project had to be abandoned by us since subsequent extended investigations of a large number of heterozygous CF carriers failed to substantiate a significant correlation between CF heterozygosity and the occurrence of fast isoamylases.

More promising results were reported by *Bardoń and Shugar* [28] who found, after investigation of 29 CF children and 45 CF heterozygotes, that 73% of the latter showed in their mixed saliva 3–5 times higher activities of acid- and heat-stable alkaline RNase than controls. CF homozygotes had increased RNase levels [409] in 62% of cases [28]. The purified alkaline RNase of both homo- and heterozygotes also hydrolyzed double-stranded RNA at twice the rate observed in 'healthy' controls [28]. The level of RNase activity was independent of the flow rate.

Chronic Pancreatitis

A safe diagnosis of chronic pancreatitis (cP) is still largely dependent on the application of the time-consuming and expensive pancreozymin-secretin test, restricted to greater gastroenterologic centers. Since several morphological and physiological aspects indicate that the pancreas and the parotid are similar glands [94, 263], there have been attempts to develop a fast, cheap and reliable screening test for cP utilizing compository changes of parotid secretion. Thus it was found that secretion of amylase was reduced in cP patients [325, 385] whereas acute pancreatitis was accompanied by increased amylase levels [325]. Basal secretion rates, too, were diminished in cP although the volume of stimulated parotid saliva did not differ between balanced groups of healthy persons and cP patients [87]. All these attempts in which changes of single parameters were observed have more or less failed, since the same changes may also be found in other diseases or physiological disorders.

Simultaneous evaluation of a variety of parameters seems therefore better suited for a cP screening test. *Kakizaki* et al. [169] proposed a test for the diagnosis of pancreatic diseases on the basis of findings from animal and human studies. These investigations had disclosed diminutions in volume, maximal hydrogen carbonate and amylase content concomitant with pancreatitis and other pancreatic diseases. The authors claimed that pilocarpine-stimulated parotid saliva output of 48 persons with pancreatic disorders, as well as its maximum hydrogen carbonate concentration and amylase content were significantly lower than those of 82 patients with nonpancreatic disorders. An abnormal saliva test was found in 83.3% of patients with pancreatic disorders. Comparison with the pancreozymin-secretin test made in 44 subjects (each 22 with pancreatic and nonpancreatic disorders) with regard to diagnostic reliability indicated an accuracy of 88.6% of the abnormal parotid saliva test for the diagnosis of pancreatic disorders. The corresponding figure for the pancreozymin-secretin test was only 66% [169]. These results were partially confirmed using other stimulation procedures, and partially debated [for references see 201].

Studying 31 patients with chronic relapsing pancreatitis and 31 healthy controls matched for sex and age, *Lankisch* et al. [201] were unable to confirm the positive results reported by the Japanese group [169]. Diagnosis of cP was established by means of the pancreozymin-secretin test. The parotid saliva test failed to detect cP in 48–87% of the patients examined. None of the parameters measured was statistically different from the controls; the most valuable parameter was HCO_3^- output which was diminished in 52% of patients. The value of abnormal parotid saliva composition, at least in the diagnosis of cP, thus remains doubtful.

Tumors of the Salivary Glands

Diagnostic attempts concerning tumorous changes of the human salivary glands have repeatedly been undertaken, but present knowledge in this field does not by a long way encourage replacement of histologic or cytologic examination of tissue samples. Although many differences between the compositions of secretions or homogenates of healthy and tumor-affected human parotid glands were noted, these pioneer investigations suffer partly from low numbers of patients examined and partly from the rather unspecific changes observed. Extended studies seem indicated to improve this situation, and comparative investigations of a combination of characteristics, for instance altered or newly encountered enzyme activities, qualitatively and quantitatively different electrophoretic patterns, and changes in the composition or levels of specific proteins, should be conducted in larger numbers of patients and controls. Even if in this way more reliable information could be obtained on clearly defined patterns of tumor-induced salivary changes, it remains doubtful if such data would be superior to the well-established histologic examination procedures, not only in accuracy but also in time required for making a diagnosis. However, biochemical studies could be of corroborative value.

Salivary changes observed in a number of parotid tumors include the appearance on gel electrophoretograms of additional protein bands due to membrane damage caused by cystadenolymphoma and parotid carcinoma which facilitates transudation of serum proteins into parotid saliva [100], decrease of protein and muramidase content but unaltered IgA levels in cystadenolymphoma [101] and pleomorphic adenoma [103], and diminished flow rates in malignant carcinoma [104], probably owing to tumor growth obstructing salivary ducts. On the other hand, parotid protein, sIgA and muramidase concentrations were increased in malignant carcinoma while benign carcinoma showed opposite changes in these three parameters. Based on the results obtained in 7, 12, and 28 patients it was concluded that the pattern of changes in protein, muramidase and IgA content permitted differentiation between pleomorphic adenoma, cystadenolymphoma and parotid malignoma [104].

The presence of malignant parotid tumors was also accompanied by an increase of cGMP in parotid saliva over the levels of healthy persons and by a simultaneous decrease of cAMP [11]. Measurement of ionic constituents revealed an iron deficiency in saliva concomitant with parotid mixed tumors [327].

Reports on salivary changes accompanying neoplasms of other glands are rare. The increased activity of acid phosphatase in parotid saliva of patients with untreated metastatic prostatic cancer was not considered of diagnostic value for the early stage of this disease [154].

Non-Tumorous Diseases of the Salivary Glands

Sialadenosis, sialadenitis, parotitis and Sjögren's syndrome were already discussed in detail in the other contributions to this volume. These non-tumorous diseases of the salivary glands of the head cannot be safely diagnosed biochemically although some of them are accompanied by characteristic salivary changes.

The typical increase of K^+ and decrease of Na^+ in parotid saliva of *sialadenosis* patients was first observed by *Rauch* [287] and since then confirmed in several investigations [40, 104, 367]. The measurement of organic salivary constituents, however, does not yield such clear-cut results. The values for protein and amylase content as well as flow rate, although showing considerable variations, were all in the range determined for normal parotid saliva [40, 76]. Based on measurements of flow rate and enzyme activities, *Skurk* et al. [326] distinguished between two types (A and B) of human sialadenosis which were not related to neurogenic or endocrine forms of this disease. The report lacks histological verification of the diagnosis. Type A was characterized by much reduced flow rates of 'resting' parotid saliva, compared to controls, and by increased protein concentrations and considerably higher activities of the enzymes amylase, kallikrein and muramidase in unstimulated secretion. The specific activity of the latter two enzymes was significantly elevated and remained high during subsequent stimulation. Type B exhibited normal unstimulated flow rates and protein concentrations but significantly reduced enzyme activities. Stimulation enhanced these changes, the flow rate being reduced together with enzyme activities except kallikrein. It was found possible to distinguish between type B of sialadenosis and chronic parotitis by 'resting' amylase secretion per minute and stimulated muramidase secretion per minute. Pending confirmation of these results it remains to be studied whether the A and B types of sialadenosis are related to the morphologically distinguishable dark, light or mixed forms of sialadenosis (cf. *Chilla*, this volume).

The inflammatory processes in *parotitis* were reflected by a number of changes that could be attributed to damaged parotid parenchyma, acini and membranes. Thus flow rate reductions in adults [40, 326] were paralleled by decreased enzyme (amylase, muramidase) and protein levels [107, 326]; response to stimulation was abolished [40]. Chronic parotitis in children was accompanied by increased muramidase and kallikrein secretion [326]. Electrolyte changes were characterized by elevated salivary levels of sodium [40] and magnesium [327] while the concentration of zinc was reduced [327]. The increased permeability of membranes facilitated transudation of albumin and other proteins from serum as shown by the higher albumin content of parotid saliva in parotitis [107] and by the appearance on electrophoretograms of several additional protein bands [100]. *Mandel* [442] documented the dramatic changes in salivary protein composition that accompanied an acute flare-up of chronic recurrent parotitis. On the first day of recurrence immense increases of total protein, lactoferrin, muramidase, albumin, 7 S IgA, IgG, IgM and transferrin were noted, owing to increased leakage from serum into saliva caused by the inflammatory process. This was followed by at first sharp (on day 5 after onset) and then gradual decline until after about 80 days normal levels were reached again. *Sialadenitis* studied in 12 patients was characterized, similar to malignant carcinoma, by reduced flow rates and increased levels of sIgA, muramidase and protein [104].

Of the various autoimmune diseases in man, *Sjögren's syndrome* afflicts the salivary glands in whose secretions elevated amounts of IgM were found to be a diagnostic criterion [118]. The syndrome is occasionally accompanied by other diseases with a similar etiology, not affecting the salivary glands, e.g., progressive systemic sclerosis [for references see 118] and rheumatoid arthritis [95], where similar changes in various Igs could be observed [95,

118]. Increased levels of IgM and IgA were found in 11 out of 17 patients with progressive systemic sclerosis [118], and IgA as well as IgM rheumatoid factors were present not only in serum (where their levels were increased) but also in saliva of patients with rheumatoid arthritis and Sjögren's syndrome [95]. A relationship between the two diseases was also apparent by the parallel changes in uric acid content of parotid saliva [392]. The observed decrease ought to be regarded with caution since salicylates, often used in the treatment of arthritics, may reduce blood levels of uric acid [392]. Apart from changes concerning immunoglobulins, increases were noted in Sjögren's syndrome for cGMP [11], potassium and calcium [385] while sodium and amylase levels were diminished [385]. Calcium reabsorption by the duct epithelia was disturbed in glands with the syndrome [385]. On the other hand, *Benedek-Spät* [40] reported reduced 'resting' potassium and stimulated sodium levels in the saliva of Sjögren's syndrome which was also distinguished from normal salivary glands by lowered flow rates.

Other Diseases

The possible contribution of *diabetes mellitus* to sialadenosis was already discussed elsewhere in this volume. Possible correlations between the function of the salivary glands and this disease were noted rather early [for references see 364]. *Varletzidis* et al. [364] reported significantly higher amylase activities, compared to 57 controls, in the parotid saliva of 112 diabetics, regardless of insulin or antidiabetic tablet treatment. Sex- and age-specific differences claimed by *Vogt and Zahl* [367] to exist between diabetics, concerned sodium content of unstimulated parotid saliva which was reduced with advancing age in diabetic women ('maturity-onset diabetes'). This decrease was all the more pronounced the less parotid potassium content differed from normal values. This change was attributed to the effect of ACTH and cortisol on the salivary glands, influencing saliva production in the striated ducts [367]. Compared with 150 controls, flow rates were increased and protein as well as potassium concentrations were decreased in unstimulated parotid secretions of all 140 diabetics investigated [367]. The authors unfortunately did not analyze their data with respect to mode of distribution. Statistical analysis was based on $\bar{x} \pm SD$ tacitly assuming normal distribution of data.

A significantly increased level of parotid salivary cAMP may be regarded as pathognomonic for *arterial hypertonicity;* such patients had higher than normal plasma-renin activities [303]. Calcium concentrations of stimulated parotid saliva in *essential hypertonicity* behaved ambiguously; while total

Ca was elevated, the level of Ca^{2+} dropped [215]. Increased levels of total salivary Ca were also shown to accompany *uremia, Conn's syndrome, glycoside intoxication* [for references see 216], and sometimes digoxin-treated *cardiac failure* [32]. Since only 16 out of 29 so-treated patients had higher than normal salivary calcium and potassium concentrations, the electrolyte modifications were not attributed to the drug but rather to the well-known adrenergic stimulation in patients with cardiac failure, because retrospective clinical studies had shown a good correlation between clinical signs of cardiac failure and increased levels of salivary calcium and potassium [32].

The presence of *inflammatory or neoplastic oral disease* led to elevated levels of leucine aminopeptidase activity in mixed saliva [270]; amylase and kallikrein concentrations as well as flow rate were reduced in the majority of 40 patients with *sarcoidosis* [50]. This fall in enzyme activities was neither associated with any apparent clinical involvement of the salivary glands nor did it correlate with volume change. Circulating antibodies from serum were found to leak into saliva of 14 patients with *subacute sclerosing panencephalitis* where antimeasles antibody could be identified [86]. Constantly high phosphate levels in female patients with *sore tongue* were attributed to hormonal imbalance since phosphate was otherwise only elevated close to mid-cycle [36]. Hormonal changes were also involved in 17 infertility patients (14 of whom were hirsute) with *polycystic ovarian syndrome;* their free androgen (testosterone) concentrations in whole saliva were significantly higher than in the controls [332]. In *congenital adrenal hyperplasia* which is characterized by deficiency of an enzyme (C-21 hydroxylase) involved in steroid metabolism, monitoring of parotid and whole saliva levels of 17α-hydroxyprogesterone by means of a radioimmunoassay could replace measurement of free plasma levels due to a close correlation between the concentrations of the free hormone in plasma and saliva [372]. In 14 patients receiving cortisol replacement therapy, the range in 17α-hydroxyprogesterone observed in saliva was about 20-fold that seen in 32 healthy children [372]. Estrone and progesterone were metabolized by whole saliva of patients with *chronic gingival inflammation* [108]; no metabolites were found in saliva of subjects with clinically normal gingiva, suggesting involvement in gingival inflammation of oral leukocytes [108]. Salivary changes accompanying a number of other diseases were summarized by *Mason and Chisholm* [225].

Compositional changes of saliva ensuing after operations or concomitant with paralyzed or disrupted nerves are only occasionally reported. The proportion of sIgA relative to total protein concentration in saliva of children was raised slightly above control levels immediately after *tonsill-ectomy* but then continuously dropped, reaching values below the normal range 8 weeks after the operation [165]. Decrease of sIgA was reversible and never attained pathologically low levels. In *paralysis of the facial nerve* the submandibular saliva of the involved side contained significantly increased amounts of the electrolytes sodium and calcium as well as of the enzyme amylase [62]. The elevated Na^+ concentrations which depended on the severity of the paresis were interpreted as being due to disorders in the reabsorption of this ion in the epithelium of the glandular duct. The disturbed ion transport in the submandibular duct system was considered a simple model well suited for the detection of a parasympathetic lesion. The sub-mandibular gland, parasympathetically denervated by *iatrogenic damage to chorda tympani nerve*, served as another model for the study of the influence of its vegetative innervation on the secretion of water and protein [77]. While flow rates dropped sharply on the involved side, protein concentrations were very much increased but amylase concentrations remained unaltered. These results pointed to the greater importance of the sympathetic nervous system for protein secretion from the human submandibular gland although this possibly did not apply to amylase secretion which did not increase despite decreased flow rates.

Monitoring of Salivary Components

Normally Occurring Components

Apart from the pathodiagnostic purposes discussed in the preceding section, compositional salivary changes are also being employed for the assessment of different physiological states of healthy persons since it is well known that the composition of saliva may reflect quite a number of internal and external influences. The latter were already described here in some detail (cf. section on collection of saliva) together with possible consequences affecting the usefulness of salivary investigations. Internal influences are exerted for instance by nutritional conditions, body weight, hormonal status, physical activity, and age. This section will be confined to internal influences owing to hormonal control, studied by investigating salivary levels of hormones, electrolytes, and enzymes. Compositional changes showing good correlations between saliva and serum levels are especially well suited for this purpose.

Estimation of endocrine activity may be performed by direct determina-tion of hormone levels in saliva (cf. section on hormones) or by monitoring the changes of other salivary constituents evoked by hormonal cycles. Salivary hormone concentrations permitted to assess adrenocortical status [316, 419] or gonadal function [199, 363, 371] and their rhythms.

Variations in several salivary constituents and their relation to different phases of the menstrual cycle were repeatedly studied [36, 49, 217, 285]. Thus the constant finding of a phosphate peak at mid-cycle pointed towards hormonal regulation and was suggested to be used as an indicator of ovulation [36]. No such changes were found in the salivary phosphate concentration of women at other hormonal stages of their life, puberty and menopause; women taking contraceptives and one male showed only minor variations throughout the investigation period [36]. Ovulatory peak values for salivary free and total calcium, sodium, chloride and again phosphate could be measured in a study from another laboratory [217]; all these parameters showed a preovulatory increase and a postovulatory decrease. Potassium exhibited completely opposite behavior while total protein and amylase reached their highest values during ovulation and in the premenstrual phase [217]. Significant electrolyte changes in submandibular saliva could be attributed to hormonal effects on salivary composition by *Puskulian* [285]. In contrast to parotid saliva from which pronounced changes were absent, submandibular calcium and sodium were characterized by marked decrease at mid-cycle while potassium levels were significantly enhanced. Studying the influence of endocrine rhythms on the content of salivary kallikrein and amylase in 220 girls (14–18 years old) throughout the menstrual cycle, *Bhoola* et al. [49] noted a significantly greater activity of kallikrein in the perimenstrual phase (days 28–32 and 1–4) compared to the mid-menstrual values (days 4–28) and to those of girls without regular cycles (>32 days). The kallikrein peak was considered statistically significant since it occurred both in the morning and afternoon samples; no such peaks were apparent for amylase and total protein [49].

Drugs

Although attempts aimed at the quantitative determination of ingested drugs in saliva rather than in serum were made very early [for references see 166, 341], serum (plasma) is still by far the preferred matrix for monitoring drug levels as a means of pharmacokinetic control and as a guide to therapy. This situation may have several reasons. In order to make correct assessments of uptake (effectivity) and possibly toxic levels of drugs used in the treatment of certain diseases, the protein-bound and free fractions of the total serum concentration of the therapeutic agent have to be known. Any drug may only unfold its activity by transportation with the blood stream to the target organs or tissues. Monitoring in saliva, rather than withdrawal of blood by venipuncture, has the great advantage of being an easy and repeatedly to perform, noninvasive stress-free procedure, but it can only reliably predict drug concentration in plasma or serum if there exists a linear relationship between serum-free and salivary drug levels. This relationship has to be established first as the prerequisite of any successful monitoring of drugs in saliva. The premise that saliva may be regarded as equivalent to an ultrafiltrate of serum with respect to the drug to be determined is not a safe one [4] since not all drugs behave alike in their distribution between serum (protein-bound and free fractions) and saliva [247, 341].

Another reason for the long-time preference of serum for control of drug availability may have been the sensitivity of the assay procedures employed. Since the freely soluble form of many drugs will be present at a higher concentration in plasma, their determination in saliva requires techniques sensitive enough to permit correct measurement in saliva. In the last decade or so such techniques were further developed (gas chromatography, high-performance liquid chromatography, fluorimetric methods) and adjusted for application to salivary samples [61, 84, 89, 134, 198, 231, 247, 356, 387]. Consequently, drug monitoring in saliva is becoming widely accepted as shown by the increasing number of positive reports. Since clinical application of such techniques requires the development of time-saving routine procedures, whole saliva is mostly investigated although for certain drugs (antibiotics) measurement in separate secretions was recommended [341].

Drug concentration in saliva does not always provide a reliable index of plasma levels. This seems largely to depend on ionization of the substance investigated [247], which is strongly influenced by salivary pH. The wide inter- and intraindividual variation of salivary pH depending on differences in flow rate makes this parameter the chief variable in the estimation of ionizable drugs in saliva. For very weakly acidic or basic drugs this is of no concern since they will behave in the same way as neutral drugs, but the appearance in saliva of acidic drugs with a pK_a below 7 and of basic drugs with a pK_a over 5.5 is profoundly affected by minor alterations in salivary flow rate and pH [247].

Mucklow et al. [247], investigating the excretory behavior of a variety of ionized and nonionized drugs, concluded from their experimental results that plasma concentration of drugs can be reliably predicted by saliva monitoring of drugs largely nonionized at normal plasma pH (e.g., phenytoin, phenobarbital, antipyrine) while ionized substances (e.g., chlorpropamide, tolbutamide, propranolol, meperidine) did not lend themselves for routine measurement in saliva. These findings could explain the various reports in which the investigators failed to establish a linear relationship between salivary and plasma drug levels [188, 227, 336, 340] while others were quite successful [4, 26, 84, 89, 134, 136, 139, 166, 190, 198, 231, 262, 293, 356, 387].

Antimicrobial agents such as sulfonamides and antibiotics have long been preferred substances for determination in saliva [37, 88, 117, 151, 152]. By studying salivary levels of a number of antibiotics it was found that the majority (phenoxymethylpenicillin, ampicillin, cloxacillin, cephalexin, erythromycin stearate, sodium fusidate, tetracycline hydrochloride, prostinamycin and lincomycin hydrochloride) obviously were not secreted in sufficient amounts to exhibit antibacterial activity in mixed or parotid saliva [336, 340, 341]. The broad-spectrum antibiotic chloramphenicol was found to be another drug not suited for monitoring in saliva [188]. Rifampicin, and to a lesser extent clindamycin, were present in mixed, parotid, submandibular and minor gland saliva and also in gingival fluid [212, 340]. Gingival fluid was a better matrix for antibiotics than whole saliva; phenoxymethylpenicillin, ampicillin, cephalexin, tetracycline hydrochloride and erythromycin estolate were secreted into this fluid as shown by a variable degree of antibacterial activity detected for at least 3 h after medication [212, 340].

A large number of other substances permitted the safe prediction of plasma levels from saliva. Very good to excellent correlations were found for the antiepileptic drug phenytoin (diphenylhydantoin) in whole [4, 247, 262] and parotid saliva [4, 331] which appeared to be the best predictor of serum ultrafiltrate phenytoin concentrations [4]. *Brügmann* et al. [61] also found close correlations between phenytoin concentrations in plasma, serum, plasma or serum dialyzate and saliva but advised caution in the interpretation of results since in a number of cases extremely high concentrations were present in saliva compared with plasma and dialyzate. Further positive results were obtained for two other antiepileptics, phenobarbital [262] and lithium [26]. Anticholinergic supplementation of lithium therapy was of only small concern [26] but an inacceptible high individual variation was noted by others [227] causing the statement that salivary lithium assessment would be of little clinical use.

The necessity to maintain therapeutic and nontoxic blood levels of certain alkaloids in the treatment of apnea of prematurity was the starting point for the development of a rapid method for the simultaneous determination of caffeine and theophylline from the serum, saliva or spinal fluid of neonates [356]. Samples (50 μl) were analyzed by high-pressure liquid chromatography with a lowest sensitivity limit of 0.1 mg/l. Although saliva was subject to slightly higher variation than the other fluids, good overall correlations were observed. A similar technique was successfully applied in the determination of the bronchodilator dyphylline (dihydroxypropyl theophylline) in saliva [134].

Comparative studies of blood and salivary alcohol (ethanol) concentrations showed that saliva is a practical medium for noninvasive determination of this habitual drug [231], provided that the saliva sample is not obtained within 20 min of alcohol ingestion [231]. Pure parotid and mixed saliva were equally suitable sources for ethanol estimation [231]. The ethanol concentration in saliva was found to be generally slightly higher than in capillary blood. This was expected because the equilibrium concentrations in various tissues and fluids are proportional to their water content [166]. On the basis of these results it was concluded that salivary ethanol analysis could well serve as supporting evidence in clinical and medicolegal assessment of ethanol intoxication [166]. Expert opinion on this proposal from the side of the police exercising traffic control is anxiously awaited.

Close correlations between blood and salivary concentration were also ascertained for many other drugs employed for diverse clinical purposes; these substances include antipyrine [235], p-aminosalicylic acid [190], salicylate [139, 293], salicylamide [84], dapsone and acetylated dapsone [198], misonidazole [387], diazepam [89], tolbutamide [228], and paracetamol [136]. Methotrexate was successfully determined in parotid but not in whole saliva [337]. The excretion into parotid saliva of pertechnetate ($^{99m}TcO_4^-$) clinically administered for scintigraphic purposes was already mentioned in the section on salivary anions [2, 143, 203].

Age-Dependent Salivary Changes

The level of many salivary constituents is not constant throughout the entire life span of an individual but shows age-specific differences. A few examples, applying to the secretions of apparently healthy people, shall be given here to illustrate this fact. These changes concern ions as well as proteins including enzymes.

Comparing the whole salivary levels of sodium and potassium in 92 infants (0–6 months) and young adults, *Paulsen and Kröger* [273] found that potassium was only slightly increased in infants while sodium was present in infants' saliva at about twice the concentration measured in adults. This was explained by the still incompletely maturated glandular duct system in infants which would thus be more permeable to ions, eliminating or diminishing the effect of reabsorption. Since salivary electrolyte rhythms were also shown to be connected with endocrine factors [83, 115, 116], maturation-dependent hormonal deficiencies could also have accounted for the observed difference between infants and adults.

Whereas the albumin concentration in parotid saliva is independent of age since the protein is probably not synthesized by the salivary glands but transudes into saliva from serum [159, 266], and in submandibular saliva will only increase in caries-resistant persons [470], secretory immuno-globulin A was shown to rise from low levels to higher ones during matura-tion [165]. Measuring sIgA content in mixed saliva of 127 children between 2 and 14 years old, *Jeschke and Ströder* [165] demonstrated a steady increase with age of the proportion of sIgA in total salivary protein which was about twice as high in the group of 13- to 14-year olds compared to the children between 2 and 4 years of age.

The two components making up the lactoperoxidase-thiocyanate sali-vary defense system are characterized by opposite age-dependent changes. In newborn infants' saliva the thiocyanate concentration was only one third that of adults' saliva but the amounts of this anion and of lactoperoxidase were found to be quite sufficient for inhibition of bacterial growth in in vitro systems [138]. While the concentration of thiocyanate ion was demonstrated to be significantly and positively correlated with age, the activity of salivary (lacto)peroxidase was distinguished by opposite changes and significantly decreased with advancing age [16]. Although there was no apparent bias in the selection process by which the donors of different ages were chosen, the author admonished that these results be interpreted with caution. The group of older persons contained more smokers than that of younger ones, and it is known that smoking reduces salivary peroxidase activity and augments salivary thiocyanate concentration [16, 460]. The subjects chosen for the study were mostly laboratory and nursing personnel associated with a medical school and it cannot be excluded that such a selected population reflects differ-ent professional and generational attitudes towards the smoking habit [16].

The main enzyme of human salivary secretions, α-amylase, exhibits age-dependent changes apparent on different levels. Salivary amylase is hardly detectable in newborns but its secretion is induced later by adaptation to starch-containing foodstuffs [286]. While total amylase activity of unstimu-lated and stimulated parotid saliva did not significantly differ [8, 75] between three sex-balanced age groups tested (0–30, 31–60, 61–90 years), it was found to be distinctly higher in stimulated submandibular saliva [7] of young persons (4–16 years) than in that of old persons (60–79 years). Total protein content of submandibular secretion showed parallel changes [7]. Such age-dependent differences may reflect various differentiation patterns during maturation of the glands involved. It was found in animal experiments that the levels of RNase and amylase in the rat parotid and submandibular glands rise pre-embryonically until birth and continue to do so in the parotid gland while the enzyme activities in the submandibular gland constantly decline with increasing age down to the low levels of an early embryonic stage [for references see 7]. This is accompanied by differentiations in the rat submandibular gland; the human submandibular gland also changes in its histological structure parallel to aging [for references see 7].

Another type of age-dependent changes may be encountered on the isoenzyme level. Amylase 'aging' occurring in vitro was severally reported, for instance by *Kauffman* et al. [179] who observed the formation of additional isoenzymes after prolonged standing of parotid amylase preparations in the cold, a process that could be accelerated by exposure to elevated temperature, particularly in an alkaline medium [181]. Incubation of saliva for 10 h at 37°C resulted in the occurrence of multiforms of amylase upon electrophoresis on cellulose acetate membranes which had revealed only one amylase zone when fresh saliva had been used [348]. Proteolysis by bacterial contamination was very unlikely in both reported cases and the observed alteration was attributed to autodigestion in the second report [348]. Investigation of salivary amylase by electrophoresis in more efficient media such as polyacrylamide gel invariably results in the separation of several isoenzymes from freshly collected parotid and submandibular saliva specimens. A basic pattern reported to consist of 5 [181] or 6 isoamylases [6, 7, 75, 176, 238] is found in nearly all members of the Caucasian race [176, 238]. This pattern is derived from the primary product of the amylase gene by a number of posttranslational and postsecretory conversions [176, 238] already discussed in detail in this chapter (fig. 3).

While these conversions do not in themselves reflect autodigestive modifications, the same processes may be at work in experimentally induced isoenzyme formation and under the physiological conditions prevailing in the oral cavity, namely, enzymatic deglycosylation [175, 176] and non-enzymatic deamidation [176, 181, 208].

The basic isoamylase pattern of human submandibular and parotid saliva is occasionally supplemented by the occurrence of additional, mostly fainter, bands of isoamylases migrating further towards the anode in an alkaline (pH>8.0) gel system. Their greater mobility characterizes those

Table XVIII. Distribution of isoamylase patterns in parotid saliva from test persons of three age groups[a]

Isoamylase pattern	Age of the test persons		
	<30 years	31–60 years	>60 years
Only basic pattern	37	30	10
Basic pattern + fast isoamylases	63	70	90

[a] The numbers refer to the percentage of patterns observed in each age group.

additional isoenzymes as 'fast isoamylases'. We have found that their number in parotid saliva is positively correlated with age [6, 75]; identical patterns were identified in stimulated and unstimulated saliva samples collected from the same donors at different times, confirming other reports on the composition of saliva with regard to several components [127, 179, 180, 205] where qualitative compositional differences were only observed between (but not in) individuals.

Besides the basic pattern predominantly found in younger persons (12–30 years) we could identify three more types of isoamylase patterns, especially in older persons (61–79 years), distinguished by the occurrence of up to six new, fast isoamaylases [6]. While the middle age group (31–60 years) showed an intermediate behavior with respect to the patterns encountered, the group of the oldest persons had a lower incidence of basic pattern but exhibited significantly higher numbers of fast isoamylase patterns (table XVIII), particularly of those comprising 3 and 6 additional amylase isoenzymes [6]. No such changes could be found in submandibular saliva although amylase from this source did contain fast isoenzymes and otherwise always showed the basic six isoenzyme pattern [7] confirming the general assumption of electrophoretic identity of parotid and submandibular amylase [110, 180, 197].

The described findings provoke questions about the mechanisms involved in the age-dependent increase of fast isoamylases and their possible implications in individual aging. The principal processes responsible for the evolvement of new isoamylases in vitro can also be conceived to operate in the human organism where they may be subject to age-specific alterations in intensity. Since it was shown that deamidation of exposed asparagine residues may result in an individually timed aging of proteins [294], the possible effects of such a 'biological timer' on the basic pattern of human parotid isoamylases can be discussed as follows. By an age-dependent and individually timed process of deamidation additional isoamylases are generated from the six isoamylases of the basic pattern which remains constant. Depending on the number of newly formed isoenzymes, a variety of additional isoamylase patterns results. The appearance of fast isoamylases certainly has no dangerous consequences but may be regarded as an indicator of aging which could point to the importance of deamidation in other proteins necessary for the maintenance of life.

To obtain direct experimental instead of statistical proof for the observed changes in the human parotid isoamylase patterns it would, however, be necessary to constantly follow the development of the actual isoamylase patterns in single individuals throughout their entire life span.

Saliva as a Source of Genetic Markers

Many proteins of human saliva are subject to genetically controlled polymorphism, that is, depending on the presence or absence of certain alleles determining phenotypic expression, different patterns of certain protein species may be detected in human salivary secretions by suitable procedures such as PAGE and subsequent staining. Due to different allelic frequencies, the appearance of such different patterns varies within and between races, and certain proteins can therefore serve as genetic markers. With this technique it is for instance possible to estimate the extent of racial admixture which may be of interest in ethnographic studies [352]. *Tan and Teng* [353] have compiled a comprehensive list of genetic markers found in human saliva and included a survey of experimental procedures for their identification. The number of genetic markers identified in human saliva is still rather small compared to blood [353] but new proteins exhibiting genetic polymorphism continue to be detected.

While many genetic markers of saliva are unique to this fluid, some of them also occur in blood where their presence and genetic distribution was investigated first, e.g., blood group specific substances. Interracial distribution of blood groups belonging to different systems is beyond the scope of this article and may be found in the pertaining literature. Antigenic specificity, conferred to BGRS by inherited specific glycosyltransferases, is always the same in one particular individual regardless of source, but genetic control by the ABH(O) blood group system of salivary agglutinin presence and levels may have functional implications. Thus it was shown that carriers of blood group A_2 had higher salivary anti-B agglutinin titers than A_1 individuals; the presence of salivary agglutinins varied with blood group and race [30]. The lowest incidence was observed for anti-A agglutinin in individuals of blood group B, both in whites (29%) and blacks (35%), while blood group O was distinguished by the occurrence of salivary anti-A and anti-B agglutinins in 64–79% of its carriers in both races. Blacks always showed a higher incidence of the ABH(O) blood group reactive salivary agglutinins [30]. The possible involvement of socioeconomic conditions in salivary agglutinin titers has been discussed [30].

The presence of inherited variants of human salivary amylase was first demonstrated by *Kamaryt and Laxová* [170, 171] and confirmed by a different laboratory [54]. On the basis of extended family studies conducted in various races (white Americans, whites from Kuwait, black Americans, black Nigerians, Orientals), *Karn* et al. [176] and *Merritt and Karn* [238] have given detailed accounts on the different alleles existing and their resulting phenotypes. After autosomal-dominant inheritance was demonstrated by *Ward* et al. [374], altogether 12 different phenotypes originating from 2 homozygous and 10 heterozygous genotypes could be identified. They differ from each other by number and migratory behavior of the isoamylases evolving from the primary Amy_1 gene product by the postsecretory modifications already discussed. (Salivary and pancreatic amylases are derived from two closely linked loci, Amy_1 for salivary and Amy_2 for pancreatic amylase [176].)

The most common Amy_1 allele in all races is allele *A*, while alleles *B* through *K* and R^n occur only rarely but show different racial distribution [238]. Amy_1 *F* variants were only detected among orientals (Koreans, Chinese and Japanese) and the variant alleles *G* and *K* were only present, at very low phenotypic frequencies, in black Americans and whites from Kuwait, respectively [238]. Caucasians have the highest allelic frequency for Amy_1 *A* resulting in homozygosity and thus appearance of phenotype A (corresponding to the basic pattern of six isoamylases) in 98.7% of individuals. Heterozygosity of allele *A* with other alleles (except R^n) leads to the occurrence of additional, more cathodal isoenzymes [176, 238] suggesting dominance for the *non-A* alleles. A tabulation of racial distribution of Amy_1 phenotypes and a diagram depicting the respective isoenzyme patterns they represent may be found in the review article of *Merritt and Karn* [238]. Several studies recording new and confirming established phenotypes have appeared [283, 335].

A number of other enzymes, e.g., salivary peroxidase [15, 16], carboxyl esterase [349], G-6-PDH [351] and acid phosphatase [350, 352] are also characterized by genetic polymorphisms which were already discussed under the appropriate headings. Studying the interracial distribution of the variant alleles determining salivary acid phosphatase phenotypes (isoenzyme patterns) in different ethnic groups, *Tan and Teng* [352] made an anthropologically interesting observation by noting the complete absence of one certain allele in Malays that was present in Chinese. This finding was remarkable since Malays, being of Mongoloid stock, are thought to be genetically closely related to Chinese [352]. The utilization of salivary genetic markers in anthropology and population genetics may open up a promising field of research.

A review of the various genetic polymorphisms reveals that very pronounced differences in the occurrence of various nonenzymatic, saliva-specific proteins seem to exist between races. Thus acidic protein (Pa) is found among Orientals two times as often (allelic frequency for $Pa^1 = 0.42$) as in Caucasians ($Pa^1 = 0.21$); it is even rarer in American blacks ($Pa^1 = 0.14$) as demonstrated by *Friedman* et al. [128]. The results of *Azen* [15] confirmed this observation. Double-band protein (Db), on the other hand, is much more frequent in American blacks ($Db^+ = 0.56$) than in Caucasians ($Db^+ = 0.12$) and Orientals ($Db^+ = 0.07$) while the proline-rich proteins (Pr) do not show such prominent interracial differences [19]. The observed significantly lower incidence of Pr proteins in Amerindians compared to whites may be an exception [330]. Parotid basic protein (Pb) coded for by two different alleles shows predominance of one allele in Caucasians while in American blacks these alleles are not quite so unevenly distributed [13]. Some genetically polymorphic salivary proteins are characterized by co-dominance of two or more alleles capable of expression (e.g., acid phosphatase, G-6-PDH, carboxyl esterase) while others with only two alleles (Pa, Db) are distinguished by the presence of a 'null allele' that does not give rise to polypeptide synthesis, resulting in either the presence or in complete absence of phenotypic expression [for review see 18]. Factors possibly involved in the 'appearance' of a null phenotype as part of a protein polymorphism may include suppression of translation or transcription of polypeptides, control of rate of synthesis of the protein, enhanced degradation, partial gene deletion, or frameshift or terminal mutations [23]. In some instances the normal protein may be present in greatly reduced amounts, appearing as a faint band after electrophoresis [23]. *Balakrishnan and Ashton* [23] have pointed out that further research may disclose that a null phenotype may be due to the epistatic action of an independent locus causing interference with the production of the normal protein.

Extensive lists in which the various genetic polymorphisms were tabulated with respect to number of loci and alleles, allelic frequencies in different human races (Caucasians, American and Nigerian blacks, Indians, Orientals such as Chinese, Japanese, Malays, and oriental Americans) and the resulting polymorphic phenotypes may be found in the literature [18, 23, 128, 238, 350, 351, 415, 448]. A new genetic marker termed Pm (salivary parotid middle-band protein) was described for Japanese [for references see 18]. The issue is unfortunately somewhat confused by the as yet non-standardized and occasionally conflicting notation used in designating symbols to the various alleles and their phenotypic expressions [415]. This situation may be regarded as typical for a rapidly expanding field of research.

Conclusion and Outlook

It is hoped that this chapter on the biochemistry of human saliva has succeeded in conveying more than but glimpses of the remarkable complexity by which the secretions from the various salivary glands are characterized. This complexity does not only concern salivary composition with regard to number and amounts of constituents encountered, it also concerns marked differences between glands, variations due to different sampling procedures, internal rhythms, changes in disease, race and age, and last but not least the various defense mechanisms operating in the oral cavity through the action of saliva. Understanding of the rules adhered to in the eternal 'cops and robbers' game between the salivary defense mechanisms and viral as well as microbial invaders is becoming more and more profound, but many more tricks remain to be learnt from friend and foe alike.

Saliva, a stepchild of research for a long time, is being increasingly accepted as a scientific tool which has even led to its investigation after return from orbit where it was safely ensconced inside the glands of the Skylab crew members [60]. The saliva obviously enjoyed the trip since mostly minor compositional changes could be noted with only sIgA making an exception. Most regrettably no comparison is possible with the behavior of saliva from crew members of the Sojus mission.

Saliva has at last been recognized as one of nature's richest sources, actually a veritable pool. This pool may still hold many more precious, and at the same time useful, fish only waiting to be caught.

References

1 Aarli, J.A.: Phenytoin-induced depression of salivary IgA. Acta oto-lar. *82:* 199–201 (1976).

2 Alexander, W.D.; Harden, R.McG.; Mason, D.K.; Shimmins, J.; Kostalas, H.: Comparison of the concentrating ability of the human salivary gland for bromine, iodine and technetium. Archs oral Biol. *11:* 1205–1207 (1966).

3 Amsterdam, A.; Schramm, M.; Ohad, I.; Salomon, Y.; Selinger, Z.: Concomitant synthesis of membrane protein and exportable protein of the secretory granule in rat parotid gland. J. Cell Biol. *50:* 187–200 (1971).

4 Anavekar, S.N.; Saunders, R.H.; Wardell, W.M.; Shoulson, I.; Emmings, F.G.; Cook, C.E.; Gringeri, A.J.: Parotid and whole saliva in the prediction of serum total and free phenytoin concentrations. Clin. Pharmacol. Ther. *24:* 629–637 (1978).

5 Andrew, W.: Comparative aspects of structure and function of the salivary glands; in Sreebny, Myer, Salivary glands and their secretion, pp. 3–11 (Pergamon Press, New York 1964).

6 Arglebe, C.; Chilla, R.; Opaitz, M.: Age-dependent distribution of isoamylases in human parotid saliva. Clin. Otolaryngol. *1:* 249–256 (1976).

7 Arglebe, C.; Flaam, B.; Chilla, R.: Amylase activity, protein concentration and isoamylase patterns of human submandibular saliva. ORL *40:* 199–205 (1978).

8 Arglebe, C.; Opaitz, M.; Chilla, R.: Amylaseaktivität im unstimulierten Parotisspeichel des Menschen unter Berücksichtigung von Flussrate und Proteinkonzentration. Lar. Rhinol. Otol. *58:* 700–705 (1979).

9 Armstrong, S.H., Jr.; Budka, M.J.E.; Morrison, K.C.; Hasson, M.: Preparation and properties of serum and plasma proteins. XII. The refractive properties of the proteins of human plasma and certain purified fractions. J. Am. chem. Soc. *69:* 1747–1753 (1947).

10 Arneberg, P.: Partial characterization of five glycoprotein fractions secreted by the human parotid glands. Archs oral Biol. *19:* 921–928 (1974).

11 Asakura, K.; Kataura, A.: cAMP and cGMP in the human parotid saliva. Archs Oto-Rhino-Lar. *226:* 145–154 (1980).

12 Aw, S.E.; Hobbs, J.R.; Wootton, I.D.P.: Chromatographic purification of isoenzymes of human α-amylases. Biochim. biophys. Acta *168:* 362–365 (1968).

13 Azen, E.A.: Genetic polymorphism of basic proteins from parotid saliva. Science *176:* 673–674 (1972).

14 Azen, E.A.: Properties of salivary basic proteins showing polymorphism. Biochem. Genet. *9:* 69–85 (1973).

15 Azen, E.A.: Salivary peroxidase (SAPX): genetic modification and relationship to the proline-rich (Pr) and acidic (Pa) proteins. Biochem. Genet. *15:* 9–29 (1977).

16 Azen, E.A.: Salivary peroxidase activity and thiocyanate concentration in human subjects with genetic variants of salivary peroxidase. Archs oral Biol. *23:* 801–805 (1978).

17 Azen, E.A.: Phosphorylation of proline-rich, double band, acidic and post-Pb proteins of human saliva. Archs oral Biol. *23:* 1173–1176 (1978).

18 Azen, E.A.: Genetic protein polymorphisms in human saliva: an interpretive review. Biochem. Genet. *16:* 79–99 (1978).

19 Azen, E.A.; Denniston, C.L.: Genetic polymorphism of human salivary proline-rich proteins: further genetic analysis. Biochem. Genet. *12:* 109–120 (1974).

20 Azen, E.A.; Oppenheim, F.G.: Genetic polymorphism of proline-rich human salivary proteins. Science *180:* 1067–1069 (1973).

21 Baenziger, J.; Kornfeld, S.: Structure of the carbohydrate units of IgA immuno-globulin. I. Composition, glycopeptide isolation, and structure of the asparagine-linked oligosaccharide units. J. biol. Chem. *249:* 7260–7269 (1974).

22 Baenziger, J.; Kornfeld, S.: Structure of the carbohydrate units of IgA immuno-globulin. II. Structure of the O-glycosidically linked oligosaccharide units. J.biol. Chem. *249:* 7270–7281 (1974).

23 Balakrishnan, C.R.; Ashton, G.C.: Polymorphisms of human salivary proteins. Am. J. hum. Genet. *26:* 145–153 (1974).

24 Balekjian, A.Y.; Longton, R.W.: Histones isolated from human parotid fluid. Biochem. biophys. Res. Commun. *50:* 676–682 (1973).

25 Balekjian, A.Y.; Hoerman, K.C.; Berzinskas, V.J.: Lysozyme of the human parotid gland secretion: its purification and physicochemical properties. Biochem. biophys. Res. Commun. *35:* 887–894 (1969).

26 Bannet, J.; Avni, J.; Weissenberg, E.; Ebstein, R.P.; Belmaker, R.H.: Salivary lithium. Br. J. Psychiat. *134:* 446 (1979).

27 Baratieri, A.; Picarelli, A.; Piselli, D.: Zinc distribution in human saliva. J. dent. Res. *58:* 540–541 (1979).

28 Bardoń, A.; Shugar, D.: Properties of purified salivary ribonuclease, and salivary ribonuclease levels in children with cystic fibrosis and in heterozygous carriers. Clinica chim. Acta *101:* 17–24 (1980).

29 Barman, T.E.: Enzyme handbook, vol. I, II (Springer, Berlin 1969).

30 Barrantes, R.; Salzano, F.M.: Genetic and nongenetic variation in the ABO agglu-tinin levels of plasma, saliva and milk. Acta Genet. med. Gemell. *27:* 31–38 (1978).

31 Battistone, G.C.; Burnett, G.W.: The free amino acid composition of human saliva. Archs oral Biol. *3:* 161–170 (1961).

32 Bauer, F.; Balant, L.; Zender, R.; Humair, L.: Electrolytes salivaires, digitale et insuffisance cardiaque. Schweiz. med. Wschr. *108:* 1891–1893 (1978).

33 Baum, B.J.; Bird, J.L.; Millar, D.B.; Longton, R.W.: Studies on histidine rich polypeptides from human parotid saliva. Archs Biochem. Biophys. *177:* 427–436 (1976).

34 Behall, K.M.; Kelsay, J.L.; Holden, J.M.; Clark, W.M.: Amylase and protein in parotid saliva after load doses of different dietary carbohydrates. Am. J. clin. Nutr. *26:* 17–22 (1973).

35 Belding, M.E.; Klebanoff, S.J.; Ray, C.G.: Peroxidase-mediated virucidal systems. Science *167:* 195–196 (1970).

36 Ben-Aryeh, H.: Salivary phosphate as an indicator of hormonal status of women. J. dent. Res. *55:* D 168 (1976).

37 Bender, I.B.; Pressman, R.S.; Tashman, S.G.: Studies on excretion of antibiotics in human saliva. J. dent. Res. *32:* 287–293, 435–439 (1953).

38 Benedek-Spät, E.: The composition of unstimulated human parotid saliva. Archs oral Biol. *18:* 39–47 (1973).

39 Benedek-Spät, E.: The composition of stimulated human parotid saliva. Archs oral Biol. *18:* 1091–1097 (1973).

40 Benedek-Spät, E.: Sialochemical examinations in non-tumorous parotid enlarge-ments. Acta oto-lar. *86:* 276–282 (1978).

41 Bennick, A.: Chemical and physical characteristics of a phosphoprotein from human parotid saliva. Biochem. J. *145:* 557–567 (1975).

42 Bennick, A.; Connell, G.E.: Purification and partial characterization of four proteins from human parotid saliva. Biochem. J. *123:* 455–464 (1971).

43 Bercy, P.; Vreven, J.: Correlation between calculus index and acid and alkaline pyrophosphatase activities of dental plaque and saliva. J. Biol. buccale *7:* 31–36 (1979).

44 Bergmeyer, H.U.: Methoden der enzymatischen Analyse, vol. I, II (Verlag Chemie, Weinheim 1974).

45 Bernfeld, P.: Enzymes of starch degradation and synthesis. Adv. Enzymol. *12:* 379–428 (1951).

46 Bernfeld, P.; Staub, A.; Fischer, E.H.: Sur les enzymes amylolytiques. XI. Propriétés de l'α-amylase de salive humaine cristallisée. Helv. chim. Acta *31:* 2165–2172 (1948).

47 Bertram, U.; Kragh-Sørensen, P.; Rafaelsen, O.J.; Larsen, N.-E.: Saliva secretion following long-term antidepressant treatment with nortriptyline controlled by plasma levels. Scand. J. dent. Res. *87:* 58–64 (1979).

48 Beutler, R.; Morrison, M.: Localization and characteristics of hexose-6-phosphate dehydrogenase (glucose dehydrogenase). J. biol. Chem. *242:* 5289–5293 (1967).

49 Bhoola, K.D.; Matthews, R.W.; Roberts, F.: A survey of salivary kallikrein and amylase in a population of schoolgirls, throughout the menstrual cycle. Clin. Sci. mol. Med. *55:* 561–565 (1978).

50 Bhoola, K.D.; McNicol, M.W.; Oliver, S.; Foran, J.: Changes in salivary enzymes in patients with sarcoidosis. New Engl. J. Med. *281:* 877–879 (1969).

51 Birkhed, D.; Söder, P.-Ö.: The presence of isoamylases in human saliva. Archs oral Biol. *18:* 203–210 (1973).

52 Block, P.L.; Brotman, S.: A method of submaxillary saliva collection without cannulation. N.Y. St. dent. J. *28:* 116–118 (1962).

53 Boettcher, B.; Lande, F.A. de la: Electrophoresis of human salivary amylase in gel slabs. Analyt. Biochem. *28:* 510–514 (1969).

54 Boettcher, B.; Lande, F.A. de la: Electrophoresis of human saliva and identification of inherited variants of amylase isozymes. Aust. J. exp. Biol. med. Sci. *47:* 97–103 (1969).

55 Bowen, S.R.; Carpenter, F.G.: Morphine depression and tolerance of nerve-induced parotid secretion. Br. J. Pharmacol. *65:* 7–13 (1979).

56 Brandtzaeg, P.; Hensten-Pettersen, A.: Immunogenic properties of human and rabbit salivary albumin. Archs oral Biol. *21:* 69–71 (1976).

57 Brandtzaeg, P.; Fjellanger, I.; Gjeruldsen, S.T.: Human secretory immunoglobulins. I. Salivary secretions from individuals with normal or low levels of serum immunoglobulins. Scand. J. Haematol., suppl. 12, pp. 1–83 (1970).

58 Bratthall, D.; Carlén, A.: Salivary agglutinin and secretory IgA reactions with oral streptococci. Scand. J. dent. Res. *86:* 430–443 (1978).

59 Bratthall, D.; Gahnberg, L.; Krasse, B.: Method for detecting IgA antibodies to *Streptococcus mutans* serotypes in parotid saliva. Archs oral Biol. *23:* 843–849 (1978).

60 Brown, L.R.; Frome, W.J.; Wheatcroft, M.G.; Riggan, L.J.; Bussell, N.E.; Johnston, D.A.: The effect of Skylab on the chemical composition of saliva. J. dent. Res. *56:* 1137–1143 (1977).

61 Brügmann, G.; Kleinau, E.; Nolte, R.; Petruch, F.: Comparison of phenytoin

determinations in plasma, plasma dialysate and saliva for control of antiepileptic therapy in children. Klin. Wschr. *57:* 93–94 (1979).

62 Bumm, P.; Berg, M.; Tiedtke, M.: Speichelchemische Untersuchungen der Submandibularisdrüse bei Fazialisparesen. Archs Oto-Rhino-Lar. *226:* 269–278 (1980).

63 Bunting, R.W.; Rickert, U.G.: Dental caries. J. natn. dent. Ass. *2:* 247–269 (1915).

64 Burgen, A.S.V.; Seeman, P.: The secretion of iodine in saliva. Can. J. Biochem. Physiol. *35:* 481 (1957).

65 Cadman, E.; Bostwick, J.R.; Eichberg, J.: Determination of protein by a modified Lowry procedure in the presence of some commonly used detergents. Analyt. Biochem. *96:* 21–23 (1979).

66 Cannon, D.C.; Olitzky, I.; Inkpen, J.A.: Proteins; in Henry, Cannon, Winkelman, Clinical chemistry, principles and technics, pp. 405–434 (Harper & Row, New York 1974).

67 Caraway, W.T.: A stable starch substrate for the determination of amylase in serum and other body fluids. Am. J. clin. Path. *32:* 97–99 (1959).

68 Carlson, A.J.; Crittenden, A.L.: The relation of ptyalin concentration to the diet and to the rate of secretion of the saliva. Am. J. Physiol. *26:* 169–177 (1910).

69 Carlström, A.: The heterogeneity of lactoperoxidase. Acta chem. Scand. *19:* 2387–2394 (1965).

70 Chauncey, H.H.: Salivary enzymes. J. Am. dent. Ass. *63:* 360–368 (1961).

71 Chauncey, H.H.; Lionetti, F.; Lisanti, V.F.: Enzymes of human saliva. II. Parotid saliva total esterases. J. dent. Res. *36:* 713–716 (1957).

72 Chauncey, H.H.; Henriques, B.L.; Tanzer, J.M.: Comparative enzyme activity of saliva from the sheep, hog, dog, rabbit, rat, and human. Archs oral Biol. *8:* 615–627 (1963).

73 Chauncey, H.H.; Feller, R.P.; Henriques, B.L.: Comparative electrolyte composition of parotid, submandibular, and sublingual secretions. J. dent. Res. *45:* 1230 (1966).

74 Chauncey, H.H.; Lionetti, F.; Winer, R.A.; Lisanti, V.F.: Enzymes of human saliva. I. The determination, distribution, and origin of whole saliva enzymes. J. dent. Res. *33:* 321–334 (1954).

75 Chilla, R.; Kropp, T.; Arglebe, C.: Amylaseaktivität und Isoamylasenmuster im Parotisspeichel des Menschen. Lar. Rhinol. Otol. *56:* 912–918 (1977).

76 Chilla, R.; Opaitz, M.; Arglebe, C.: Flussrate, Amylase- und Proteingehalt des Parotisspeichels bei Sialadenose. Lar. Rhinol. Otol. *57:* 274–279 (1978).

77 Chilla, R.; Brüner, M.; Arglebe, C.: Function of submaxillary gland following iatrogenic damage to chorda tympani nerve. Acta oto-lar. *87:* 152–155 (1979).

78 Chilla, R.; Niemann, H.; Arglebe, C.; Domagk, G.F.: Age-dependent changes in the α-isoamylase pattern of human and rat parotid glands. ORL *36:* 373–382 (1974).

79 Chodirker, W.B.; Tomasi, T.B.: Gamma globulins: quantitative relationships in human serum and non-vascular fluids. Science *142:* 1080–1081 (1963).

80 Choih, S.-J.; Smith, Q.T.; Schachtele, C.F.: Modification of human parotid saliva proteins by oral *Streptococcus sanguis*. J. dent. Res. *58:* 516–524 (1979).

81 Curby, W.A.: Device for collection of human parotid saliva. J. Lab. clin. Med. *41:* 493–496 (1953).

82 Dawes, C.: The effects of flow rate and duration of stimulation on the concentrations

of protein and the main electrolytes in human parotid saliva. Archs oral Biol. *14:* 277–294 (1969).

83 Dawes, C.; Ong, B.Y.: Circadian rhythms in the concentrations of protein and the main electrolytes in human unstimulated parotid saliva. Archs oral Biol. *18:* 1233–1242 (1973).

84 De Boer, A.G.; Gubbens-Stibbe, J.M.; Koning, F.H. de; Bosma, A.; Breimer, D.D.: Assay of underivatized salicylamide in plasma, saliva and urine. J. Chromat. *162:* 457–460 (1979).

85 Demetriou, J.A.; Drewes, P.A.; Gin, J.B.: Enzymes: amylase; in Henry, Cannon, Winkelman, Clinical chemistry, principles and technics, pp. 943–949 (Harper & Row, New York 1974).

86 Derakhshan, I.; Mirchamsy, H.; Shafii, A.: Subacute sclerosing panencephalitis. Immunological findings in saliva and salivary glands. Eur. Neurol. *18:* 79–83 (1979).

87 Descos, L.; Lambert, R.; Minaire, Y.: Comparison of human salivary secretion in health and chronic pancreatitis. Digestion *9:* 76–80 (1973).

88 Devine, L.F.; Knowles, R.C.; Pierce, W.E.; Pechinpaugh, R.O.; Hagerman, C.R.; Lytle, R.I.: Proposed model for screening antimicrobial agents for potential use in eliminating meningococci from the nasopharynx of healthy carriers; in Hobby, Antimicrobial agents and chemotherapy, pp. 307–314 (American Society for Microbiology, Bethesda 1969).

89 DiGregorio, G.J.; Piraino, A.J.; Ruch, E.: Diazepam concentrations in parotid saliva, mixed saliva, and plasma. Clin. Pharmacol. Ther. *24:* 720–725 (1978).

90 Dixon, M.; Webb, E.C.: Enzymes (Longmans Green, London 1964).

91 Doering, K.M.; Arglebe, C.; Lubahn, H.; Chilla, R.: 'Fast isoamylases' in the parotid saliva of children with cystic fibrosis and heterozygous carriers. Eur. J. Pediat. *126:* 185–188 (1977).

92 Dogon, I.L.; Amdur, B.H.: Evidence for the presence of two thiocyanate-dependent antibacterial systems in human saliva. Archs oral Biol. *15:* 987–992 (1970).

93 Draus, F.J.; Tarbet, W.J.; Miklos, F.L.: Salivary enzymes and calculus formation. J. periodont. Res. *3:* 232–235 (1968).

94 Dreiling, D.A.; Noronha, M.; Nacchiero, M.; Pieroni, P.; Wolfson, P.: The parotid and the pancreas. VI. Clinical and physiologic associations between the pancreas and parotid glands. Am. J. Gastroent., N.Y. *70:* 627–634 (1978).

95 Dunne, J.V.; Carson, D.A.; Spiegelberg, H.L.; Alspaugh, M.A.; Vaughan, J.H.: IgA rheumatoid factor in the sera and saliva of patients with rheumatoid arthritis and Sjögren's syndrome. Ann. rheum. Dis. *38:* 161–165 (1979).

96 Dunnette, S.L.; Gleich, G.J.; Miller, D.R.; Kyle, R.A.: Measurement of IgD by a double antibody radioimmunoassay: demonstration of an apparent trimodal distribution of IgD levels in normal human sera. J. Immun. *119:* 1727–1731 (1977).

97 Durrant, M.L.; Royston, P.: The effect of preloads of varying energy density and methyl cellulose on hunger, appetite and salivation. Proc. Nutr. Soc. *37:* 87 A (1978).

98 Eggers Lura, H.: Investigations on the salivary phosphates and phosphatases. J. dent. Res. *26:* 203–224 (1947).

99 Eichel, H.J.; Conger, H.; Chernick, W.S.: Acid and alkaline ribonucleases of human parotid, submaxillary and whole saliva. Archs Biochem. Biophys. *107:* 197–208 (1964).

100 Eichner, H.: Elektrophoretische und immunelektrophoretische Befunde des mensch-

lichen Parotissekretes bei verschiedenen Ohrspeicheldrüsenerkrankungen. Lar. Rhinol. Otol. *55:* 897–905 (1976).

101 Eichner, H.; Hochstrasser, K.: Biochemische Befunde der Sekrete menschlicher Ohrspeicheldrüsen mit Zystadenolymphomen im Vergleich zu Sialographie und Szintigraphie. Lar. Rhinol. Otol. *55:* 833–839 (1976).

102 Eichner, H.; Münzel, M.; Bretzel, G.: Vergleichende Untersuchungen von Fluss-raten, Elektrolyt- und Gesamteiweisskonzentrationen und diskelektrophoretische Auftrennung des Sekretes an fraktioniert gewonnenem menschlichem Parotissekret. Lar. Rhinol. Otol. *54:* 19–27 (1975).

103 Eichner, H.; Bretzel, G.; Hochstrasser, K.: Simultane Bestimmungen von Flussrate, Gesamteiweiss, Lysozym und Immunglobulin A bei Drüsensekreten von menschli-chen Ohrspeicheldrüsen mit pleomorphen Adenomen. Lar. Rhinol. Otol. *55:* 586–592 (1976).

104 Eichner, H.; Bretzel, G.; Hochstrasser, K.: Biochemische Veränderungen der Sekret-zusammensetzung von menschlichen Ohrspeicheldrüsen mit malignen Tumoren, chronischen Entzündungen und Sialadenosen. Immunglobulin-A-, Lysozym-, Fluss-raten- und Gesamteiweissbestimmungen. Lar. Rhinol. Otol. *56:* 32–40 (1977).

105 Eichner, H.; Eichner, V.; Münzel, M.; Hochstrasser, K.: Simultanbestimmungen von Lysozym- und Immunglobulin-A-Gehalt von menschlichem Parotissekret im Vergleich zu Flussrate und Gesamtproteinausscheidung bei fraktionierter Ruhe- und Reizabnahme. Lar. Rhinol. Otol. *54:* 554–565 (1975).

106 Eichner, H.; Eichner, V.; Fiedler, F.; Hochstrasser, K.: Zum Sekretionsverhalten der BAEE-Esterase (Kallikrein) im gesunden menschlichen Parotissekret unter frak tionierter Abnahme bei Ruhe und Reiz. Lar. Rhinol. Otol. *55:* 239–244 (1976).

107 Eichner, H.; Bretzel, G.; Münzel, M.; Hochstrasser, K.: Über die Proteinzusammen-setzung des menschlichen Parotissekretes bei akuten und chronischen Entzündungen. Quantitative densitometrische Bestimmung der einzelnen Proteinfraktionen im Ver-gleich zu normalen Drüsensekreten. Lar. Rhinol. Otol. *55:* 499–506 (1976).

108 Elattar, T.M.A.: Metabolism of estrone and progesterone in vitro in human saliva. J. Steroid Biochem. *6:* 1455–1458 (1975).

109 Ellison, S.A.: Chemical and immunological studies of the proteins and glycoproteins of human parotid saliva; in Sreebny, Meyer, Salivary glands and their secretion, pp. 365–380 (Pergamon Press, New York 1964).

110 Ellison, S.A.: Antigenic analysis of saliva. J. dent. Res. *45:* 644–654 (1966).

111 Ellison, S.A.: Proteins and glycoproteins of saliva; in Code, Handbook of physiology, sect. 6, vol. 2, pp. 531–559 (American Physiological Society, Washington 1967).

112 Ericson, S.: The importance of sialography for the determination of the parotid flow. The normal variation in salivary output in relation to the size of the gland at stimulation with citric acid. Acta oto-lar. *72:* 437–444 (1971).

113 Faillard, H.; Schauer, R.: Glycoproteins as lubricants, protective agents, carriers, structural proteins and as participants in other functions; in Gottschalk, Glyco-proteins; their composition, structure and function. B.B.A. Library, vol. 5, part B, pp. 1246–1267 (Elsevier, Amsterdam 1972).

114 Ferguson, D.B.: Salivary glands and saliva; in Lavell, Applied physiology of the mouth, pp. 145–179 (Wright, Bristol 1975).

115 Ferguson, D.B.; Fort, A.: Circadian variations in human resting submandibular saliva flow rate and composition. Archs oral Biol. *19:* 47–55 (1974).

116 Ferguson, D.B.; Fort, A.; Elliott, A.L.; Potts, A.J.: Circadian rhythms in human parotid saliva flow rate and composition. Archs oral Biol. *18:* 1155–1173 (1973).

117 Fickling, B.W.; Pincus, P.; Boyd-Cooper, B.: M.&B. 693 in the saliva. Lancet *ii:* 1310–1311 (1939).

118 Fiessinger, J.N.; Camilleri, J.P.; Amat, C.; Ollier, M.P.; Housset, E.; Hartmann, L.: Salivary immunoglobulins in progressive systemic sclerosis. Biomedicine *28:* 298–303 (1978).

119 Findlay, D.; Lawrence, J.R.: An alternative method of assessing changes in salivary flow: comparison of the effects of clonidine and tiamenidine (HOE 440). Eur. J. clin. Pharmacol. *14:* 231–235 (1978).

120 Fiori, A.; Giusti, G.V.; Panari, G.; Porcelli, G.: Gel filtration of ABH blood group substances of human saliva. J. Chromat. *55:* 337–349 (1971).

121 Fischer, E.H.; Stein, E.A.: α-Amylase from human saliva. Biochem. Prep. *8:* 27–33 (1961).

122 Fleming, A.: On a remarkable bacteriolytic element found in tissues and secretions. Proc. R. Soc., Lond., ser. B *93:* 306–317 (1922).

123 Foot, C.H.; Wiener, K.: Phadebas amylase test kits. Clin. Chem. *25:* 818 (1979).

124 Friedman, R.D.; Allushuski, R.: An improved method for the detection of anionic polymorphic proteins in human saliva on polyacrylamide slab gels. Analyt. Biochem. *65:* 561–566 (1975).

125 Friedman, R.D.; Merritt, A.D.: Partial purification and characterization of a polymorphic protein (Pa) in human parotid saliva. Am. J. hum. Genet. *27:* 304–314 (1975).

126 Friedman, R.D.; Karn, R.C.: Immunological relationships and a genetic interpretation of major and minor acidic proteins in human parotid saliva. Biochem. Genet. *15:* 549–562 (1977).

127 Friedman, R.D.; Merritt, A.D.; Bixler, D.: Immunological and chemical comparison of heterogeneous basic glycoproteins in human parotid saliva. Biochim. biophys. Acta *230:* 599–602 (1971).

128 Friedman, R.D.; Merritt, A.D.; Rivas, M.L.: Genetic studies on human acidic salivary protein (Pa). Am. J. hum. Genet. *27:* 292–303 (1975).

129 Fujimoto, M.; Kameji, T.; Kanaya, A.; Hagihira, H.: Purification and properties of rat small intestinal arginase. J. Biochem., Tokyo *79:* 441–449 (1976).

130 Germaine, G.R.; Tellefson, L.M.; Johnson, G.L.: Proteolytic activity of *Candida albicans:* action on human salivary proteins. Infect. Immunity *22:* 861–866 (1978).

131 Gibbons, R.J.; Qureshi, J.V.: Selective binding of blood group-reactive salivary mucins by *Streptococcus mutans* and other oral organisms. Infect. Immunity *22:* 665–671 (1978).

132 Gillard, B.K.; Markman, H.C.; Feig, S.A.: Direct spectrophotometric determination of α-amylase activity in saliva, with *p*-nitrophenyl α-maltoside as substrate. Clin. Chem. *23:* 2279–2282 (1977).

133 Gilman, S.; Thornton, R.; Miller, D.; Biersner, R.: Effects of exercise stress on parotid gland secretion. Hormone metabol. Res. *11:* 454 (1979).

134 Gisclon, L.; Rowse, K.; Ayres, J.: Saliva, urine and plasma analysis of dyphylline via HPLC. Res. Commun. chem. Pathol. Pharmacol. *23:* 523–531 (1979).

135 Gitlitz, P.H.; Frings, C.S.: Interferences with the starch-iodine assay for serum amylase activity, and effects of hyperlipemia. Clin. Chem. *22:* 2006–2009 (1976).

136 Glynn, J.P.; Bastain, W.: Salivary excretion of paracetamol in man. J. Pharm. Pharmac. *25:* 420–421 (1973).

137 Gopalakrishna, R.; Nagarajan, B.: Arginase in human saliva. Indian J. Biochem. Biophys. *15:* 488–490 (1978).

138 Gothefors, L.; Marklund, S.: Lactoperoxidase activity in human milk and in saliva of newborn infants. Infect. Immunity *11:* 1210–1215 (1975).

139 Graham, G.; Rowland, M.: Application of salivary salicylate data to biopharmaceutical studies of salicylates. J. pharm. Sci. *61:* 1219–1222 (1972).

140 Grimmel, K.; Rossbach, G.; Kasper, H.: Amylase activity of parotid saliva in acute and chronic pancreatitis. Acta hepato-gastroent. *23:* 334–344 (1976).

141 Haeringen, N.J. van; Ensink, F.T.E.; Glasius, E.: The peroxidase-thiocyanate-hydrogenperoxide system in tear fluid and saliva of different species. Expl. Eye Res. *28:* 343–347 (1979).

142 Halpern, M.S.; Koshland, M.E.: Novel subunit in secretory IgA. Nature, Lond. *228:* 1276–1278 (1970).

143 Harden, R. McG.; Alexander, W.D.: The relation between the clearance of iodide and pertechnetate in human parotid saliva and salivary flow rate. Clin. Sci. *33:* 425–431 (1967).

144 Hattingh, J.: Albumins in saliva: what concentration? S. Afr. J. Sci. *75:* 184–186 (1979).

145 Hay, D.I.: The interaction of human parotid salivary proteins with hydroxyapatite. Archs oral Biol. *18:* 1517–1529 (1973).

146 Hay, D.I.: Fractionation of human parotid salivary proteins and the isolation of a histidine-rich acidic peptide which shows high affinity for hydroxyapatite surfaces. Archs oral Biol. *20:* 553–558 (1975).

147 Hay, D.I.; Oppenheim, F.G.: The isolation from human parotid saliva of a further group of proline rich proteins. Archs oral Biol. *19:* 627–632 (1974).

148 Heap, R.; Broad, S.: Oestrogens in saliva. Br. J. Hosp. Med. *11:* 471 (1974).

149 Henkin, R.I.; Lippoldt, R.E.; Bilstad, J.; Wolf, R.O.; Lum, C.K.L.; Edelhoch, H.: Fractionation of human parotid saliva proteins. J. biol. Chem. *253:* 7556–7565 (1978).

150 Herp, A.; Wu, A.M.; Moschera, J.: Current concepts of the structure and nature of mammalian salivary mucous glycoproteins. Mol. cell. Biochem. *23:* 27–44 (1979).

151 Hoeprich, P.D.: Prediction of antimeningococcic chemoprophylactic efficacy. J. infect. Dis. *123:* 125–133 (1971).

152 Hoeprich, P.D.; Warshauer, D.M.: Entry of four tetracyclines into saliva and tears. Antimicrob. Agents Chemother. *5:* 330–336 (1974).

153 Hoerman, K.C.; Englander, H.R.; Shklair, I.L.: Lysozyme: its characteristics in human parotid and submaxillo-lingual saliva. Proc. Soc. exp. Biol. Med. *92:* 875–878 (1956).

154 Hoerman, K.C.; Chauncey, H.H.; Herrold, D.: Parotid saliva acid phosphatase in prostatic cancer. Cancer *12:* 359–363 (1959).

155 Hogg, D.M.; Jago, G.R.: The antibacterial action of lactoperoxidase. The nature of the antibacterial inhibitor. Biochem. J. *117:* 779–790 (1970).

156 Holbrook, I.B.; Molan, P.C.: The identification of a peptide in human parotid saliva particularly active in enhancing the glycolytic activity of the salivary microorganisms. Biochem. J. *149:* 489–492 (1975).

157 Hsiu, J.; Fischer, E.H.; Stein, E.A.: Alpha-amylases as calcium-metalloenzymes. II. Calcium and the catalytic activity. Biochemistry 3: 61–66 (1964).

158 Hunter, R.L.; Markert, C.L.: Histochemical demonstration of enzymes separated by zone electrophoresis in starch gels. Science 125: 1294–1295 (1957).

159 Hürliman, J.; Zuber, C.: In vitro synthesis by human salivary glands. II. Synthesis of proteins specific to saliva and other excretions. Immunology 14: 819–824 (1967).

160 Hyde, R.J.; Pangborn, R.M.: Effects of visual influences and tactile stimulation on human parotid flow rates. J. dent. Res. 58: 542 (1979).

161 IUPAC–IUB: Commission on Biochemical Nomenclature 1971. The nomenclature of multiple forms of enzymes recommendations. Archs Biochem. Biophys. 147: 1–3 (1971).

162 Iwamoto, Y.; Inoue, M.; Tsunemitsu, A.; Matsumura, T.: Some properties of the salivary antibacterial factor (S.A. factor). Archs oral Biol. 12: 1009–1012 (1967).

163 Iwamoto, Y.; Nakamura, R.; Tsunemitsu, A.; Matsumura, T.: The heterogeneity of human salivary peroxidase. Archs oral Biol. 13: 1015–1018 (1968).

164 Iwamoto, Y.; Nakamura, R.; Watanabe, T.; Tsunemitsu, A.: Heterogeneity of peroxidase related to antibacterial activity in human parotid saliva. J. dent. Res. 51: 503–508 (1972).

165 Jeschke, R.; Ströder, J.: Continual observation of clinical and immunological parameters, in particular of salivary IgA, in tonsillectomised children. Archs Oto-Rhino-Lar. 226: 73–84 (1980).

166 Jones, A.W.: Distribution of ethanol between saliva and blood in man. Clin. exp. Pharmacol. Physiol. 6: 53–59 (1979).

167 Josephson, A.S.; Weiner, R.S.: Studies of the proteins of lacrimal secretions. J. Immun. 100: 1080–1092 (1968).

168 Kaiser, D.; Schöni, M.; Drack, E.: Anionen- und Kationenausscheidung der Parotis in Abhängigkeit von der Fliessrate bei Mukoviszidosepatienten und Gesunden. Helv. paediat. Acta 29: 145–150 (1974).

169 Kakizaki, G.; Saito, T.; Soeno, T.; Sasahara, M.; Fujiwara, Y.: A new diagnostic test for pancreatic disorders by examination of parotid saliva. Am. J. Gastroent., N.Y. 65: 437–445 (1976).

170 Kamaryt, J.; Laxová, R.: Amylase heterogeneity: some genetic and clinical aspects. Humangenetik 1: 579–586 (1965).

171 Kamaryt, J.; Laxová, R.: Amylase heterogeneity variants in man. Humangenetik 3: 41–45 (1966).

172 Kanamori, T.; Kuzuya, H.; Nagatsu, T.: Excretion of cyclic AMP and cyclic GMP into human parotid saliva. J. dent. Res. 53: 760 (1974).

173 Kanamori, T.; Nagatsu, T.; Matsumoto, S.: Origin of cyclic adenosine monophosphate in saliva. J. dent. Res. 54: 535–539 (1974).

174 Karn, R.C.; Rosenblum, B.B.; Merritt, A.D.: A biochemical explanation for the complex isozyme patterns of salivary amylase (Amy$_1$) and pancreatic amylase (Amy$_2$). Am. J. hum. Genet. 25: 39 A (1973).

175 Karn, R.C.; Shulkin, J.D.; Merritt, A.D.; Newell, R.C.: Evidence for post-transcriptional modification of human salivary amylase (Amy$_1$) isozymes. Biochem-Genet. 10: 341–350 (1973).

176 Karn, R.C.; Rosenblum, B.B.; Ward, J.C.; Merritt, A.D.: Genetic and post. translational mechanisms determining human amylase isozyme heterogeneity; in

Markert, Isozymes IV. Genetics and evolution, pp. 745–761 (Academic Press, New York 1975).

177 Karn, R.C.; Rosenblum, B.B.; Ward, J.C.; Merritt, A.D.; Shulkin, J.D.: Immunological relationships and post-translational modifications of human salivary amylase (Amy$_1$) and pancreatic amylase (Amy$_2$) isozymes. Biochem. Genet. *12:* 485–499 (1974).

178 Katz, R.L.; Mandel, I.D.: Action and interaction of isoproterenol and alpha- and beta-adrenergic blockers on parotid and submaxillary secretions in man. Proc. Soc. exp. Biol. Med. *128:* 1140–1145 (1968).

179 Kauffman, D.L.; Zager, N.I.; Cohen, E.; Keller, P.J.: The isoenzymes of human parotid amylase. Archs Biochem. Biophys. *137:* 325–339 (1970).

180 Kauffman, D.L.; Watanabe, S.; Evans, J.R.; Keller, P.J.: The existence of glycosylated and non-glycosylated forms of human submandibular amylase. Archs oral Biol. *18:* 1105–1111 (1973).

181 Keller, P.J.; Kauffman, D.L.; Allan, B.J.; Williams, B.L.: Further studies on the structural differences between the isoenzymes of human parotid α-amylase. Biochemistry *10:* 4867–4874 (1971).

182 Klebanoff, S.J.: Inactivation of estrogen by rat uterine preparations. Endocrinology *76:* 301–311 (1965).

183 Klebanoff, S.J.: Iodination of bacteria: a bactericidal mechanism. J. exp. Med. *126:* 1063–1078 (1968).

184 Klebanoff, S.J.: Myeloperoxidase-halide-hydrogen peroxide antibacterial system. J. Bact. *95:* 2131–2138 (1968).

185 Klebanoff, S.J.; Luebke, R.G.: The antilactobacillus system of saliva. Role of salivary peroxidase. Proc. Soc. exp. Biol. Med. *118:* 483–486 (1965).

186 Knauf, H.; Frömter, E.: Die Kationenausscheidung der grossen Speicheldrüsen des Menschen. Pflügers Arch. ges. Physiol. *316:* 213–237 (1970).

187 Kolb, E.: Körper- und Zellbestandteile. I. D: Verdauungssekrete; in Rauen, Biochemisches Taschenbuch, vol. II, pp. 365–366 (Springer, Berlin 1964).

188 Koup, J.R.; Lau, A.H.; Brodsky, B.; Slaughter, R.L.: Relationship between serum and saliva chloramphenicol concentrations. Antimicrob. Agents Chemother. *15:* 658–661 (1979).

189 Kousvelari, E.E.; Oppenheim, F.G.: Immunological comparison of proline-rich proteins from human and primate parotid secretion. Biochim. biophys. Acta *578:* 76–86 (1979).

190 Krakowka, P.; Izdebska-Makosa, Z.; Wareska, W.: Determination of para-aminosalicylic acid in the saliva as check-up of treatment with this drug. Pol. med. J. *5:* 895–899 (1966).

191 Kreusser, W.; Heidland, A.; Hennemann, H.; Wigand, M.E.; Knauf, H.: Mono- and divalent electrolyte patterns, pCO$_2$ and pH in relation to flow rate in normal human parotid saliva. Eur. J. clin. Invest. *2:* 398–406 (1972).

192 Kumlien, A.: Iodine metabolism and peroxidase activity in salivary glands. Acta endocr., Copenh. *70:* 239–246 (1972).

193 Kutscher, A.H.; Mandel, I.D.; Zegarelli, E.V.; Denning, C.; Eriv, A.; Ruiz, L.; Ellgood, K.; Phalen, J.: A technique for collecting the secretion of minor salivary glands: use of capillary tubes. J. oral Ther. Pharm. *3:* 391–392 (1967).

194 Lamberts, B.L.; Meyer, T.S.: Amylolytic fractions of salivary secretion; in Schneyer,

Secretory mechanisms of salivary glands, pp. 313–325 (Academic Press, New York 1967).

195 Lamberts, B.L.; Meyer, T.S.: Permeability of cellophane membranes to parotid proteins during dialysis. Experientia 35: 165–166 (1979).

196 Lamberts, B.L.; Meyer, T.S.; Losee, F.L.: Isolation of amylolytic fractions from human parotid saliva. Fed. Proc. 24: 441 (1965).

197 Lamberts, B.L.; Meyer, T.S.; Osborne, R.M.: A comparative study of human parotid and submaxillary amylase. Archs oral Biol. 16: 517–526 (1971).

198 Lammintausta, K.; Kangas, L.; Lammintausta, R.: The pharmacokinetics of dapsone and acetylated dapsone in serum and saliva. Int. J. clin. Pharmacol. Biopharm. 17: 159–163 (1979).

199 Landman, A.D.; Sanford, L.M.; Howland, B.E.; Dawes, C.; Pritchard, E.T.: Testosterone in human saliva. Experientia 32: 940–941 (1976).

200 Langmyhr, F.J.; Eyde, B.: Determination of the total content and distribution of cadmium, copper and zinc in human parotid saliva. Analytica chim. Acta 107: 211–218 (1979).

201 Lankisch, P.G.; Chilla, R.; Luerssen, K.; Koop, H.; Arglebe, C.; Creutzfeldt, W.: Parotid saliva test in the diagnosis of chronic pancreatitis. Digestion 19: 52–55 (1979).

202 Lashley, K.S.: Reflex secretion of the human parotid gland. J. exp. Psychol. 1: 461–493 (1916).

203 Lazarus, J.H.; Harden, R. McG.; Robertson, J.W.K.: Sex differences in human parotid salivary secretion of iodide, pertechnetate and bromide. Archs oral Biol. 16: 225–231 (1971).

204 Lehrner, L.M.; Malacinski, G.M.: Genetic and structural studies of chicken α-amylase isozymes and their modified forms, and structural studies of hog amylase; in Markert, Isozymes IV. Genetics and evolution, pp. 727–743 (Academic Press, New York 1975).

205 Levine, M.; Keller, P.J.: The isolation of some basic proline-rich proteins from human parotid saliva. Archs oral Biol. 22: 37–41 (1977).

206 Levine, M.J.; Ellison, S.A.; Bahl, O.P.: The isolation from human parotid saliva and partial characterization of the protein core of a major parotid glycoprotein. Archs oral Biol. 18: 827–837 (1973).

207 Lionetti, F.J.; Chauncey, H.H.; Lisanti, V.F.: Human parotid salivary acid phosphomonoesterase. Biochim. biophys. Acta 24: 496–502 (1957).

208 Lorentz, K.: Salivary isoamylases: deamidation products of amylase. Clinica chim. Acta 93: 161–162 (1979).

209 Lorentz, K.: α-Amylase assay: current state and future development. Rep. Workshop Conf. German Soc. Clinical Chemistry, Frankfurt 1978. J. clin. Chem. clin. Biochem. 17: 499–504 (1979).

210 Lowry, O.H.; Rosebrough, N.J.; Farr, A.L.; Randall, R.J.: Protein measurement with the Folin phenol reagent. J. biol. Chem. 193: 265–275 (1951).

211 Lutz, D.; Gülzow, H.-J.: Respirometric investigations into the influence of the sugar substitute xylitol on sucrose degradation in human saliva. Caries Res. 13: 132–136 (1979).

212 Macfarlane, C.B.; McCrossan, J.; Stephen, K.W.; Speirs, C.F.: Physicochemical factors influencing the presence of antibiotics in salivary secretion. J. dent. Res. 53: 1081 (1974).

213 Madsen, S.N.; Badawi, I.: Variations in the content of cyclic adenosine mono-phosphate in human mixed saliva during physiological stimulation. Archs oral Biol. *21:* 481–483 (1976).

214 Mahler, I.R.; Chauncey, H.H.: Lipolytic and esterolytic activity of saliva and salivary organisms. J. dent. Res. *36:* 338–342 (1957).

215 Maier, H.; Coroneo, M.T.; Heidland, A.; Wigand, M.E.: Ionisiertes Calcium und Totalcalcium im Parotisspeichel bei Normalpersonen und essentiellen Hypertonikern. Lar. Rhinol. Otol. *57:* 1013–1017 (1978).

216 Maier, H.; Coroneo, M.T.; Antonczyk, G.; Heidland, A.: The flow-rate-dependent excretion of ionized calcium in human parotid saliva. Archs oral Biol. *24:* 225–227 (1979).

217 Maier, H.; Geissler, M.; Heidland, A.; Schindler, J.G.; Wigand, M.E.: Beeinflussung speichelchemischer Parameter in Abhängigkeit vom Menstruationszyklus. Lar. Rhinol. Otol. *58:* 706–710 (1979).

218 Mandel, I.D.: Human submaxillary, sublingual, and parotid glycoproteins and enamel pellicle; in Horowitz, Pigman, The glycoconjugates, vol. I: Mammalian glycoproteins and glycolipids, pp. 153–179 (Academic Press, New York 1977).

219 Mandel, I.D.; Ellison, S.A.: The proteins of human parotid and submaxillary saliva. Ann. N.Y. Acad. Sci. *106:* 271–277 (1963).

220 Mandel, I.D.; Ellison, S.A.: Organic components of human parotid and submaxillary saliva. Ann. N.Y. Acad. Sci. *131:* 802–811 (1965).

221 Mandel, I.D.; Khurana, H.S.: The relation of human salivary gamma-A globulin and albumin to flow rate. Archs oral Biol. *14:* 1433–1435 (1969).

222 Mandel, I.D.; Thompson, R.H., Jr.; Ellison, S.A.: Studies on the mucoproteins of human parotid saliva. Archs oral Biol. *10:* 499–507 (1965).

223 Mandel, I.D.; Thompson, R.H., Jr.; Wotman, S.; Taubman, M.; Kutscher, A.H.; Zegarelli, E.V.; Denning, C.R.; Botwick, J.T.; Fahn, B.S.: Parotid saliva in cystic fibrosis. Am. J. Dis. Child. *110:* 646–651 (1965).

224 Marks, P.A.; Banks, J.: Inhibition of mammalian glucose-6-phosphate dehydro-genase by steroids. Proc. natn. Acad. Sci. USA *46:* 447–452 (1960).

225 Mason, D.K.; Chisholm, D.M.: Salivary glands in health and disease (Saunders, London 1975).

226 Mason, D.K.; Harden, R. McG.; Alexander, W.D.: The influence of flow rate on the salivary iodide concentration in man. Archs oral Biol. *11:* 235–246 (1966).

227 Mathew, R.J.; Claghorn, J.L.; Fenimore, D.; Davis, C.; Mirabi, M.: Red cell and salivary lithium levels. Br. J. Psychiat. *134:* 318 (1979).

228 Matin, S.B.; Wan, S.H.; Karam, J.H.: Pharmacokinetics of tolbutamide: prediction by concentration in saliva. Clin. Pharmacol. Ther. *16:* 1052–1058 (1974).

229 Mayo, J.W.; Carlson, D.M.: Protein composition of human submandibular secre-tions. Archs Biochem. Biophys. *161:* 134–135 (1974).

230 Mayo, J.W.; Carlson, D.M.: Isolation and properties of four α-amylase isozymes from human submandibular saliva. Archs Biochem. Biophys. *163:* 498–506 (1974).

231 McColl, K.E.L.; Whiting, B.; Moore, M.R.; Goldberg, A.: Correlation of ethanol concentrations in blood and saliva. Clin. Sci. *56:* 283–286 (1979).

232 McConnell, W.R.; Dewey, W.L.; Harris, L.S.; Borzelleca, J.F.: A study of the effect of delta⁹-tetrahydrocannabinol (delta⁹-THC) on mammalian salivary flow. J. Pharmac. exp. Ther. *206:* 567–573 (1978).

233 McGeachin, R.; Hay, P.; Prell, P.: Comparison of saliva in amylase-levels in the human male and female. Nature, Lond. *208:* 1211–1212 (1965).

234 McKean, F.J.; Beeley, J.A.: Immunological studies on human salivary albumin. Archs oral Biol. *19:* 103–106 (1974).

235 Meffin, P.J.; Williams, R.L.; Blaschke, T.F.; Rowland, M.: Application of salivary concentration data to pharmacokinetic studies with antipyrine. J. pharm. Sci. *66:* 135–137 (1977).

236 Mellersh, A.; Clark, A.; Hafiz, S.: Inhibition of *Neisseria gonorrhoeae* by normal human saliva. Br. J. vener. Dis. *55:* 20–23 (1979).

237 Menguy, R.; Masters, Y.F.; Desbaillets, L.: Human salivary glycosidases. Proc. Soc. exp. Biol. Med. *134:* 1020–1025 (1970).

238 Merritt, A.D.; Karn, R.C.: The human α-amylases; in Harris, Hirschhorn, Advances in human genetics, vol. 8, pp. 135–234 (Plenum Press, New York 1977).

239 Meyer, P.; Nürnberger, E.: Zur Sekretion von Amylase und saurer Phosphatase durch die Parotis des Menschen vor und nach gustatorischer Stimulation unter Berücksichtigung der Enzymkonzentration und der Enzymsekretionsrate. Lar. Rhinol. Otol. *53:* 223–229 (1974).

240 Meyer, P.; Schneider, D.: Der Albumingehalt des Parotisspeichels unter Berücksichtigung des Lebensalters. Lar. Rhinol. Otol. *54:* 551–553 (1975).

241 Mirth, D.B.; Miller, C.J.; Kingman, A.; Bowen, W.H.: Inhibition of saliva-induced aggregation of *Streptococcus mutans* by wheat germ agglutinin. Caries Res. *13:* 121–131 (1979).

242 Moriya, H.; Pierce, J.V.; Webster, M.E.: Purification and some properties of three kallikreins. Ann. N.Y. Acad. Sci. *104:* 172–185 (1963).

243 Moriya, H.; Yamazaki, K.; Fukushima, H.: Biochemical studies on kallikreins and their related substances. I. Isolation and purification of human saliva kallikrein. J. Biochem., Tokyo *58:* 201–207 (1965).

244 Morrison, M.; Hultquist, D.E.: Lactoperoxidase. II. Isolation. J. biol. Chem. *238:* 2847–2849 (1963).

245 Morrison, M.; Allen, P.Z.; Bright, J.; Jayasinghe, W.: Lactoperoxidase. V. Identification and isolation of lactoperoxidase from salivary gland. Archs Biochem. Biophys. *111:* 126–133 (1965).

246 Mosimann, W.; Sumner, J.B.: Salivary peroxidase. Archs Biochem. Biophys. *33:* 487 (1951).

247 Mucklow, J.C.; Bending, M.R.; Kahn, G.C.; Dollery, C.T.: Drug concentration in saliva. Clin. Pharmacol. Ther. *24:* 563–570 (1978).

248 Münzel, M.: Die Biochemie der menschlichen Speicheldrüsensekrete. Archs Oto-Rhino-Lar. *213:* 209–285 (1976).

249 Mutzbauer, H.; Schulz, G.V.: Die Bestimmung der molekularen Konstanten von α-Amylase aus Humanspeichel. Biochim. biophys. Acta *102:* 526–532 (1965).

250 Muus, J.: Studies on salivary amylase with special reference to the interaction with chloride ions. C. r. Lab. Carlsberg, sér. chim. *28:* 317–334 (1953).

251 Muus, J.: The amino acid composition of human salivary amylase. J. Am. chem. Soc. *76:* 5163–5165 (1954).

252 Muus, J.; Vnenchak, J.M.: Isozymes of salivary amylase. Nature, Lond. *204:* 283–285 (1964).

253 Myers, V.C.; Free, A.H.; Rosinsky, E.E.: Studies on animal diastases. VI. The determination of diastase (amylase) in blood. J. biol. Chem. *154:* 39–48 (1944).

254 Myrbäck, K.: Über Verbindungen einiger Enzyme mit inaktiverenden Stoffen. II. Hoppe-Seyler's Z. physiol. Chem. *159:* 1–84 (1926).

255 Nacchiero, M.; Biezunski, D.; Landau, S.; Dreiling, D.A.; Adler, M.; Rudick, J.: The parotid and the pancreas. V. Effects of a synthetic prostaglandin analog on parotid gland secretion. Am. J. Gastroent., N.Y. *70:* 374–378 (1978).

256 Nakamura, R.; Tsunemitsu, A.: The presence of cytidine-5'-monophosphosialic acid: glycoprotein sialyltransferase in human saliva. J. dent. Res. *54:* 188 (1975).

257 Nakamura, R.; Tsunemitsu, A.: The presence of guanosine diphosphofucose: glycoprotein fucosyltransferase in human saliva. J. dent. Res. *54:* 514 (1975).

258 Nakamura, R.; Watanabe, T.; Iwamoto, Y.; Tsunemitsu, A.: Purification and properties of acid phosphomonoesterase from human parotid saliva. J. dent. Res. *49:* 561–566 (1970).

259 Nakamura, R.; Watanabe, T.; Yasutake, A.; Tsunemitsu, A.: The presence of uridine-5'-diphosphogalactose: N-acetylglucosamine galactosyltransferase in human saliva. J. dent. Res. *53:* 937 (1974).

260 Nawrot, C.F.; Campbell, D.J.; Schroeder, J.K.; Valkenburg, M. van: Dental phosphoprotein-induced formation of hydroxylapatite during in vitro synthesis of amorphous calcium phosphate. Biochemistry *15:* 3445–3449 (1976).

261 Nickerson, J.F.; Kraus, F.W.; Perry, W.I.: Peroxidase and catalase in saliva. Proc. Soc. exp. Biol. Med. *95:* 405–408 (1957).

262 Nishihara, K.; Uchino, K.; Saitoh, Y.; Honda, Y.; Nakagawa, F.; Tamura, Z.: Estimation of plasma unbound phenobarbital concentration by using mixed saliva. Epilepsia *20:* 37–45 (1979).

263 Noronha, M.; Dreiling, D.A.; Bordalo, O.: The parotid and the pancreas. IV. Parotid secretion after secretin stimulation as a screening test of pancreatic dysfunction. Am. J. Gastroent., N.Y. *70:* 282–285 (1978).

264 Ogita, S.: Genetico-biochemical studies on the salivary and pancreatic amylase isoenzymes in the human. Med. J. Osaka Univ. *16:* 271–286 (1966).

265 Ohno, S.; Payne, H.W.; Morrison, M.; Beutler, E.: Hexose-6-phosphate dehydrogenase found in human liver. Science *153:* 1015–1016 (1966).

266 Oppenheim, F.G.: Preliminary observations on the presence and origin of serum albumin in human saliva. Helv. odont. Acta *14:* 10–17 (1970).

267 Oppenheim, F.G.; Hay, D.I.; Franzblau, C.: Proline-rich proteins from human parotid saliva. I. Isolation and partial characterization. Biochemistry *10:* 4233–4238 (1971).

268 Oram, J.D.; Reiter, B.: The inhibition of streptococci by lactoperoxidase, thiocyanate, and hydrogen peroxide. The oxidation of thiocyanate and the nature of the inhibitory compound. Biochem. J. *100:* 382–388 (1966).

269 Ornstein, L.; Davis, B.J.: Disc electrophoresis (Distillation Products Industries, distributed by Eastman Kodak Co., Rochester 1961).

270 Oya, H.; Yamamoto, T.; Nagatsu, T.: Presence of leucine aminopeptidase activity in human saliva from the parotid gland and the submaxillary-sublingual glands. Archs oral Biol. *13:* 941–948 (1968).

271 Oya, H.; Nagatsu, I.; Nagatsu, T.: Purification and properties of glycoprolyl-β-

naphthylamidase in human submaxillary gland. Biochim. biophys. Acta *258:* 591–599 (1972).

272 Patrick, R.L.; Thiers, R.E.: The direct spectrophotometric determination of protein in cerebrospinal fluid. Clin. Chem. *9:* 283–295 (1963).

273 Paulsen, K.; Kröger, H.D.: Die Natrium- und Kaliumionenkonzentration im Gesamtspeichel von Säuglingen und Erwachsenen. Arch. Ohr.-Nas.-KehlkHeilk. *201:* 136–146 (1972).

274 Pazur, J.H.; French, D.; Knapp, D.W.: Mechanism of salivary amylase action. Proc. Iowa Acad. Sci. *57:* 203–209 (1950).

275 Perlitsch, M.J.; Glickman, I.: Salivary neuraminidase. II. Its source in whole human saliva. J. dent. Res. *45:* 1239 (1965).

276 Peters, E.H.; Azen, E.A.: Isolation and partial characterization of human parotid basic proteins. Biochem. Genet. *15:* 925–946 (1977).

277 Peters, E.H.; Goodfriend, T.; Azen, E.A.: Human Pb, human post-Pb and non human primate Pb proteins: immunological and biochemical relationships. Biochem. Genet. *15:* 947–962 (1977).

278 Petit, J.F.; Jolles, P.: Purification and analysis of human saliva lysozyme. Nature, Lond. *200:* 168–169 (1963).

279 Pierce, J.V.; Webster, M.E.: Human plasma kallidins: isolation and chemical studies. Biochem. biophys. Res. Commun. *5:* 353–357 (1961).

280 Pilz, H.; O'Brien, J.S.; Heipertz, R.: Human saliva peroxidase: microanalytical isoelectric fractionation and properties in normal persons and in cases with neuronal ceroid-lipofuscinosis. Clin. Biochem. *9:* 85–88 (1976).

281 Pless, J.; Stürmer, E.; Guttman, S.; Boissonnas, R.A.: Kallidin, Synthese und Eigenschaften. Helv. chim. Acta *45:* 394–396 (1962).

282 Porembska, Z.; Barańczyk, A.; Jachimowicz, J.: Arginase isoenzymes in liver and kidney of some mammals. Acta biochim. Polon. *18:* 77–85 (1971).

283 Pronk, J.C.; Frants, R.R.: New genetic variants of parotid salivary amylase. Hum. Hered. *29:* 181–186 (1979).

284 Pu, F.S.; Chiou, W.L.: Creatinine. VII. Determination of saliva creatinine by high-performance liquid chromatography. J. pharm. Sci. *68:* 534–535 (1979).

285 Puskulian, L.: Salivary electrolyte changes during the normal menstrual cycle. J. dent. Res. *51:* 1212–1216 (1972).

286 Rapoport, S.M.: Medizinische Biochemie (VEB Verlag Volk und Gesundheit, Berlin 1977).

287 Rauch, S.: Die Speicheldrüsen des Menschen. Anatomie, Physiologie und klinische Pathologie (Thieme, Stuttgart 1959).

288 Raymond, S.; Nakamichi, M.; Aurell, B.: Acrylamide gel as an electrophoresis medium. Nature, Lond. *195:* 697–699 (1962).

289 Revis, G.J.: Immunoelectrophoretic identification of lysozyme in saliva. Proc. Soc. exp. Biol. Med. *137:* 90–96 (1971).

290 Revis, G.J.: Immunoelectrophoretic identification of peroxidase in human parotid saliva. Archs oral Biol. *22:* 155–158 (1977).

291 Rick, W.; Stegbauer, H.P.: α-Amylase. Messung der reduzierenden Gruppen; in Bergmeyer, Methoden der enzymatischen Analyse, vol. I, pp. 918–923 (Verlag Chemie, Weinheim 1974).

292 Riva, A.; Puxeddu, P.; Fiacco, M. del; Testa-Riva, F.: Ultrastructural localization

of endogenous peroxidase in human parotid and submandibular glands. J. Anat. *127:* 181–191 (1978).

293 Roberts, M.S.; Rumble, R.H.; Brooks, P.M.: Salivary salicylate secretion and flow rate. Br. J. clin. Pharmacol. *6:* 429 (1978).

294 Robinson, A.B.; McKerrow, J.H.; Cary, P.: Controlled deamidation of peptides and proteins: an experimental hazard and a possible biological timer. Proc. natn. Acad. Sci. USA *66:* 753–759 (1970).

295 Robyt, J.F.; Whelan, W.J.: The α-amylases; in Radley, Starch and its derivatives, pp. 430–476 (Chapman & Hall, London 1968).

296 Rose, G.A.; Kerr, A.C.: The amino acids and phosphoethanolamine in salivary gland secretions of normal men and of patients with abnormal calcium, phosphorus and amino acid metabolism. Q. Jl. exp. Physiol. *43:* 160–168 (1958).

297 Rosenblum, B.B.; Karn, R.C.; Merritt, A.D.: A model for the pleiotropic isozyme expression of human salivary amylase. Fed. Proc. *34:* 676 (1975).

298 Roukema, P.A.; Nieuw Amerongen, A.V.: Sulphated glycoproteins in human saliva; in Kleinberg, Ellison, Mandel, Proc. 'Saliva and Dental Caries'. Microbiology Abstracts, suppl., pp. 67–80 (Information Retrieval, New York 1979).

299 Ruhwinkel, B.; Münzel, M.: Der Immunglobulingehalt des menschlichen Parotis-sekretes. Lar. Rhinol. Otol. *54:* 361–365 (1975).

300 Sachs, L.: Angewandte Statistik. Planung und Auswertung, Methoden und Modelle (Springer, Berlin 1974).

301 Saito, S.; Kizu, K.: Phosphatase activity in whole and parotid saliva and its relationship to dental caries. J. dent. Res. *38:* 500–505 (1959).

302 Schaeffer, L.D.; Sproles, A.; Kradowski, A.: Detection of cyclic AMP in parotid saliva of normal individuals. J. dent. Res. *52:* 629 (1973).

303 Schmid, G.; Hempel, K.; Fricke, L.; Wernze, H.; Heidland, A.: Erhöhte cAMP-Konzentration im Parotisspeichel des Menschen bei arterieller Hypertonie. Dt. med. Wschr. *100:* 1435–1437 (1975).

304 Schneyer, L.H.: Method for the collection of separate submaxillary and sublingual salivas in man. J. dent. Res. *34:* 257–261, 275–281 (1955).

305 Schneyer, L.H.: Source of resting total mixed saliva of man. J. appl. Physiol. *9:* 79–81 (1956).

306 Schneyer, L.H.: Amylase content of separate salivary gland secretions of man. J. appl. Physiol. *9:* 453–455 (1956).

307 Schneyer, L.H.; Pigman, W.; Hanahan, LaBr.; Gilmore, R.W.: Rate of flow of human parotid, sublingual, and submaxillary secretions during sleep. J. dent. Res. *35:* 109–114 (1956).

308 Schultz, J.; Felberg, N.; John, S.: Myeloperoxidase. VIII. Separation into ten components by free-flow electrophoresis. Biochem. biophys. Res. Commun. *28:* 543–549 (1967).

309 Sewell, H.F.; Matthews, J.B.; Flack, V.; Jefferis, R.: Human immunoglobulin D in colostrum, saliva and amniotic fluid. Clin. exp. Immunol. *36:* 183–188 (1979).

310 Shannon, I.L.: Parotid fluid flow rate as related to whole saliva volume. Archs oral Biol. *7:* 391–394 (1962).

311 Shannon, I.L.: Climatological effects on human parotid gland function. Archs oral Biol. *11:* 451–453 (1966).

312 Shannon, I.L.: Reference table for human parotid saliva collected at varying levels of exogenous stimulation. J. dent. Res. *52:* 1157 (1973).

313 Shannon, I.L.; Chauncey, H.H.: Hyperhydration and parotid flow in man. J. dent. Res. *46:* 1028–1031 (1967).

314 Shannon, I.L.; Suddick, R.P.: Effects of light and darkness on human parotid salivary flow rate and chemical composition. Archs oral Biol. *18:* 601–608 (1973)

315 Shannon, I.L.; Feller, R.P.: Effects of lights of specific spectral characteristics on human resting parotid gland function. Archs oral Biol. *19:* 1077–1088 (1974).

316 Shannon, I.L.; Prigmore, J.R.; Beering, S.C.: Effect of graded doses of ACTH on parotid fluid corticosteroid levels. Archs oral Biol. *10:* 461–464 (1965).

317 Shannon, I.L.; Suddick, R.P.; Dowd, F.J., Jr.: Saliva: composition and secretion (Karger, Basel 1974).

318 Shaw, C.R.: Glucose-6-phosphate dehydrogenase. Homologous molecules in deer mouse and man. Science *153:* 1013–1015 (1966).

319 Shaw, C.R.; Koen, A.L.: Glucose-6-phosphate dehydrogenase and hexose-6-phosphate dehydrogenase of mammalian tissues. Ann. N.Y. Acad. Sci. *151:* 149–156 (1968).

320 Shinowara, G.Y.; Jones, L.M.; Reinhart, H.L.: The estimation of serum inorganic phosphate and 'acid' and 'alkaline' phosphatase activity. J. biol. Chem. *142:* 921–933 (1942).

321 Siepmann, R.; Stegemann, H.: Enzym-Elektrophorese in Einschluss-Polymerisaten des Acrylamids. A. Amylasen, Phosphorylasen. Z. Naturf. *22b:* 949–955 (1967).

322 Simons, K.; Weber, P.; Stiel, M.; Gräsback, R.: Immunoelectrophoresis of human saliva. Acta med. scand., suppl. 412, pp. 257–264 (1964).

323 Skurk, A.; Mlynski, G.; Fendel, K.: Methoden der quantitativen Eiweissbestimmung im menschlichen Parotisspeichel. Acta oto-lar. *71:* 71–74 (1971).

324 Skurk, A.; Fritsche, D.; Fendel, K.: Variation in the amylase isoenzyme of human parotid saliva in health and disease. Archs oral Biol. *20:* 429–435 (1975).

325 Skurk, A.; Fendel, K.; Albrecht, R.: Enzymdiagnostik im menschlichen Parotisspeichel und ihre Probleme. Acta oto-lar. *81:* 315–322 (1976).

326 Skurk, A.; Krebs, S.; Rehberg, J.: Flow rate, protein, amylase, lysozyme and kallikrein of human parotid saliva in health and disease. Archs oral Biol. *24:* 739–743 (1979).

327 Skurk, A.; Winnefeld, K.; Leifer, M.; Fendel, K.: Die Konzentration zweiwertiger Kationen (Ca, Mg, Fe, Cu und Zn) im menschlichen Parotisspeichel. Lar. Rhinol. Otol. *53:* 863–867 (1974).

328 Skurk, A.; Winnefeld, K.; Tiedt, H.-J.; Schmidt, A.; Fendel, K.: Spurenelemente in Speichelsteinen. Die Bestimmung von Ca, Mg, Fe, Cu, Zn, Mn und P. Z. Lar. Rhinol. Otol. *52:* 822–824 (1973).

329 Slowey, R.R.; Eidelman, S.; Klebanoff, S.J.: Antibacterial activity of the purified peroxidase from human parotid saliva. J. Bact. *96:* 575–579 (1968).

330 Smith, Q.T.; Shapiro, B.L.; Hamilton, M.J.: Polyacrylamide gel patterns of parotid saliva proteins in Caucasoids and Amerindians. Archs oral Biol. *20:* 369–373 (1975).

331 Smith, Q.T.; Hamilton, M.J.; Biros, M.H.; Pihlstrom, B.L.: Salivary and plasma IgA of seizure subjects receiving phenytoin. Epilepsia *20:* 17–23 (1979).

332 Smith, R.G.; Besch, P.K.; Dill, B.; Buttram, V.C., Jr.: Saliva as a matrix for mea-

suring free androgens: comparison with serum androgens in polycystic ovarian disease. Fert. Steril. *31:* 513–517 (1979).

333 Somogyi, M.: Micromethods for estimation of diastase. J. biol. Chem. *125:* 399–414 (1938).

334 Somogyi, M.: Diastatic activity of human blood. Archs intern. Med. *67:* 665–679 (1941).

335 Soyza, K. de: Polymorphism of human salivary amylase. A preliminary communication. Hum. Genet. *45:* 189–192 (1978).

336 Speirs, C.F.; Stenhouse, D.; Stephen, K.W.; Wallace, E.T.: Comparison of human serum, parotid and mixed saliva levels of phenoxymethyl penicillin, ampicillin, cloxacillin and cephalexin. Br. J. Pharmacol. *43:* 242–247 (1971).

337 Steele, W.H.; Stuart, J.F.B.; Whiting, B.; Lawrence, J.R.; Calman, K.C.; McVie. J.G.; Baird, G.M.: Serum, tear and salivary concentrations of methotrexate in man, Br. J. clin. Pharmacol. *7:* 207–211 (1979).

338 Stefanovich, V.; Wells, H.: Cyclic AMP in human saliva. Fed. Proc. *30:* 565 (1971).

339 Stegemann, H.: Apparatur zur thermokonstanten Elektrophorese und Focussierung und ihre Zusatzteile. Z. analyt. Chem. *261:* 388–391 (1972).

340 Stephen, K.W.; Speirs, C.F.: Oral environmental source of antibacterial drugs – the importance of gingival fluid; in McPhee, Host resistance to commensal bacteria, pp. 76–83 (Churchill-Livingstone, Edinburgh 1972).

341 Stephen, K.W.; Speirs, C.F.: Methods for collecting individual components of mixed saliva: the relevance to clinical pharmacology. Br. J. clin. Pharmacol. *3:* 315–319 (1976).

342 Stephen, K.W.; Harden, R. McG.; Mason, D.K.: Effect of duration of stimulus on iodide concentration in human parotid saliva. Archs oral Biol. *16:* 581–586 (1971).

343 Stephen, K.W.; Lamb, A.B.; McCrossan, J.: A modified appliance for the collection of human submandibular and sublingual salivas. Archs oral Biol. *23:* 835–837 (1978).

344 Stiefel, D.J.; Keller, P.J.: Preparation and some properties of human pancreatic amylase including a comparison with human parotid amylase. Biochim. biophys. Acta *302:* 345–361 (1973).

345 Street, H.V.; Close, J.R.: Determination of amylase activity in biological fluids. Clinica chim. Acta *1:* 256–268 (1956).

346 Strickland, R.D.; Mack, P.A.; Gurule, F.T.; Podleski, T.R.; Salome, O.; Childs, W.A.: Determining serum proteins gravimetrically after agar electrophoresis. Analyt. Chem. *31:* 1410–1413 (1959).

347 Takeuchi, T.; Matsushima, T.; Sugimura, T.: Separation of human α-amylase isozymes by electrofocusing and their immunological properties. Clinica chim. Acta *60:* 207–213 (1975).

348 Takeuchi, T.; Matsushima, T.; Sugimura, T.; Kozu, T.; Takeuchi, T.; Takemoto, T.: Occurrence of multiforms of α-amylase, new isozymes or autodigested forms? Clinica chim. Acta *60:* 205–206 (1975).

349 Tan, S.G.: Human saliva esterases: genetic studies. Hum. Hered. *26:* 207–216 (1976).

350 Tan, S.G.; Ashton, G.C.: Saliva acid phosphatases: genetic studies. Hum. Hered. *26:* 81–89 (1976).

351 Tan, S.G.; Ashton, G.C.: An autosomal glucose-6-phosphate dehydrogenase

(hexose-6-phosphate dehydrogenase) polymorphism in human saliva. Hum. Hered. *26:* 113–123 (1976).

352 Tan, S.G.; Teng, Y.S.: Saliva acid phosphatases in Malaysians: report of a new variant. Hum. Hered. *29:* 61–63 (1979).

353 Tan, S.G.; Teng, Y.S.: Human saliva as a source of biochemical genetic markers. I. Techniques. Hum. Hered. *29:* 69–76 (1979).

354 Taylor, E.A.; Kaspi, T.L.; Turner, P.: The pH dependent absorption of propranolol and indomethacin by parafilm, a stimulant of salivary secretion. J. Pharm. Pharmac. *30:* 813–814 (1978).

355 Theorell, H.; Paul, K.G.: Dissociation constants and their relations to the activity in peroxidases. Ark. Kemi Mineral. Geol. *18A:* 1–23 (1944).

356 Tin, A.A.; Somani, S.M.; Bada, H.S.; Khanna, N.N.: Caffeine, theophylline and theobromine determinations in serum, saliva and spinal fluid. J. anal. Toxicol. *3:* 26–29 (1979).

357 Tomana, M.; Mestecky, J.; Niedermeier, W.: Studies on human secretory immunoglobulin A. IV. Carbohydrate composition. J. Immun. *108:* 1631–1636 (1972).

358 Tomasi, T.B.: Structure and function of mucosal antibodies. Annu. Rev. Med. *21:* 281–298 (1970).

359 Tomasi, T.B.: Secretory immunoglobulins. New Engl. J. Med. *287:* 500–506 (1972).

360 Tomasi, T.B.; Tan, E.M.; Solomon, A.; Prendergast, R.A.: Characteristics of an immune system common to certain external secretions. J. exp. Med. *121:* 101–125 (1965).

361 Trautschold, I.; Werle, E.; Schweitzer, G.: Kallikrein; in Bergmeyer, Methoden der enzymatischen Analyse, vol. I, pp. 1071–1080 (Verlag Chemie, Weinheim 1974).

362 Truelove, E.L.; Bixler, D.; Merritt, A.D.: Simplified method for collection of pure submandibular saliva in large volumes. J. dent. Res. *46:* 1400–1403 (1967).

363 Turkes, A.; Turkes, A.O.; Joyce, B.G.; Read, G.F.; Riad-Fahmy, D.: A sensitive solid phase enzyme immunoassay for testosterone in plasma and saliva. Steroids *33:* 347–359 (1979).

364 Varletzidis, E.; Ikkos, D.; Paleologou, G.; Pantazopoulos, P.; Miras, K.; Adamopoulos, G.: Salivary amylase activity in diabetes mellitus. Panminerva med. *20:* 255–262 (1978).

365 Vogel, J.J.; Naujoks, R.; Brudevold, F.: The effective concentrations of calcium and inorganic phosphate in salivary secretions. Archs oral Biol. *10:* 523–534 (1965).

366 Vogt, K.; Semmann, W.M.: Zur physiologischen Beeinflussung der Gesamtproteinsekretion der grossen Kopfspeicheldrüsen durch Tageszeit, Alter und Geschlecht. Z. Lar. Rhinol. Otol. *49:* 611–620 (1970).

367 Vogt, K.; Zahl, J.: Über Einflüsse von Diabetes mellitus und Geschlecht auf die Sekretion der Glandula parotis des Menschen. Arch. Ohr.-Nas.-KehlkHeilk. *203:* 310–324 (1973).

368 Vreven, J.; Frank, R.M.: Activités pyrophosphatasiques acide et alcaline de la plaque dentaire humaine. Archs oral Biol. *19:* 203–208 (1974).

369 Wadström, T.; Nord, C.-E.; Kjellgren, M.: A rapid method for separation and detection of human salivary amylase isoenzymes by isoelectric focusing in polyacrylamide gel. Scand. J. dent. Res. *84:* 234–239 (1976).

370 Wainwright, W.W.: Human saliva. II. A technical procedure for calcium analysis. J. dent. Res. *14:* 425–434 (1934).

371 Walker, R.F.; Read, G.F.; Fahmy, D.R.: Salivary progesterone and testosterone concentrations for investigating gonadal function. J. Endocr. *81:* 164 P (1979).

372 Walker, R.F.; Read, G.F.; Hughes, I.A.; Riad-Fahmy, D.: Radioimmunoassay of 17α-hydroxyprogesterone in saliva, parotid fluid, and plasma of congenital adrenal hyperplasia patients. Clin. Chem. *25:* 542–545 (1979).

373 Wallenfels, K.; Földi, P.; Niermann, H.; Bender, H.; Linder, D.: The enzymic synthesis, by transglucosylation of a homologous series of glycosidically substituted malto-oligosaccharides, and their use as amylase substrates. Carbohyd. Res. *61:* 359–368 (1978).

374 Ward, J.C.; Merritt, A.D.; Bixler, D.: Human salivary amylase: Genetics of electrophoretic variants. Am. J. hum. Genet. *23:* 403–409 (1971).

375 Watanabe, T.; Nakamura, R.; Iwamoto, Y.; Tsunemitsu, A.: Isolation and characterization of β-N-acetylglucosaminidase from human parotid saliva. J. dent. Res. *52:* 783–790 (1973).

376 Watkins, W.M.: Blood-group specific substances; in Gottschalk, Glycoproteins; their composition, structure and function. B.B.A. Library, vol. 5, part B, pp. 830–891 (Elsevier, Amsterdam 1972).

377 Weinstein, E.; Mandel, I.D.: Facts and artifacts in acid phosphatase and esterase localization in disc electrophoresis of human saliva. Archs oral Biol. *14:* 1–6 (1969).

378 Weinstein, E.; Khurana, H.; Mandel, I.D.: Lactate dehydrogenase isoenzymes in human saliva. Archs oral Biol. *16:* 157–160 (1971).

379 Werle, E.; Rodin, P.: Über das Vorkommen von Kallikrein in den Speicheldrüsen und im Mundspeichel. Biochem. Z. *286:* 219 (1936).

380 Werle, E.; Trautschold, I.; Leysath, G.: Isolierung und Struktur des Kallidins. Hoppe-Seyler's Z. physiol. Chem. *326:* 174–176 (1961).

381 Wermus, G.; Adams, T.; Menson, R.: A stoichiometric method for the determination of serum amylase; in Lorentz, α-Amylase assay: current state and future development. Rep. Workshop Conf. German Soc. Clinical Chemistry, Frankfurt 1978, p.503 (J. clin. Chem. clin. Biochem. *17:* 499–504, 1979).

382 Weymes, C.: Sterilization with ethylene oxide at sub-atmospheric pressure. Br. Hosp. J. soc. Serv. Rev. *66:* 1745–1750 (1966).

383 Whitlow, K.J.; Gochman, N.; Forrester, R.L.; Wataji, L.J.: Maltotetraose as a substrate for enzyme-coupled assay of amylase activity in serum and urine. Clin. Chem. *25:* 481–483 (1979).

384 Wiener, K.; Foot, C.H.: A study of some factors affecting the Phadebas amylase test. Clinica chim. Acta *75:* 177–180 (1977).

385 Wigand, M.E.; Winckler, J.; Heidland, A.: Speichelchemie und Katecholamingehalt adrenerger Nerven der Parotisdrüse bei chronischer Parotitis und Sjögren-Syndrom. Arch. Ohr.-Nas.-KehlkHeilk. *205:* 109–113 (1973).

386 Wolf, R.O.; Taylor, L.L.: Isoamylases of human parotid saliva. Nature, Lond. *213:* 1128–1129 (1967).

387 Workman, P.; Wiltshire, C.R.; Plowman, P.N.; Bleehen, N.M.: Monitoring salivary misonidazole in man: a possible alternative to plasma monitoring. Br. J. Cancer *38:* 709–718 (1978).

388 Yip, M.C.M.; Knox, W.E.: Function of arginase in lactating mammary gland. Biochem. J. *127:* 893–899 (1972).

389 Yosizawa, Z.: Sulphated glycoproteins; in Gottschalk, Glycoproteins; their composition, structure and function. B.B.A. Library, vol. 5, part B, pp. 1000–1018 (Elsevier, Amsterdam 1972).

390 Zacharski, L.R.; Rosenstein, R.: Reduction of salivary tissue factor (thromboplastin) activity by warfarin therapy. Blood *53:* 366–374 (1979).

391 Zahradnik, R.T.; Propas, D.; Moreno, E.C.: Effect of salivary pellicle formation time on in vitro attachment and demineralization by *Streptococcus mutans*. J. dent. Res. *57:* 1036–1042 (1978).

392 Zipkin, I.; Hawkins, G.R.; Mazzarella, M.: The tyrosine, tryptophan and protein content of human parotid saliva in oral and systemic disease. Use of ultraviolet absorption technics; in Sreebny, Meyer, Salivary glands and their secretion, pp. 331–350 (Pergamon Press, New York 1964).

393 Zöllner, E.J.; Klepsch, D.M.; Zahn, R.K.: Different deoxyribonuclease in human submandibular saliva. J. dent. Res. *53:* 1499 (1974).

394 Zöllner, E.J.; Klepsch, D.M.; Zahn, R.K.; Knepper, R.: Deoxyribonucleases in human parotid saliva. Enzyme *19:* 60–64 (1974).

395 Allars, H.M.; Blomfield, J.; Rush, A.R.; Brown, J.M.: Colloid and crystal formation in parotid saliva of cystic fibrosis patients and non-cystic fibrosis subjects. I. Physicochemistry. Pediat. Res. *10:* 578–584 (1976).

396 Allars, H.M.; Cockayne, D.J.H.; Blomfield, J.; Rush, A.R.; Lennep, E.W. van; Brown, J.M.: Colloid and crystal formation in parotid saliva of cystic fibrosis patients and non-cystic fibrosis subjects. II. Electron microscopy and electrophoresis. Pediat. Res. *10:* 584–594 (1976).

397 Baig, M.M.; Winzler, R.J.; Rennert, O.M.: Isolation of mucin from human submaxillary secretions. J. Immun. *111:* 1826–1833 (1973).

398 Beisenherz, G.; Boltze, H.J.; Bücher, T.; Czok, R.; Garbade, K.H.; Meyer-Arendt, E.; Pfleiderer, G.: Diphosphofructose-Aldolase, Phosphoglycerinaldehyd-Dehydrogenase, Milchsäuredehydrogenase und Pyruvat-Kinase aus Kaninchenmuskel in einem Arbeitsgang. Z. Naturf. *8b:* 555–577 (1963).

399 Belcourt, A.: Etude d'une glycoprotéine salivaire humaine précipitable par les ions calcium. Eur. J. Biochem. *53:* 185–191 (1975).

400 Bennick, A.; Wong, R.: Salivary acidic proline-rich phosphoproteins: structure and possible function in the oral cavity; in Kleinberg, Ellison, Mandel, Proc. 'Saliva and Dental Caries'. Microbiology Abstracts, suppl., pp. 59–65 (Information Retrieval, New York 1979).

401 Blomfield, J.; Rush, A.R.; Allars, H.M.; Brown, J.M.: Parotid gland function in children with cystic fibrosis and child control subjects. Pediat. Res. *10:* 574–578 (1976).

402 Blomfield, J.; Lennep, E.W. van; Shorey, C.D.; Malin, A.S.; Dascalu, J.; Brown, J.M.: Ultrastructure of the *in vitro* formation of hydroxyapatite in submandibular saliva of children with cystic fibrosis. Archs oral Biol. *19:* 1153–1160 (1974).

403 Blumberger, W.; Glatzel, H.: Über Variabilität von Speichelsekretion und Speichelbeschaffenheit des gesunden Menschen und ihre Beziehungen zur Kostform. Dt. Z. Verdau.-StoffwechsKrankh. *23:* 210–225 (1963).

404 Boat, T.F.; Wiesman, U.N.; Pallavicini, J.C.: Purification and properties of the

calcium-precipitable protein in submaxillary saliva of normal and cystic fibrosis subjects. Pediat. Res. *8:* 531–539 (1974).

405 Caldwell, R.C.; Pigman, W.: The carbohydrates of human submaxillary glyco-proteins in secretors and non-secretors of blood group substances. Biochim. biophys. Acta *101:* 157–165 (1965).

406 Callow, A.B.: The heat-stable peroxidase of bacteria. Biochem. J. *20:* 247–252 (1926).

407 Ceska, M.; Brown, B.; Birath, K.: Ranges of α-amylase activities in human serum and urine and correlations with some other α-amylase methods. Clinica chim. Acta *26:* 445–453 (1969).

408 Chatterjee, R.; Kleinberg, I.: Aggregation of salivary proteins; in Kleinberg, Ellison, Mandel, Proc. 'Saliva and Dental Caries'. Microbiology Abstracts, suppl., pp. 155–173 (Information Retrieval, New York 1979).

409 Chernick, W.S.; Eichel, H.J.; Barbero, G.J.: Submaxillary salivary enzymes as a measure of glandular activity in cystic fibrosis. J. Pediat. *65:* 694–700 (1964).

410 Cole, C.H.; Sella, G.: Inhibition of ouabain-sensitive ATPase by the saliva of patients with cystic fibrosis of the pancreas. Pediat. Res. *9:* 763–766 (1975).

411 Dirksen, T.R.: Salivary lipids; in Kleinberg, Ellison, Mandel, Proc. 'Saliva and Dental Caries'. Microbiology Abstracts, suppl., pp. 113–122 (Information Retrieval, New York 1979).

412 Doggett, R.G.; Harrison, G.M.: Cystic fibrosis: reversal of ciliary inhibition in serum and saliva by heparin. Tex. Rep. Biol. Med. *31:* 685–689 (1973).

413 Edelman, G.M.; Cunningham, B.A.; Gall, W.E.; Gottlieb, P.D.; Rutishauser, U.; Waxdal, M.J.: The covalent structure of an entire gamma-G immunoglobulin molecule. Proc. natn. Acad. Sci. USA *63:* 78–85 (1969).

414 Eggers Lura, H.: Die Enzyme des Speichels und der Zähne (Hanser, München 1949).

415 Ellison, S.A.: The identification of salivary components; in Kleinberg, Ellison, Mandel, Proc. 'Saliva and Dental Caries'. Microbiology Abstracts, suppl., pp. 13–29 (Information Retrieval, New York 1979).

416 Fujimoto, Y.; Moriwaki, C.; Moriya, H.: Studies on human salivary kallikrein. II. Properties of purified salivary kallikrein. J. Biochem., Tokyo *74:* 247–252 (1973).

417 Gillard, B.K.; Markman, H.C.; Feig, S.A.: Differences between cystic fibrosis and normal saliva α-amylase as a function of age and sex. Pediat. Res. *12:* 868–872 (1978).

418 Gottschalk, A.: Glycoproteins; their composition, structure and function. B.B.A. Library, vol. 5, parts A, B (Elsevier, Amsterdam 1972).

419 Greaves, M.S.; West, H.F.: Cortisol and cortisone in saliva of pregnancy. J. Endocr. *26:* 189–195 (1963).

420 Greengard, O.; Sahib, M.K.; Knox, W.E.: Developmental formation and distribu-tion of arginase in rat tissues. Archs Biochem. Biophys. *137:* 477–482 (1970).

421 Hay, D.I.: The isolation from human parotid saliva of a tyrosine-rich acidic peptide which exhibits high affinity for hydroxyapatite surfaces. Archs oral Biol. *18:* 1531–1541 (1973).

422 Hay, D.I.; Moreno, E.C.: Macromolecular inhibitors of calcium phosphate precipi-tation in human saliva. Their roles in providing a protective environment for the teeth; in Kleinberg, Ellison, Mandel, Proc. 'Saliva and Dental Caries'. Microbiology Abstracts, suppl., pp. 45–58 (Information Retrieval, New York 1979).

423 Heidelberger, M.; Pederson, K.O.: The molecular weight of antibodies. J. exp. Med. *65:* 393–414 (1937).

424 Herzfeld, A.; Raper, S.M.: The heterogeneity of arginases in rat tissues. Biochem. J. *153:* 469–478 (1976).

425 Hilschmann, N.; Craig, L.C.: Amino acid sequence studies with Bence-Jones proteins. Proc. natn. Acad. Sci. USA *53:* 1403–1409 (1965).

426 Hine, M.K.; O'Donnell, J.F.: Incidence of urease producing bacteria in saliva. J. dent. Res. *22:* 103–106 (1943).

427 Holbrook, I.B.; Molan, P.C.: A further study of the factors enhancing glycolysis in human saliva. Archs oral Biol. *18:* 1275–1282 (1973).

428 Hopkinson, D.A.; Spencer, N.; Harris, H.: Genetical studies on human red cell acid phosphatase. Am. J. hum. Genet. *16:* 141–154 (1964).

429 Horowitz, M.I.; Pigman, W.: The glycoconjugates, vol. I: Mammalian glycoproteins and glycolipids (Academic Press, New York 1977).

430 Jenkins, G.N.: Physiology of the mouth (Blackwell, Oxford 1970).

431 Jenkins, G.N.: Salivary effects on plaque pH; in Kleinberg, Ellison, Mandel, Proc. 'Saliva and Dental Caries'. Microbiology Abstracts, suppl., pp. 307–322 (Information Retrieval, New York 1979).

432 Kabat, E.A.: Blood-group substances (Academic Press, New York 1956).

433 Kauffman, D.L.; Watanabe, S.; Keller, P.J.: The relationship of flow rate to glycosylation of human parotid amylase. Archs oral Biol. *19:* 597–599 (1974).

434 Kilsheimer, G.S.; Axelrod, B.: Phylogenetic distribution of acid phosphatase inhibited by (+)-tartrate. Nature, Lond. *182:* 1733–1734 (1958).

435 Kleinberg, I.; Ellison, S.A.; Mandel, I.D.: Proc. 'Saliva and Dental Caries'. Microbiology Abstracts, suppl. (Information Retrieval, New York 1979).

436 Kleinberg, I.; Kanapka, J.A.; Chatterjee, R.; Craw, D.; D'Angelo, N.; Sandham, H.J.: Metabolism of nitrogen by the oral mixed bacteria; in Kleinberg, Ellison, Mandel, Proc. 'Saliva and Dental Caries'. Microbiology Abstracts, suppl., pp. 357–377 (Information Retrieval, New York 1979).

437 Köstlin, A.; Rauch, S.: Zur Chemie des Ruhespeichels einzelner Speicheldrüsen. Helv. med. Acta *24:* 600–621 (1957).

438 Kuhn, R.: Der Wirkungsmechanismus der Amylasen; ein Beitrag zum Konfigurationsproblem der Stärke. Ann. Chem. *443:* 1–71 (1925).

439 Leuchs, E.F.: Über die Verzuckerung des Stärkemehls durch Speichel. Arch. Chem. Meteorol. *3:* 105 (1831).

440 Leuchs, E.F.: Die Wirkung des Speichels auf Stäkre. Ann. phys. Chem. *22:* 623 (1831).

441 Lundsgaard-Hansen, P.: Der Einsatz von Albumin in der Klinik. Die gelben Hefte (Immunbiologische Informationen, Behringwerke, Marburg) *18:* 8–13 (1978).

442 Mandel, I.D.: In defense of the oral cavity; in Kleinberg, Ellison, Mandel, Proc. 'Saliva and Dental Caries'. Microbiology Abstracts, suppl., pp. 473–491 (Information Retrieval, New York 1979).

443 Mandel, I.D.; Eisenstein, A.: Lipids in human salivary secretions and salivary calculus. Archs oral Biol. *14:* 231–233 (1969).

444 Mandel, I.D.; Hampar, B.; Thompson, R.H., Jr.; Ellison, S.A.: The carbohydrates of human parotid saliva. Archs oral Biol. *3:* 278–282 (1961).

445 Marmar, J.; Barbero, G.J.; Sibinga, M.S.: The pattern of parotid gland secretion in cystic fibrosis of the pancreas. Gastroenterology *50:* 551–555 (1966).

446 Mayo, J.M.; Wallace, W.M.; Matthews, L.W.; Carlson, D.M.: Quantitation of

submandibular proteins resolved from normal individuals and children with cystic fibrosis. Archs Biochem. Biophys. *175:* 507–513 (1976).

447 Morris, J.G.: Oxygen and growth of the oral bacteria; in Kleinberg, Ellison, Mandel, Proc. 'Saliva and Dental Caries'. Microbiology Abstracts, suppl., pp. 293–306 (Information Retrieval, New York 1979).

448 Oppenheim, F.G.; Kousvelari, E.; Troxler, R.F.: Genetic, immunological and structural relationships of anionic proline-rich proteins from salivary secretions; in Kleinberg, Ellison, Mandel, Proc. 'Saliva and Dental Caries'. Microbiology Abstracts, suppl., pp. 31–44 (Information Retrieval, New York 1979).

449 Payen, Persoz: Mémoire sur la diastase, les principaux produits de ses réactions, et leurs applications aux arts industriels. Annls Chim. Phys. *53:* 73–92 (1833).

450 Pigman, W.: General aspects; in Horowitz, Pigman, The glycoconjugates, vol. I, pp. 1–11 (Academic Press, New York 1977).

451 Pigman, W.: Introduction: mucous glycoproteins; in Horowitz, Pigman, The glycoconjugates, vol. I, pp. 131–135 (Academic Press, New York 1977).

452 Pigman, W.: Blood group glycoproteins; in Horowitz, Pigman, The glycoconjugates, vol. I, pp. 181–188 (Academic Press, New York 1977).

453 Pollock, J.J.; Goodman Bicker, G.; Katona, L.I.; Cho, M.I.; Iacono, V.J.: Lysozyme bacteriolysis; in Kleinberg, Ellison, Mandel, Proc. 'Saliva and Dental Caries'. Microbiology Abstracts, suppl., pp. 429–447 (Information Retrieval, New York 1979).

454 Pusztai, A.; Morgan, W.T.J.: Studies in immunochemistry. 22. The amino acid composition of the human blood-group A, B, H and Le^a specific substances. Biochem. J. *88:* 546–555 (1963).

455 Rabinowitz, J.; Shannon, I.L.: Lipid changes in human male parotid saliva by stimulation. Archs oral Biol. *20:* 403–406 (1975).

456 Rolla, G.; Bonesvoll, P.; Opermann, R.: Interactions between oral streptococci and salivary proteins; in Kleinberg, Ellison, Mandel, Proc. 'Saliva and Dental Caries'. Microbiology Abstracts, suppl., pp. 227–241 (Information Retrieval, New York 1979).

457 Rosan, B.; Jenkins, G.N.; Kanapka, J.A.: Report on Session II: influence of saliva on bacteria, substrate and host; in Kleinberg, Ellison, Mandel, Proc. 'Saliva and Dental Caries'. Microbiology Abstracts, suppl., pp. 557–565 (Information Retrieval, New York 1979).

458 Schachter, M.: Kinins – a group of active peptides. A. Rev. Pharmacol. *4:* 281–292 (1964).

459 Schlesinger, D.H.; Hay, D.I.: Complete covalent structure of statherin, a tyrosine-rich acidic peptide which inhibits calcium phosphate precipitation from human parotid saliva. J. biol. Chem. *252:* 1689–1695 (1977).

460 Tenovuo, J.; Mäkinen, K.K.: Concentration of thiocyanate and ionizable iodine in saliva of smokers and nonsmokers. J. dent. Res. *55:* 661–663 (1976).

461 Theorell, H.: The iron-containing enzymes. B. Catalases and peroxidases: 'hydroperoxidases'; in Sumner, Myrbäck, The enzymes; chemistry and mechanism of action, vol. II, part 1, pp. 397–427 (Academic Press, New York 1951).

462 Tiedemann, F.; Gmelin, L.: Recherches expérimentales physiologiques et chimiques sur la digestion (Baillière, Paris 1826).

463 Tiselius, A.; Kabat, E.A.: An electrophoretic study of immune sera and purified antibody preparations. J. exp. Med. *69:* 119–131 (1939).

464 Tomasi, T.B., Jr.; Bienenstock, J.: Secretory immunoglobulins. Adv. Immunol. *9:* 1–96 (1968).

465 Ward, M.; Politzer, I.; Laseter, J.: Gas chromatographic mass spectrometric evaluation of free organic acids in human saliva. Biomed. Mass Spectrometry *3:* 77–80 (1976).

466 Wasserman, R.L.; Capra, J.D.: Immunoglobulins; in Horowitz, Pigman, The glycoconjugates, vol. I, pp. 323–348 (Academic Press, New York 1977).

467 Webb, E.C.: Nomenclature of multiple enzyme forms. Nature, Lond. *203:* 821 (1964).

468 Windeler, A.S.; Shannon, I.L.: The precipitation of protein from parotid fluid. J. dent. Res. *45:* 1784–1787 (1966).

469 Wolf, R.O.; Taylor, L.L.: Concentration of blood group substances in parotid, sublingual and submaxillary saliva. J. dent. Res. *43:* 272–276 (1964).

470 Zengo, A.N.; Mandel, I.D.; Goldman, R.; Khurana, H.S.: Salivary studies in human caries resistance. Archs oral Biol. *16:* 557–560 (1971).

Akadem. Rat Christian Arglebe, PhD, Universitäts-HNO-Klinik Göttingen, Geiststrasse 5/10, D-3400 Göttingen (FRG)

Subject Index

ABH(O) blood group system 147–149,
206
Acetylcholine 137
esterase 137
N-Acetylgalactosamine 140, 148, 149, 154
N-Acetylglucosamine 140, 143, 148–150,
153, 182
β-N-Acetyl-D-glucosaminidase 139
N-Acetylneuraminic acid 119–121, 143,
146, 148–150, 152–157, 160, 167
Acid α_1-glycoprotein 141, 153
Acid phosphatase 111, 127–129, 190, 194,
208
activity 127–129
blood type 128
isoenzymes 129, 208
parotid 128, 194
prostatic type 128
purification 128
submandibular 190
substrate specificity 127, 128
Acidic protein, see Pa protein
Acinar cells 22, 23, 125, 141, 146, 177
cytoplasm 146
dark 22
human parotid 177
light 22, 23
rat parotid 6, 141
serous 125
Acinar diameter 55–58
cytological 57
histological 57
sialadenosis 55, 56, 58

Acinar lumen 7, 191
Acquired pellicle 98, 156, 158, 183, 184,
186
formation 183, 184
ACTH 168, 196
Adenosine triphosphatase 137, 138, 191
Adenovirus 181
Adrenocortical status 168, 199
Age 11, 99, 103–106, 178, 191, 193, 196,
198, 203–205, 209
Age-dependent changes 105, 107, 202–206,
209
amylase 107, 203, 204
electrolytes 202, 203
isoamylases 204–206
lactoperoxidase 203
protein 105, 107, 204
secretory IgA 203
thiocyanate 203
Age-specific differences 104, 105, 107,
191, 195, 196, 202, 204, 205
Agglutination 147, 158, 182
Agglutinin 181, 182, 206, 207
wheat germ 182
Aging 21, 204
Alanine 154, 166
Albinos 166
Albumin 108–111, 195, 203
biological role 109
plasma 109–111, 195
salivary 108–111, 203
Alcohol 127, 202
dehydrogenase 175